Treatment and Care of the Geriatric Veterinary Patient

Treatment and Care of the Geriatric Veterinary Patient

Edited by Mary Gardner and Dani McVety

WILEY Blackwell

Registered Offices
John Wiley & Sons, Inc., 111 River Street, Hoboken, NJ 07030, USA
John Wiley & Sons Ltd, The Atrium, Southern Gate, Chichester, West Sussex, PO19 8SQ, UK

Editorial Office
John Wiley & Sons, Inc., 111 River Street, Hoboken, NJ 07030, USA

For details of our global editorial offices, customer services, and more information about Wiley products visit us at www.wiley.com.

Wiley also publishes its books in a variety of electronic formats and by print-on-demand. Some content that appears in standard print versions of this book may not be available in other formats.

Library of Congress Cataloging-in-Publication Data

Names: Gardner, Mary, 1973– editor. | McVety, Dani, 1981– editor.
Title: Treatment and care of the geriatric veterinary patient / edited by Mary Gardner, Dani McVety.
Description: 1st edition. | Hoboken, NJ : John Wiley & Sons, 2017. | Includes bibliographical references.
Identifiers: LCCN 2017013228 (print) | LCCN 2017014319 (ebook) | ISBN 9781119187233 (pdf) |
    ISBN 9781119187226 (epub) | ISBN 9781119187219 (pbk.)
Subjects: | MESH: Veterinary Medicine–methods | Geriatrics–methods | Dogs–physiology |
    Cats–physiology | Aging–physiology
Classification: LCC SF745 (ebook) | LCC SF745 (print) | NLM SF 768.5 | DDC 636.089–dc23
LC record available at https://lccn.loc.gov/2017013228

Cover design: Wiley
Cover image: Courtesy of Mary Gardner

Set in 10/12pt Warnock by SPi Global, Pondicherry, India

10 9 8 7 6 5 4 3 2 1

Contents

List of Contributors

Laura Devlin Bacon, DVM, DABVP

Faith Banks, DVM

Brad Bates, VMD, MS

Cheryl A. Braswell, DVM, DACVECC, CHT-V

Melanie Hasson Cohen, DVM

Shea Cox, DVM, CHPV, CVPP, CPLP

Steve Dale, CABC

Mary Gardner, DVM

Amanda Grant, DVM

Heidi B. Lobprise, DVM, DAVDC

Dani McVety, DVM

Tammy Perkins Johnson, DVM, CCRP, CERP, CVA, cVSMT

Michael Petty, DVM, CVPP, CMAV, CCRT, DAAPM

Sheilah Robertson, BVMS (Hons), PhD, DACVA, DECVA, CVA, MRCVS

Carlo Siracusa, DVM, MS, PhD, Dip. ACVB, Dip. ECAWBM

Meredith Voyles, DVM, DACVO, MS

Kayla Waler, DVM

Dawnetta Woodruff, DVM

About the Companion Website

This book is accompanied by a companion website:

www.wiley.com/go/gardner/geriatric

The website provides videos, client education handouts, and images.

Part I

They Just Don't Live Long Enough

"It's paradoxical that the idea of living a long life appeals to everyone, but the idea of getting old doesn't appeal to anyone."

— Andy Rooney

1

Introduction

Mary Gardner

My heart tightens as I watch her "spaghetti legs" quiver as she drinks happily at her bowl and washes down her dinner. The menu tonight was …"whatever she wants." It's only a matter of time when the chapter of my story with Serissa ends abruptly and the companion that acted as my shadow for 14.5 years will leave my world. The thought brings tears to my eyes and that pesky lump to my throat.

"Hey baby girl, you want to go outside?" I say in the sweetest voice I can muster up and she looks at me with adoration, wags her pathetically haired tail and gives me a weak and croaky "BARK" as if to say "Heck yeah!" Serissa navigates the bathmats that I laid down for her and struts to the door like a runway model. At one time she was a majestic beauty of a Samoyed and even worked as a therapy dog in nursing homes (Figure 1.1) – now she was a thin, patchy haired, skinny, old girl with hot garbage breath. She was a frail geriatric herself.

But, before we could get to the door, she pops a squat and urinates on the bathmat. In past years, this would be a naughty thing, but today, I could care less! Her legs quiver harder and she almost tumbles over. She finds her balance, quickly finishes, and Serissa's thoughts go back to being outside with mom. Nothing brings more joy to my face than seeing her sweet face turn to look at me as if to say, "You coming?" (Figure 1.2).

I was taught many things in veterinary school, but dealing with an aging and terminally ill pet was left out of the classroom lectures. In fact, most of the textbooks we read and lectures we sat through did not cover the process of aging and death. Instead, we were taught the mantra that "Old age is not a disease!" But, aging *does* change quality of life for the pet and the owner. We did discuss senior wellness and preventative medicine but really digging into why the body ages and what happens as things fall apart was not covered in detail. At the time, even the education of euthanasia was left to a two-hour discussion. Luckily, now at my alma mater the University of Florida (Go Gators) a comprehensive 'end of life' course is offered.

The lifespan of companion animals continues to get longer and longer. Just a few decades ago, a pet over the age of 10 years was an anomaly – it was not "normal". But as we advance in technology, as the pet–parent bond grows stronger and more intimate and our societal views on companion animals shift, we are seeing a much larger population of pets reaching a much higher age and many sail into their "twilight" years with a lot of

Treatment and Care of the Geriatric Veterinary Patient, First Edition. Edited by Mary Gardner and Dani McVety.
© 2017 John Wiley & Sons, Inc. Published 2017 by John Wiley & Sons, Inc.
Companion Website: www.wiley.com/go/gardner/geriatric

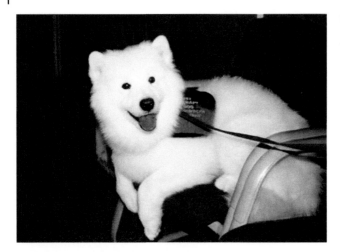

Figure 1.1 Serissa, 2 years old, in her therapy dog vest, waiting to visit residents in a nursing home.

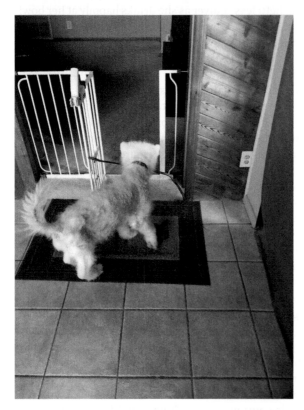

Figure 1.2 Serissa, 14 years old, attempting to get a stick through the baby gate that is in place for her safety.

vigor. But, what we are fighting against is still "not normal" – our bodies will eventually fail, no matter how many patch jobs we put in place.

I remember clearly as a new veterinarian when a colleague looked at radiographs of a 15-year-old cat and said "Ehh – it's just old cat lungs." He flipped off the light and boldly walked into the room to deliver the "good news". I sat there thinking, "but that isn't good … it must possess some problem for the cat and what does it mean for him to have areas of fibrosis in his lungs?." But my deep thoughts were cut off quickly when my next patient came in, Abagail, a 13-year-old FBD ("Florida Brown Dog" or, as others would just call her, a "mixed breed"). She had a three-month history of staring into space, acting as if she is lost, and is often found in odd places. I internally sigh because I know how frustrating cognitive disorders can be and how limited our options currently are at this time. But, I still cannot wait to see Abagail and her parents.

As much as I love a bunch of kittens and the rubbing of a puppy belly, there is absolutely nothing better than a gray muzzle. I adore hearing the stories of how they came to be in the family, the memories the pet was present for, and how great their loss will be when it comes time to say goodbye. I left general practice in 2010 and since then have exclusively helped families with home-based veterinary hospice, geriatric consultations and end of life care. I have sat on many couches, on hundreds of master beds, have wormed my way behind toilets and scaled many a cat tree in my practice – and I love it. The conditions I see may range from mobility to organ failure or simply "old age" (yes, I said it), but one thing always remains the same, the enormous love the family has for their aging pets. It is an honor to help those families through the aging process, the disease progression and finally, the moment they say goodbye.

This book was inspired by my desire to learn on a practical level why pets age, how each body system is effected by the aging process and how owners and the veterinary staff can manage the changes that occur. There is a plethora of fantastic textbooks about each of the body systems and the disease they encounter, but this book is meant to be a reference manual specific to the aging process, the care of the geriatric pet and a guide to help you with the most precious time owners have with their pets.

Fourteen and a half years seemed to have flown by as I laid next to Serissa and snuggled with her one last time while she drifted off to a peaceful sleep. Her presence in my heart will always remain. I will miss that smile, her smell, the scratching on the wall as she ran in her sleep, and even that whining in the middle of the night as her mind became more confused with cognitive impairments. How blessed I was to have such a wonderful companion who was with me through veterinary school and would bring joy to me in a millisecond. Caring for her as she aged was extremely difficult for me financially, physically and emotionally, but I would do it for 20 more years if possible. Although terribly missed, thoughts of her now only bring a smile to my face (Figure 1.3).

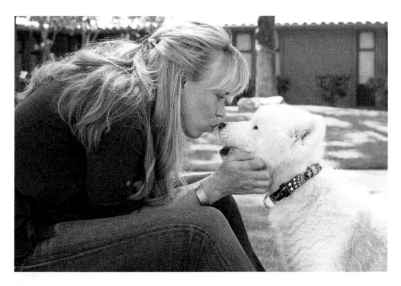

Figure 1.3 Serissa and Mary.

Serissa's story lives on throughout my work, where her conditions and experiences helped me to further research and dig deeper into the body system. I am sure she is smiling, too, with her geriatric cohorts, as they realize that their experiences will offer insight to the veterinary community and ease the distress of pet owners when dealing with their pet's twilight years.

2

Maintaining the Human–Animal Bond
Dani McVety

The industry of veterinary medicine started in a much different place than we find ourselves today; we started as mechanics. In a world where horses and cattle accounted for the vast majority of our transportation, keeping these animals healthy was an important role. As the animal population has moved closer and closer to our homes, and even into our beds, the responsibility of keeping these pets healthy has more in common with a pediatrician than any other aspect of medicine.

Pets are not just animals that happily coexist with humans in a mutually friendly way; for more than half of the population, pets are family members. A survey conducted by the American Veterinary Medical Association (2012) found that of 63.2% considered their pets to be family members. Another 35.8% considered their pets to be pets or companions and only the remaining 1% considered their pets to be property. Furthermore, similar to the human caregiving model, women are typically the primary caregivers of pets; the study showed that 74.5% of pet owners with primary responsibility for their pets were female. It is easy to see how our industry has undergone such a drastic change from caring for animals in the barnyard to the family members that share the homes and beds with their "mom" or "dad."

Maintaining the human animal bond is just as important at the end of a pet's life as it is at any other time. In a 2012 survey at the Lap of Love Veterinary Hospice, about 25% of over 1000 respondents reported that they would not return to the clinic that euthanized their pet, mostly because it was "simply too hard to return." Similarly, every veterinary professional can account for the clients with "do not put in exam room 2" written on their client file because one of their pets was euthanized in that room.

Losing any family member can be traumatizing and heartbreaking. And of course we usually do not chose the human family members we have in our life (aside from our spouse), nor do we choose to add another after one has been lost. We do, however, actively make the choice to bring a pet into our heart and home, and the probability of making that choice again when the loss of a previous pet has been stressful and harrowing goes way down. Therefore, given that we know that pet owners can be traumatized by the loss of a pet and that this trauma may lead to a disconnect from their veterinary office, it makes sense that our profession would take great care with our geriatric

Treatment and Care of the Geriatric Veterinary Patient, First Edition. Edited by Mary Gardner and Dani McVety.
© 2017 John Wiley & Sons, Inc. Published 2017 by John Wiley & Sons, Inc.
Companion Website: www.wiley.com/go/gardner/geriatric

patients and the people that love them through the entire end of life phase. Starting by practicing conscientious geriatric care (which is an underlying purpose of this book) and ending with a peaceful death process, the support of the human–animal bond through the loss of a pet will ensure that these families will open their hearts and homes to another animal when the time is right.

As veterinary hospice practitioners, we can give you story after story of the immense emotions that come with the loss of a pet. And, for most of us, we realize at some point that this loss represents something very important in their life: The old man whose wife died a year ago, and now, as his dog dies, he is losing the last connection he had to her; the mother whose son was killed in a motorcycle accident month before, and now must say goodbye to his cat; the woman whose dog woke her up seven years ago in a house fire, saving her life, and now due to old age, she feels like she is not returning the favor by making the decision to euthanize. Their pet represents something major in their life, or a series of events, and perhaps that is the case for any major loss in our life.

It is not uncommon for us to hear these phrases in a home:

> "This is worse than the death of my parents."
> "I feel like I don't have a reason to live without my pet."
> "He was the only one that got me through that part of my life."
> "She was the only one I trusted."
> "This is the hardest thing I've ever been through."

It is clear to anyone in the veterinary or pet profession that the human–animal bond moves our industry. It is, in a large way, the product that we are selling to the consumer. They are in our clinics because of the bond they have with their pet. Without that bond, there is no reason to keep their pet healthy, buy him or her good food, purchase toys, or buy them clothes!

It takes just a few minutes to walk down the aisle of a large pet store to realize how differently that human animal bond can be supported. To some, it is rhinestone-studded collars; to others, it is mentally stimulating toys, and to still others, it is a safety jacket worn while hunting with his owner. The important part is that all of them love their pet. And just as differently as we choose to entertain and "dress" our animals, our clients will choose different ways of medically caring for them. The barn dog or cat may not have the same consistent veterinary care that we provide for our own pet, but that does not mean that pet is less loved; he is simply differently loved.

A second underlying theme of this book is how to support each of those families and pets through this geriatric phase. You will find many helpful tips, ideas, exercises, medical protocols, and much more to help you connect with and support the clients who need just a little more help at this important time. This may come in the form of extra time spent in the exam room to explain exactly why their geriatric cat is not hearing them shake the food bowl any more (see Chapter 5 on auditory changes) or why their dog's bark has changed (see Chapter 13 on the respiratory system). Use these tips to connect with your clients and find news ways to support the bond they have with their own pets.

Just as some veterinarians will go mentally blank when needing to make medical decisions for their own personal pets, our clients are already starting from "zero" when it comes to this kind of knowledge. And in the case of geriatric pets, some of us forget that this 12-year-old, 80-lb mixed-breed dog is more like an 85-year-old person. We tend to understand more readily why our fellow humans are aging and what they are going through, but are not as easily able to connect with the natural aging process in pets (or we simply do not want to accept it).

Let this book be a guide for you and your clients. Use these tools to help connect with, describe, and assist the families we are privileged to help at a time when they are most confused about the wellbeing of their animal family member. We hope that it brings additional support to all parties involved.

Reference

American Veterinary Medical Association. *US Pet Ownership and Demographics Sourcebook.* Schaumburg, IL: 2012.

3

Geriatrics and Fragility

Mary Gardner (Research Assistant Stacy Glass)

Introduction

Determining who was going to pick up Margaret, the 89-year-old matriarch of the Gardner family, for Thanksgiving was usually more of a debate than what type of pies we would bake that year. You see, Grandma Gardner was fragile – we often compared her to an egg – and she needed special assistance in many facets of her life. She still lived alone in a small condo in South Florida, but this New Jersey transplant was in no way fully independent. Grandma Gardner was a shadow of her younger self, muscle atrophied, age-spots dotting her hands and face, thick glasses, thin skin and extremely wobbly. She needed help rising from a chair, assistance into the car, and could only lift about three pounds; with her, everything involved extra consideration, even purchasing milk. We had to buy a quart instead of a gallon, as the gallon was too heavy for her to lift unassisted. We also had to help cut her food into smaller pieces, as her ability to swallow properly became a challenge, and we certainly could not tell her too many jokes while she ate, as she had a boisterous laugh which predisposed her to aspiration! Regardless, she still had most of her wits about her, and honestly, she was a delight to be around, the member of the family with the least drama and the best advice!

Fetching Grandma Gardner for an outing was no small feat. The person appointed to this task had to have the "right" car: One large enough to fit her walker with enough room in the front seat for her to stretch out, yet just the right height and size for her to easily get into, with a steady arm assisting her, of course. She also had to be comfortable enough to properly handle her cherished homemade apple cake (a secret family recipe which she tightly held on to). When picking her up, it was imperative to remember her sweater as even with the 85-degree Florida weather and 90 percent humidity, she still became easily chilled. Plus, this person had to be willing to leave early to take her home in the event she tired before everyone else.

I was always the appointed one, as I had the perfect car. Frankly, I genuinely enjoyed the opportunity to pick her up. I loved being in her condo, seeing the pictures she dearly treasured (especially of her and my late Grandfather, Figure 3.1), hearing the sound of the grandfather clock, and the unique, yet pleasant smell. I don't know what it was – but

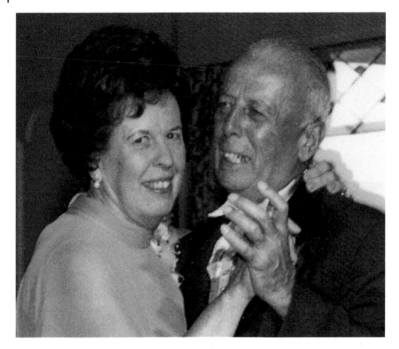

Figure 3.1 Margaret and Edward Gardner dancing in the 1970s.

the smell of Grandma's house was one that I adored. Of course, the candies she kept fully stocked in the dish on the end table were also a plus!

Grandma Gardner (Figure 3.2) was not in the best of "health." Most of the ailments she had trouble managing were from the natural declining progression of life; nonetheless, in no way was she ready for hospice. Apart from something drastic happening, she had years left, and it was safe to say that she also was not your "normal" older person – or senior citizen. She was what I consider a "geriatric," a term that is often unclear, generating multiple questions: What exactly is a geriatric? What graduates someone from a senior to a geriatric? Is there technically a difference between the two terms? Does "geriatric" relate to the need for much greater care, being at risk for more disasters, or is it simply a term used once someone has made it to a certain age?

As a veterinarian who concentrates exclusively on geriatric pets, hospice and euthanasia, I can see the parallels that our companion animals have to humans as they mature, age and inevitably decline. A nine-year-old Labrador may fit the criteria of a "senior" while still functioning perfectly fine in the home. However, a 12-year-old Labrador with no terminal disease looming might have a much harder time managing the ailments that plague the advanced aged pet. Thus, the family must care for the elder pet differently. Think back to the reference of picking up Grandma Gardner (in her late 80s); this experience involves much different efforts than picking up my father who is a bit younger, in his mid-60s. As extra assistance was required for Grandma Gardner, the advanced aged Labrador may also need the same type of consideration. For instance, the food bowl may need to be raised, the floor lined in bath mats, nightlights added to the dark hallway, and a ramp installed to get up the back steps or into the car. Although there is evidently more care taken for the further aged Labrador the question is raised: Is there

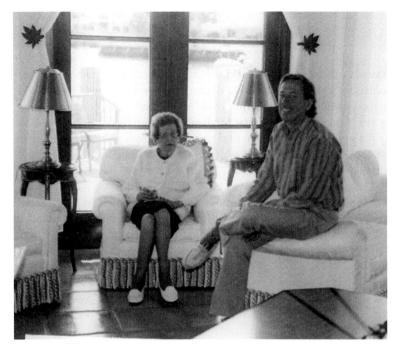

Figure 3.2 Grandma Gardner (and her youngest son, my father, Allan) at Thanksgiving dinner 1995.

technically a difference between senior and geriatric pets? Are they treated differently in terms of veterinary medicine? Regardless of the definition, I believe that they should be treated differently because they indeed, are different.

Senior or Geriatric … It's All in a Name – or Is It?

My journey into understanding geriatrics began with seniors and was relatively basic, with the goal of answering broad questions such as: what does "senior" mean, and how do human and veterinary medicine define it? The word "senior" arose in the late thirteenth century from Latin *seniores* meaning "older." Its original use in the English language dates back to the 1510s as a definition of rank, suggesting "higher in rank, longer in service." It was also used at this time as an addition to a personal name indicating "the father" when father and son had the same name (for example, Allan Senior and Allan Junior). The term "senior citizen" was first recorded in 1938 to define an elderly person, one who is past the age of retirement; however, the term had nothing to do with the individual's medical state.

An article titled "Ageism in Language" in a newsletter from the American Society of Aging (ASA, 2007) presented the following question to readers, "What term(s) do you think are appropriate when referring to people aged 65-plus?" The most commonly used expressions and percentage of individuals considering each term 'appropriate' were:

- older adults = 80%
- elders = 41%

- seniors = 33%
- senior citizens = 11%
- elderly = 10%.

Based on these statistics, is the word "senior" becoming a word of the past? Are more people beginning to use the term "older adult" to define those over the age of 65? Should we, as veterinarians, be saying "older pet" rather than "senior pet?" This concept led me to researching how the American Veterinary Medical Association (AVMA) uses the term "senior." In my research, I was unable to find an actual definition; nonetheless, the AVMA does offer a page on their website that addresses the question, "When does a pet become 'old'?" Their answer:

> It varies, but cats and small dogs are generally considered "senior" at seven years of age. Larger breed dogs tend to have shorter life spans compared to smaller breeds and are often considered senior when they are 5 to 6 years of age. Contrary to popular belief, dogs do not age at a rate of seven human years for each year in dog years." (AVMA, 2017).

Both the AVMA and the ASA offer no clear definition of what a "senior" is; however, I learned that the term does not relate as much to "biology" as I thought it would, which led me to wonder, what is a "geriatric?"

Geriatric Medicine for Humans

The US elderly population is expected to dramatically rise over the coming decades (the same can be said for the elderly pet population); thus, increasing the need for more focus by physicians on geriatrics. Since advancements in human medicine most often precede veterinary medicine, I decided to take a look into the history of human geriatrics to get an understanding of how it came to fruition, what a geriatrician does, and if there are parallels we can make in veterinary medicine. Accordingly, a human geriatrician must first be a family medicine physician or internal medicine physician to qualify for the certification of geriatrics. The certification is referred to as a certificate of added qualifications (CAQ). Fewer than 10,000 of the 120,000 practicing general internists and family physicians in the United States have earned a CAQ in geriatric medicine (Warshaw et al., 2003). To get their CAQ, the physician must first complete a fellowship program and then sit for the exam. The five most reputable schools offering a fellowship program for geriatric medicine are:

1) John Hopkins
2) University of California, Los Angeles
3) Icahn School of Medicine at Mount Sinai
4) Duke University
5) Harvard Medical School Teaching Hospital.

While geriatric medicine cares for the older population, the specialty itself is quite young. Box 3.1 shows a timeline of the growth of human geriatric medicine (Forciea, 2014).

In May 2016, I attended a conference for human geriatricians in Long Beach, California. It was quite eye opening on many levels, although two primary themes were

---

Box 3.1 The Growth of Human Geriatric Medicine

1943	The American Geriatric Society was organized and held its first annual meeting.
1945	The Gerontological Society of America was established in the United States.
1965	President Lyndon Johnson signed the legislation establishing Medicare, a health insurance program for the elderly.
1966	Dr Leslie Libow developed the first fellowship training experience in geriatric medicine at City Hospital Center in New York.
1974	National Institute on Aging was founded, sponsoring training at many levels.
1976	Congress authorized the first Geriatric Research, Education, and Clinical Center (GRECC).
1976	The Veterans' Administration began to sponsor innovation in the care of the elderly through its Geriatric Research and Education Clinical Centers.
1977	The first professorship in geriatrics in the United States was established at Cornell University.
1982	The first department of geriatrics at a major teaching center, Mount Sinai Medical School (Dr Libow's institution) was started.
1988	The American Boards of Internal Medicine and Family Practice jointly offered a certifying examination for a Certificate of Added Qualifications in Geriatric Medicine (CAQGM). At this time, there were 62 fellowship programs in internal medicine and 16 in family practice.
1995	The initial geriatric fellowship programs had a two-year requirement, but in 1995 it was reduced to one year. While there are a few institutions that offer a second and third year of additional geriatric training, most of the fellows in geriatrics prefer the one-year fellowship.

---

accentuated. First, the care-givers themselves are a major concern when caring for a geriatric. At the conference, much emphasis was placed on their mental and physical wellbeing. Recognizing that family members comprise a majority of the care-giving team, a primary goal of human geriatrics is to find new ways of educating and supporting that team and to alleviate care-giver fatigue.

Second, dementia is a massive and widespread ailment in human health. I was thoroughly shocked at the severity of this problem within our society and, consequently, how difficult it is on the care-giving unit. My uncle recently passed away from early onset Alzheimer's disease, and I personally witnessed how extremely taxing it was on my aunt. Thankfully, she was a nurse, but that did not discount the fact that she was first a wife. I often felt exhausted just from looking at how consumed she was with the care of Uncle Gene.

A woman I chatted with at the conference was a mental health counselor, and was very interested in how our families deal with their aging pets. I spoke with her about anticipatory grief, care-giver fatigue and pet loss grief, all very similar in both of our worlds. As we sipped our morning coffee I told her that I was still confused as to what a "geriatrician" really does and asked if she could help to clarify. I knew that they "cared for elderly people," but how is that different from a family physician? Fortunately, she laid it out quite simply for me. First, the family physician refers the patient to a geriatrician. The geriatrician then has two main roles: 1) To monitor all of the medications the patient is on (since many see multiple specialists, polypharmacy is a huge concern); and 2) To deal with dementia – and there it was, another reference to that awful ailment!

> Geriatrics, from *geras*, old age, and *iatrikos*, relating to the physician, is a term I would suggest as an addition to our vocabulary, to cover the same field in old age that is covered by the term pediatrics in childhood, to emphasize the necessity of considering senility and its disease apart from maturity and to assign it a separate place in medicine.
>
> (Forciea, 2014).

Would a specialty in geriatrics make sense in veterinary medicine? Do we have as much of a problem with polypharmacy? Do many of our patients suffer from a form of dementia? I can only answer "yes" to the third question, as I see it in over 50% of my patients, but I feel that the primary care physician (as well as the internist, oncologist, cardiologist and neurologist) are skilled at handling that illness in our companion animals.

Many of the paths that veterinary specialties take are modeled after human specialties, often coming to fruition decades after the human medicine program. With that, I do not believe that veterinary medicine has to *always* follow human medicine. Although we often have similarities and fundamentals that are in line with each other, the two professions do not have to function in exactly the same way. Veterinary medicine does not have a pediatric specialty, so why would we need one for geriatrics? At this point, I do not think we do; however, with the continued improvement of veterinary medicine, and as technology becomes more advanced, the elderly pet population is going to continue to expand. It is imperative that veterinarians, technicians and students understand the aging process, what it means to have old-age symptoms, how families can manage these symptoms, and how we, as veterinarians, can offer support to families. Better education in these avenues is necessary, and should start in veterinary schools. After reaching out to all of the veterinary schools in the United States, I was unable to find a single school that offered a course specifically in geriatrics. Veterinary programs incorporated "senior" content in many of their classes, but a course specific to geriatrics may unfortunately be in the distant future.

Fragility

Regardless of the label we use (senior or geriatric) I am mainly concerned with those pets that are fragile and need extra consideration, like my grandmother – the "fragile egg." Fragility is one of those complex terms that has a multitude of definitions, meanings and criteria. The concept itself is fragile!

Fragility is a syndrome where one has increased vulnerability and decreased physical function; thus, increasing the probability for adverse outcomes. In humans, the prevalence of fragility in older populations (65 years and older) is about 9.9%, and 25–50% in people aged 85 and older. (Liu et al., 2012). So, what classifies one as "fragile?"

Classifiers of the fragility syndrome for humans include various combinations of the following indicators:

- weakness (including grip strength)
- fatigue/exhaustion

- weight loss
- impaired balance
- decreased physical activity
- slowed motor performance (gate speed)
- social withdrawal
- mild cognitive dysfunction
- increased vulnerability to physiological stresses.

It has been proposed that, to be classified as geriatric, one must exhibit at least three of the following criteria:

- weakness
- weight loss
- slowed mobility
- fatigue
- low levels of activities.

I can easily link this to a multitude of older pets presenting at least three of those conditions, thus raising the question of when pets (or humans) are considered "fragile" are they also "geriatric?" The answer remains unclear.

The criteria of "slowed mobility" interested me, as I always thought that my geriatric patients, as well as Grandma Gardner, had a turtle's pace because of some underlying disease, like arthritis or sarcopenia. Yet, my grandmother never expressed pain or weakness when walking. One lecture I attended at the geriatric conference discussed gait speed (the "normal" pace of a person's walking) in relation to fragility, as well as dementia. To better clarify this phenomenon, I spoke with the presenter (Manuel Montero-Odasso, MD) afterwards. He explained that, based on studies, in the absence of pathologic issues resulting in gait disorders, pace may slow down as a person ages for no physical reason. Individuals experiencing this slowed mobility are completely unconscious of the decrease in speed. Additionally, he described the theory that the part of the brain indicating our normal pace is in the same location where pathology is found in many humans with dementia; thus, the person possibly is not aware of their slower walking speed. Consequently, he concluded that a slower gait pace not only indicates a greater risk of falling but it could also be a predictor of upcoming dementia (Montero-Odasso et al., 2012).

After learning this, I hightailed it to the next lecture at a speed no one could keep up with! Exhausted from my fast clip to the next lecture, I sat in the back and waited eagerly to learn more about our aging human population. Speaking of exhaustion, it also happens to be a criterion for fragility. Exhaustion is the perception of inadequate energy levels to meet one's demand. Measuring levels of exhaustion in humans varies. Some studies ask questions like, "How often have you had a hard time getting going?" and "How often does everything seem an effort?" A response of "Most of the time," or 'A moderate amount of time" would classify that individual as exhausted. The trouble with exhaustion is that it is self-reporting and it is therefore a difficult criterion to assess in our companion animals.

Interestingly, observational data have suggested that exhaustion and weight loss tend to develop later than other components of fragility, and may identify people at greater risk for subsequent rapid decline (Whitson et al., 2011). Not to anthropomorphize, but in my own observation, those pets with unexplained weight loss and whom seem to have a "lack of energy" decline much faster than those animals not exhibiting those concerns.

Table 3.1 Age chart (courtesy of Fred L. Metzger, DVM, DABVP).

Years	1	2	3	4	5	6	7	8	9	10	11	12	13	14	15	16	17	18	19	20
Small dog breed/cats (1–20 lb)	7	13	20	26	33	40	44	48	52	56	60	64	68	72	76	80	84	88	92	96
Medium dog breed (20–50 lb)	7	14	21	27	34	42	47	51	56	60	68	69	74	78	83	87	92	96	101	105
Large dog breed (50–90 lb)	8	16	24	31	38	45	50	55	61	66	72	77	82	88	93	99	104	109	115	120
Extra-large dog breed (>90 lb)	9	18	26	34	41	49	56	64	71	78	86	93	101	108	115	123	131	139		
			Adult				Senior					Geriatric								

The process of decline, vulnerability and fragility is unfortunately not well defined, and there is little research in fragility in animals – most that has been done was in mice, to help determine the effects of fragility for humans; however, considering and treating certain advanced aged pets as fragile may provide new opportunities for prevention, health promotion and improved care for both the pet and the family unit.

The Geriatric Life Stage in Dogs and Cats

As mentioned earlier, the AVMA does not have a defined set of rules to include a pet in the senior category. Furthermore, they do not provide classification on the geriatric life stage. In fact, they often use the two terms interchangeably. Although I have yet to find a clear distinction between the two, I do believe, in theory, that they are different and we should approach each pet individually. If signs of advanced ageing, fragility and vulnerability exist, we should handle the treatment and care of the pet differently.

Pet parents may be more open to assistance if they felt that we as a profession understood the changes in their pet as well as the struggles they face physically and emotionally during the twilight years of their pets. Table 3.1 is a chart that I find useful to give to all my clients with advanced aged pets. It helps them to appreciate the stage their pet may be at, and opens the door to better conversations about care. There is a great deal of information in Chapter 22 of this textbook on how you can market, manage, handle and treat geriatric pets in your clinic.

Summary

In my research for this textbook, and for my own personal growth and education, I have learned a large amount about the aging process, not only biologically, but also socially. One may begin to think more about decline as one ages themselves. But I do not believe that to be the reason I am so intrigued. My own mortality is not my leading concern. It is my deep desire to not only help our aging, frail geriatric pets, but the families that love them so dearly as well. They want to know why their pet only lives to a certain age, while other species may live four times as long. They want to know why their pet sleeps most of the day, why their bark has changed, why their legs start to quiver more often, why they stare off into the corner of the room and become startled easily. Most important, are the questions my clients ask about how to manage these symptoms.

None of the symptoms alone is difficult, but as they start to mount up, it becomes a struggle for the entire family. No one wants to give up on their pet. They make a promise the day they get them to care for them to the best of their abilities. How can we as the veterinary team help them keep that promise? Understanding the vulnerability in our older pets allows us to support the family as the primary care-giving unit and offers them the education and tools to successfully care for their geriatric pet. This textbook provides insight into many aspects of the geriatric pet. Although old age is technically not a disease, it certainly can diminish quality of life if decline takes hold of the pet. In short, most can agree that our pets simply do not live long enough, but we can make the last life stage a little easier – and quite possibly, help them live a longer, better life.

References

American Society on Aging. (2007) "Ageism in Language." *ASA Connection*, June.

American Veterinary Medical Association. Senior Pets. (2017) Available at www.avma.org/public/PetCare/Pages/Senior-Pets.aspx.

Forciea, M. A. (2014) "Geriatric Medicine: History of a Young Specialty." *AMA Journal of Ethics*, **16**(5): 385–389.

Liu, H., Graber, T. G., Ferguson-Stegall, L., Thompson, L. V. (2012) "Gait and Cognition: A Complementary Approach to Understanding Brain Function and the Risk of Falling." *Journal of the American Geriatric Society*, **60**(11): 2127–2136.

Montero-Odasso, M., Verghese, J., Beauchet, O., Hausdorff, J. M. (2012) "Gait and Cognition: A Complementary Approach to Understanding Brain Function and the Risk of Falling." *Journal of the American Geriatric Society*, **60**(11): 2127–2136.

Warshaw, G. A., Thomas, D. C., Callahan, E. H., Bragg, E. J., Shaull, R. W., Lindsell, C. J., and Goldenhar, L. M. (2003) "A National Survey on the Current Status of General Internal Medicine Residency Education in Geriatric Medicine" *Journal of General Internal Medicine*, **18**: 679–684.

Whitson, H. E., Thielke, S., Diehr, R., O'Hare, A. M., Chaves, P. H., Zakai, N. A., Arnold, A., Chaudhry, S., Ives, D., Newman, A. B. (2011) "Patterns and Predictors of Recovery from Exhaustion in Older Adults: The Cardiovascular Health Study." *Journal of the American Geriatric Society*, **59**(2): 207–213.

Part II

The Aging Body Systems

"Never tease an old dog; he might have one bite left."

— Robert A. Heinlein

4

Vision Changes
Kayla Waler and Meredith Voyles

Introduction and Description

Vision is a fundamental sense that plays a critical role in our patient's lives. Whether it be playing ball outside or chasing a laser in the house, vision plays an important role in the quality of life for our patients and in the bond between a pet and an owner. The eye is a complex organ which requires many factors to function correctly in order to achieve the desired result: vision. In all species, vision affords a survival advantage and most animals rely on their vision to help them communicate, locate food, and avoid predators. The eye is composed of three layers:

1) The outer fibrous tunic layer (cornea and sclera).
2) The middle uveal layer (iris, ciliary body, choroid).
3) The inner nervous layer (retina and optic nerve).

The eye is also composed of three chambers: the anterior chamber, posterior chamber and vitreous (Figure 4.1). Each of these structures is specifically designed to play a unique role in the function of the eye and in vision. During the aging process, these different structures of the eye lose function just as any other aging part of the body. Luckily, aging pets do not always go blind, and the ocular changes attributed solely to age do not usually affect functional vision. Therefore, if a patient appears to have trouble seeing, other pathologic disease processes should be considered and ruled out. This chapter discusses "normal" age-associated ocular conditions that occur in the geriatric animal. Because many of these changes present similarly to pathologic disease processes, it is important to ensure that they are differentiated from one another. Differentiation may be difficult, so performing a thorough and complete ocular examination combined with patient history and signalment is critical.

Treatment and Care of the Geriatric Veterinary Patient, First Edition. Edited by Mary Gardner and Dani McVety.
© 2017 John Wiley & Sons, Inc. Published 2017 by John Wiley & Sons, Inc.
Companion Website: www.wiley.com/go/gardner/geriatric

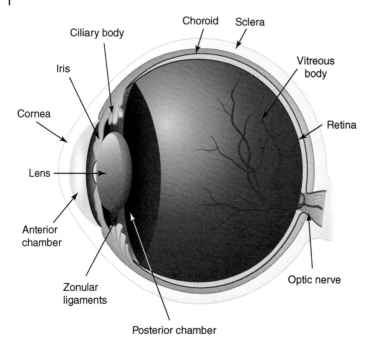

Figure 4.1 Normal ocular anatomy (reproduced with permission from John Wiley & Sons, Inc.).

Nuclear/Lenticular Sclerosis

Nuclear sclerosis is a common aging change seen in all dogs, which manifests at approximately six to seven years of age. The lens comprises an inner nucleus and outer cortex encased in an exterior capsule. It consists of about 65% water and 35% proteins, both of which decrease with age (Samuelson, 2013). The proportion of insoluble proteins increases in an old lens and becomes greater in the nucleus, which is the older portion of the lens. As the lens becomes older, the proteins become compacted together, causing the lens fibers to lose their flexibility and ability to change shape (Samuelson, 2013). This loss of elasticity is what accounts for the inability in humans to accommodate, which necessitates the use of bifocal glasses. The combination of growth of the lens, together with protein changes in the lens, creates an increase in the density of the lens nucleus and in the reflection of light (Martin, 2010a). The growth of the lens has been compared to that of the growth of an onion's layers. As new layers of protein are added, the older, inner layer becomes compacted together and becomes harder with age. This creates a central hazy, whitish, blue-gray appearance to the center of the lens, which is oftentimes confused with a cataract.

Differentiation of nuclear sclerosis from a cataract is only possible through examination of the lens. Pupil dilation is important in this process and can be accomplished with application of a short acting mydriatic agent, such as topical tropicamide (0.5% or 1%). One drop is administered and then application is repeated once after 5–10 minutes. This will produce adequate dilation for visualization of the lens and will allow for differentiation between nuclear sclerosis and cataracts. With nuclear sclerosis, the outline

Figure 4.2 Nuclear sclerosis in a dog. Note the outline of the lens nucleus, often described as a "lens within a lens". This dog has no visual deficits (courtesy of the ophthalmology department, University of Illinois).

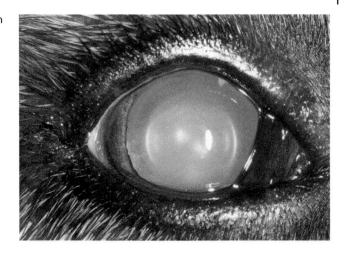

of the lens nucleus, which has been described as a "lens within a lens" can be visualized (Figure 4.2). Light will also be able to shine through, allowing examination of the fundus, whereas with cataracts, light will be unable to pass and funduscopic examination will not be possible (Maggs *et al.*, 2013a). Experience with the evaluation of lens density can even be used to age an animal as accurately as dental examination (Martin, 2010a). Determination of specific age with this technique can be difficult; however, if nuclear sclerosis is determined to be present upon lens examination, it can be approximated that the patient be at least eight to nine years of age. It is important to note that dilation of the pupil should not be performed if lens luxation or an increase in intraocular pressures (glaucoma) are suspected. In most animals, except for the most severe cases, vision is not affected with nuclear sclerosis and the patient is not considered a surgical candidate, nor is medical therapy necessary. However, older dogs with nuclear sclerosis may also develop subsequent cataracts (Bromberg, n.d.).

Senile Cataracts

The term cataract refers to a loss of transparency of the lens or its capsule (Maggs *et al.*, 2013a). The opacities may vary in extent, location within the lens, cause, rate of progression, and age of onset. Senile cataracts are part of the aging process that occurs in animals older than eight or nine years of age. One study reported that by 13.5 years of age, all dogs had some degree of cataract formation (Williams *et al.*, 2004). However, it should be noted that the age of onset in which cataracts can be considered to be age related is arbitrary and breed related (Gelatt, 2014a). It is difficult to determine whether a cataract is truly age related and difficult to distinguish a non-heritable from a heritable cataract. Hereditary cataracts often develop in the young or middle aged dog and involve the cortex or capsule region of the lens. In cats, the majority of cataracts are formed secondary to intraocular inflammation, but senile cataracts have been noted to develop in the late teen years (Moore, 2001). Senile cataracts most often affect the inner portion of the lens, called the nucleus, and are typically preceded by dense nuclear sclerosis. The pathogenesis of senile cataracts is unknown; however, in people, oxidative

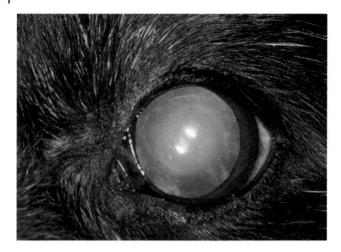

Figure 4.3 Direct illumination of a senile cataract in a dog. Note the dense nuclear sclerosis and the presence of multifocal opacities in the lens cortices (courtesy of the ophthalmology department, University of Illinois).

injury to the lens secondary to solar radiation and ultraviolent light is thought to play a role (Gelatt, 2014a). The location and stage of cataract formation can be used to help determine the cause of the cataract. The stages of cataract formation include incipient (<10% of lens involvement), immature (>10% but < 100% lens involvement), mature (100% lens involvement), and hypermature (100% or less lens involvement and wrinkled capsule).

Evaluation of cataracts can be performed by visualizing the lens after pupil dilation. This can be achieved by the application of a short-acting mydriatic agent such as tropicamide, followed by direct illumination or retroillumination. With direct illumination, light is localized directly over the lens and the cataract appears white (Figure 4.3). In contrast, retroillumination directs the light towards the back of the eye from afar and the cataract appears dark. This helps to distinguish not only between different stages of cataracts but between the presence of a cataract and nuclear sclerosis. Mature cataract formation results in total vision loss and thus no tapetal refraction will be present upon examination. In contrast, some tapetal refraction will be seen with incipient and immature cataracts, as they do not cause 100% vision loss. In patients that present with cataracts or the complaint of visual deficits, a menacing gesture should be performed to assess vision. It is important that an air current not be created when performing this gesture, as a falsely positive response can result. An obstacle course can also be set up in the exam room to evaluate the patient's navigation in a new and unfamiliar place. It may be helpful to assess the patient's navigation through the obstacle course in both dim and bright light. A cotton ball test can also be performed to assess vision, in which a cotton ball is dropped in front of the animal's field of vision. The patient is then observed for tracking of the cotton ball as it falls. Typically, senile cataracts are slowly progressive and take years to reach full maturity. However, over time, cataracts can produce inflammation inside of the eye, called lens-induced uveitis. Performing tonometry in every patient with cataracts is therefore an important part of the ocular examination. It is important to realize that other systemic disease processes, most notably diabetes mellitus, can cause the formation of cataracts. Therefore, the etiology of the cataract must be differentiated before being attributed solely to age.

Cataracts can be managed medically, surgically with phacoemulsification, and through observation; however, management is dependent on several factors. If the cataract is causing significant lens-induced uveitis, medical management with a topical nonsteroidal anti-inflammatory agent such as ketorolac, diclofenac, or flurbiprofen may be selected. Surgical case selection is also multifactorial and is dependent on visual deficit, stage of the cataract, presence and control of lens-induced uveitis, retinal health and function, anesthetic risk, and owner compliance (Maggs *et al.*, 2013a). It is important to consider the anesthetic risk associated with surgery, especially in geriatric patients. If the anesthetic risk is high, withholding surgery may outweigh the benefit of correcting visual deficits. If vision is not significantly affected by the cataract and lens-induced uveitis is not present, observation of the rate of progression through serial recheck examinations may be the best option.

There is currently no medical therapy to dissolve or diminish cataracts; however, an antioxidant nutritional supplement called Ocu-Glo™ may be used to support lens health after diagnosis of cataracts. This product was formulated by board-certified ophthalmologists with the primary goal of supporting canine eye health. The three main ingredients include grapeseed extract, lutein, and omega 3 fatty acids, with lutein being important for lens health. Use of this product will not eliminate current cataract formation, but may prevent cataract progression while supporting the current health of the lens. It should be noted that although Ocu-Glo is recommended as a supplement for existing ocular health after diagnosis of cataracts, it cannot be used to prevent cataract formation prior to diagnosis.

Counseling and educating owners is immensely important with cataracts and their management. Signs associated with cognitive dysfunction, such as pacing, circling and panting, are often interpreted by owners as being caused by blindness. Therefore, for older patients, owners should be counseled about senility and cognitive dysfunction (Maggs *et al.*, 2013a). It should be discussed that although cataract removal may be successful, it may not result in the expectation sought, owing to concurrent disease processes that occur with age. Discussion about cataract surgery and the time, cost, effort, and compliance associated with its success should also be discussed. Cataract surgery is not the best option for every patient, or every owner, and it is not without risk. Risk factors such as the development of postoperative glaucoma, uveitis, and retinal detachment should be discussed with owners. Significant postoperative care, hands-on medicating, and time are also required to ensure the success of cataract surgery. The decision to pursue surgical removal of cataracts should therefore be one that is made jointly with the client, with their expectations and capabilities in mind.

Iris Atrophy

Iris atrophy is characterized by thinning of the stroma or pupillary margin of the iris and occurs in older animals of all species. It is commonly seen in toy and miniature Poodles, miniature Schnauzers and Chihuahuas, although it can occur in any breed (Maggs *et al.*, 2013b). Iris atrophy is most commonly observed in dogs, although blue-eyed cats will manifest both congenital hypoplasia and atrophy of the iris with age (Martin, 2010b). Iris atrophy can take many different forms, and can cause the iris to appear moth eaten and scalloped, or even create holes in the iris, known as stromal iris

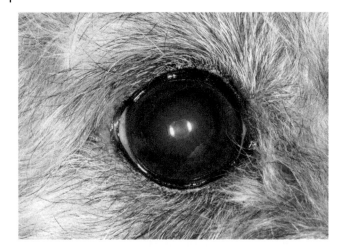

Figure 4.4 Iris atrophy of the pupillary margin with subsequent dyscoria (misshaped pupil) in a geriatric dog (courtesy of the ophthalmology department, University of Illinois).

atrophy. The most common location for iris atrophy is in the iris sphincter muscle, which involves the pupillary margin (Figure 4.4). This margin defines the shape of the pupil, so the presence of iris atrophy can result in dyscoria (abnormal pupil shape) or mydriasis (pupil dilation; Figure 4.4). This may lead to reduced or absent normal pupillary light responses, although vision is unaffected (Gelatt, 2014b). Pupillary light responses are tested by shining a bright light into the eye, such as with a transilluminator. The completeness and briskness of pupil constriction is then noted. The response noted in the eye in which the light source was directed is termed the direct reflex, while the response in the fellow eye is called the consensual reflex. This absence of a normal pupillary light response causes an inability of the eye to control how much light is entering it and may cause the affected animal to be sensitive to bright light (Bromberg, n.d.).

The atrophy may also not be present symmetrically in both eyes and anisocoria (different pupil sizes) may be noted. This normal aging change should be differentiated from pathologic disease processes, such as glaucoma, Horner's syndrome, uveitis, and other cranial nerve abnormalities that can cause alterations to normal pupil size (Bromberg, n.d.). Other aspects of the ophthalmic examination, such as tonometry and a neurologic examination, can help to differentiate this normal aging change from a pathologic disease process. There is no treatment or medical therapy for iris atrophy, and the onset of this normal aging change should not affect quality of life for the patient or the owner. However, if patients are extremely sensitive to light, owners can be counseled on avoiding exposure of their pets to bright sunlight. Going on walks at dusk or at night is an option that can be recommended to owners to prevent exposure of their pets to bright light.

Retinal Degeneration

The retina is responsible for converting light into signals that are eventually perceived as a visual image via the visual cortex in the brain. The retina is thus an important structure for vision. The photoreceptor cells in the retina of dogs and cats comprise rods and cones, each of which have different functions. Rods are more sensitive than cones to low levels of light and function in dim environments and at night (scotopic vision). Cones are less sensitive to small changes in light levels and function predominately in bright light (photopic vision) (Maggs *et al.*, 2013c). The dog and cat retina is composed predominately of rods; thus, as the retina thins in the aging animal, some decrease in night vision may result. The predominant differential for this age-related retinal thinning is progressive retinal atrophy, which is an inherited condition most commonly seen in Poodles and resulting in blindness (Bromberg, n.d.). Progressive retinal atrophy can be diagnosed definitively with an electroretinogram, which is similar to an echocardiogram for the heart. As the retina thins, it absorbs less light and more light is reflected back. Hyperreflectivity may therefore be noted upon fundic examination. Owners may notice their pet hesitating when going out at night or in dark areas of the house, so it may be helpful to recommend that they turn on more lights in the house or add nightlights throughout the house to aid the pet in visualization and navigation.

There is no treatment for age-associated retinal changes, although Ocu-Glo antioxidant nutritional supplements may be found to be beneficial. Ocu-Glo contains lutein, which is important for retinal health, as well as omega 3 fatty acids, which act to enrich the normal function of retinal photoreceptors. Although this supplement will not correct or reverse the changes already present, it will act to support the current health of the retina and prevent progression. Typically, this aging change of the retina does not progress to complete blindness and the quality of life for the patient is not significantly affected.

Vitreal Degeneration/Asteroid Hyalosis

The vitreous is the transparent, gel-like substance that occupies the posterior segment of the eye. The vitreous maintains ocular volume and helps to maintain the lens and the retina in their correct locations (Maggs *et al.*, 2013d). Vitreal degeneration is the term used to describe the changes consistent with the breakdown of the vitreous. Signs of vitreal degeneration include liquefaction, called syneresis, and opacities, termed asteroid hyalosis (Gelatt, 2014c). When the vitreous degenerates, it loses its jelly-like consistency and become more liquefied in nature. Because the vitreous plays a major role in supporting the retina and keeping it in its appropriate anatomic location, retinal detachment becomes a concern secondary to vitreal degeneration. Vitreal degeneration is difficult to diagnose and is most commonly diagnosed with ocular ultrasound during preoperative screening of surgical cataract candidates (Maggs *et al.*, 2013d). Retinopexy is a surgical procedure that can be performed prophylactically to prevent retinal detachment secondary to vitreal degeneration. During the procedure, a laser is used to "spot-weld" or fuse the retina to the underlying tissues. The procedure requires the use of general anesthesia, so retinopexy may not be the best option for our geriatric patients. Each patient should be assessed on an individual basis and the risks of performing the procedure should be discussed in detail with the client. Referral to a veterinary ophthalmologist is recommended if this procedure is elected.

Asteroid hyalosis is another manifestation of vitreal degeneration which increases in frequency with age. It is bilateral in 50% of patients and is characterized by the appearance of numerous small calcium and lipid opacities scattered throughout the vitreous (Figure 4.5; Martin, 2010c). When the eye moves, these refractive bodies can be seen

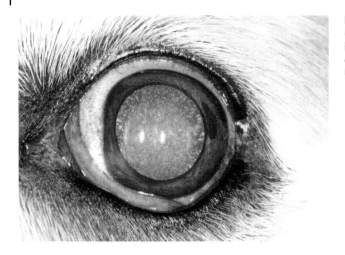

Figure 4.5 Asteroid hyalosis (form of vitreal degeneration) in a dog (courtesy of the ophthalmology department, University of Illinois).

moving or vibrating concurrently. The appearance is oftentimes described as similar to that of the falling snow that is seen when a snow globe is shaken. Examination of the vitreous is often performed with a bright light following pupil dilation through ophthalmoscopy or through indirect illumination with a strong penlight or transilluminator. With indirect illumination, the vitreal opacities will appear dark against the tapetal reflection (Moore, 2001). It should also be noted that asteroid hyalosis can occur secondary to episodes of inflammation, but occurs most frequently in geriatric animals (Townsend, 2009). The pathogenesis of asteroid hyalosis is unknown, but it has been hypothesized that because the vitreous is high in calcium content, precipitation with age can result in the changes seen (Bromberg, n.d.). Typically, no major visual impairments are caused by vitreal degeneration, with the exception of some cloudiness to vision. No treatment or management options exist for this age-associated condition of the vitreous and quality of life for the patient is unaffected.

Corneal Endothelial Degeneration/Dystrophy

The cornea is the transparent, avascular, anterior portion of the outer fibrous coat of the eye. It is composed of an outer epithelium, inner endothelium and middle stoma, which is made up of collagen. The endothelium acts as the major contributor to the control of corneal stromal fluid, as it contains a sodium potassium ATPase-associated pump mechanism (Cook *et al.*, 2009). This pump acts to regulate fluid and maintain the transparency of the cornea and its relative dehydration. Control of water entry into the cornea and maintenance of a state of dehydration is critical to corneal transparency and therefore to vision. With age, senile degeneration of the endothelium occurs causing the endothelial cells to enlarge and decrease in number. Endothelial cells have a limited capacity to replicate in most species and therefore, with age, endothelial cell numbers decrease (Maggs *et al.*, 2013e). This, in turn, results in an insufficient pump, which causes leakage. An opaque, blue-gray, diffuse corneal edema results, which is slowly progressive, starting in one eye and eventually becoming bilateral (Figure 4.6; Martin, 2010d). The edema starts in a temporal location and eventually progresses to cover the

Figure 4.6 Diffuse corneal edema in a dog with advanced corneal endothelial degeneration. Note the blue color to the cornea caused by diffuse edema (courtesy of the ophthalmology department, University of Illinois).

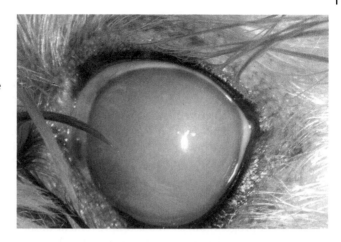

entire surface of the cornea. When fluid accumulates between the stroma and the epithelium, small bullae may develop which can subsequently rupture and cause superficial corneal ulceration. This condition is termed bullous keratopathy and can cause significant discomfort for the patient. Although corneal endothelial degeneration can occur in any breed, Boston terriers, Chihuahuas, Poodles, Basset Hounds, Chow Chows and Dalmatians are breeds that are predisposed (Martin, 2010d).

It is important to note that the endothelium can be damaged secondary to trauma, lens luxation, glaucoma, and uveitis (Maggs *et al.*, 2013e). Tonometry should therefore be performed in every patient with corneal edema. When a patient presents with corneal edema, the following algorithm can be followed to help determine the cause. First, assessment of whether the edema is diffuse or focal in nature should be made. Diffuse corneal edema is typically marked and fluorescein stain is not retained when applied. Focal corneal edema is milder and retains fluorescein stain, owing to the loss of epithelial cells secondary to corneal ulceration (Maggs *et al.*, 2013e). If focal edema is noted, the cause of ulceration must be found. If diffuse edema is present, underlying causes must be distinguished. This can be done by assessing the level of discomfort and pain in the patient, as well as intraocular pressure measurement. A non-painful eye with marked diffuse edema and normal intraocular pressure will most likely have endothelial degeneration or dystrophy present. If the patient is demonstrating pain and has abnormal intraocular pressures, glaucoma, uveitis, and lens luxation must be ruled out. A thorough intraocular examination and assessment of intraocular pressures will aid in determining the cause. However, it should be noted that if the edema present is severe, evaluation of the structures inside of the eye may be difficult, resulting in a limited intraocular examination. Normal intraocular pressures for a dog are $20 \pm 5\,\text{mmHg}$. Lower than normal pressures will be obtained in a patient with uveitis and higher than normal pressures will be obtained in a patient with glaucoma or with anterior lens luxation. Pupil size can also be used to distinguish between glaucoma and uveitis. Glaucoma is typically associated with a mydriatic pupil whereas a miotic pupil is typically noted with uveitis. The presence of iris atrophy should also be taken into consideration when evaluating the pupil size of a geriatric patient. The summation of ocular examination findings will aid in distinguishing a condition secondary to aging versus a pathologic disease process. If endothelial degeneration is diagnosed, the patient must be monitored for corneal bullae formation and secondary ulceration. This can be extremely painful and affect quality of life for the patient as well as the human animal bond between the patient and owner.

Because the end result of severe corneal endothelial degeneration is blindness, therapy is palliative. Hypertonic salt solutions, such as 5% sodium chloride ointment, can be used to draw water out of the cornea, although its effect has been shown to be minimal (Martin, 2010d). Topical antibiotics should also be applied if the bullae rupture, causing secondary ulceration. Placement of a thin, conjunctival graft, as well as thermokeratoplasty procedures have been used to prevent and reduce bullae formation (Maggs *et al.*, 2013e). During thermokeratoplasty, multiple small, superficial stromal burns are created with cautery to prevent recurrent ulcerations (Martin, 2010d). The patient should be referred to a veterinary ophthalmologists for these procedures.

As there is no cure for this condition, the goal in treatment should be aimed towards prevention of progression, as well as improvement of the comfort level and quality of life for the patient. Clients should be informed and prepared that this condition affects vision and, if severe, will ultimately result in blindness. Coping strategies for having a blind pet should then be discussed with the client, as hearing this news can be devastating and unexpected.

Coping Mechanisms for Owners with Blind Pets

The transition to owning a blind pet can be overwhelming, unexpected, and devastating for owners. Counseling clients on coping with having a newly blind pet is thus of immense importance. There are several coping techniques and strategies that owners can adopt to help their blind pet adjust to this new lifestyle. For example, using scent markers, such as Tracerz® (Innovet), which can be affixed to walls, furniture, flooring, and appliances, can help pets to find important locations and avoid obstacles in the house. Halos and visors such as the Optivizor are custom-designed products that can be used to help protect blind dogs from bumping into walls and objects. Small bells can also be attached to the collars of other pets in the household to alert and signal the blind pet of their whereabouts.

It is important that pools, steps, stairs, and any other unsafe areas of the house be blocked off to prevent blind animals from injuring themselves. Spontaneous rearrangement of furniture in the house should also be avoided, as blind pets adapt to the current layout of their home to navigate safely. If rearrangement of furniture is performed, it is recommended that it be done gradually. Blind pets adjust to using their other senses of hearing and smell quite well and verbal cues can be used as warnings, such as "watch", "wait", or "slow down" when approaching steps, corners, or other potentially unsafe areas. Blind pets can also continue to engage in the activities they enjoyed prior to becoming blind, such as throwing ball and playing fetch. Selecting balls and toys with sounds and scents for these activities may help blind pets to locate them more easily. A KONG filled with smelly treats such as peanut butter is another great play toy for blind pets. Establishing schedules and routines may also be helpful such as feeding at the same time and place each time. *Living With Blind Dogs* by Caroline Levin is a reputable resource book and training guide that can also be recommended to owners of blind pets to help aid them during this process.

Owners should be reassured that the success rate for animals adapting to being blind is extremely high and that most animals are able to live normal and happy lives. Sharing success stories with clients of other patients that have recently become blind may provide emotional support and reassurance that they are not alone in the process. Thankfully, the age-associated ocular conditions that affect our geriatric patients are ones that are not painful and do not cause significant morbidity or mortality. Although blindness cannot typically be reversed, the lifestyle changes discussed above can help to make the adjustment and transition for a blind pet easier and less stressful. It is important to discuss with clients that being blind alone does not warrant euthanasia for their pet. Owners should be reminded that vision is not a domestic animal's primary sense and that blind pets continue to function well, and will adjust with their other senses of hearing and smell. However, concurrent disease processes may be present in a geriatric animal in addition to being blind, which may significantly alter their quality of life. Each patient and their quality of life must be assessed on an individual basis and end of life decisions must be made based on the patient as a whole. Please refer Chapter 23 for more information concerning end of life decisions.

References

Bromberg, N. M. (n.d.) *"Your Dog Needs Bifocals' Geriatric Changes in the Eyes of Dogs and Cats."* Meridian, ID: American College of Veterinary Ophthalmology.

Cook, C. S., Peiffer, R. L., Jr., and Landis, M. L. (2009). "Clinical Basic Science." In Peiffer, R., and Petersen-Jones, S. *Small Animal Ophthalmology: A Problem-Oriented Approach.* 4th ed., pp. 1–12. St Louis, MO: Elsevier Saunders.

Gelatt, K. N. (2014a) "Canine Lens: Cataract, Luxation and Surgery." In *Essentials of Veterinary Ophthalmology.* 3rd ed., p. 312. Hoboken, NJ: John Wiley & Sons, Inc.

Gelatt, K. N. (2014b) "Canine Anterior Uvea: Diseases and Surgery." In *Essentials of Veterinary Ophthalmology.* 3rd ed., p. 279. Hoboken, NJ: John Wiley & Sons, Inc.

Gelatt, K. N. (2014c) "Canine Posterior Segment: Diseases and Surgery." In *Essentials of Veterinary Ophthalmology.* 3rd ed., pp. 329–330. Hoboken, NJ: John Wiley & Sons, Inc.

Levine, C. D. (2003) *Living With Blind Dogs: A Resource Book and Training Guide for the Owners of Blind and Low-Vision Dogs.* 2nd ed. Lantern Publications.

Maggs, D. J., Miller, P. E., and Ofri, R. (2013a) "Lens." In *Slatter's Fundamentals of Veterinary Ophthalmology.* 5th ed., pp. 276–287. St Louis, MO: Elsevier Saunders

Maggs, D. J., Miller, P. E., and Ofri, R. (2013b) "Uvea." In *Slatter's Fundamentals of Veterinary Ophthalmology.* 5th ed., p. 246. St Louis, MO: Elsevier Saunders.

Maggs, D. J., Miller, P. E., and Ofri, R. (2013c) "Retina." In *Slatter's Fundamentals of Veterinary Ophthalmology.* 5th ed., p. 303. St Louis, MO: Elsevier Saunders.

Maggs, D. J., Miller, P. E., and Ofri, R. (2013d) "Vitreous." In *Slatter's Fundamentals of Veterinary Ophthalmology.* 5th ed., pp 291–294. St Louis, MO: Elsevier Saunders.

Maggs, D. J., Miller, P. E., and Ofri, R. (2013e) "Cornea and Sclera." In *Slatter's Fundamentals of Veterinary Ophthalmology.* 5th ed., pp. 184–189. St Louis, MO: Elsevier Saunders.

Martin, C. L. (2010a) "Lens." In *Ophthalmic Disease in Veterinary Medicine*, pp. 369–395. Boca Raton, FL: CRC Press.

Martin, C. L. (2010b) "Anterior Uvea and Anterior Chamber." In *Ophthalmic Disease in Veterinary Medicine*, pp. 298–336. Boca Raton, FL: CRC Press.

Martin, C. L. (2010c) "Vitreous and Ocular Fundus." In *Ophthalmic Disease in Veterinary Medicine*, p. 404. Boca Raton, FL: CRC Press.

Martin, C. L. (2010d) "Cornea and Sclera." In *Ophthalmic Disease in Veterinary Medicine*, pp. 251–252. Boca Raton, FL: CRC Press.

Moore, P. A. (2001) "Examination Technique and Interpretation of Ophthalmic Findings." *Clinical Techniques in Small Animal Practice*, **16**(1): 1–12.

Samuelson, D. A. (2013) "Ophthalmic Anatomy." In Gelatt, K. N., Gilger, B. C., and Kern, T. J. (eds) *Veterinary Ophthalmology*, 5th ed., pp.124–125. Ames, IA: Wiley-Blackwell.

Townsend, W. M., Bedford, P. G. C., and Jones, R. G. (2009). "Abnormal Appearance." In Peiffer, R. and Petersen-Jones S. (eds). *Small Animal Ophthalmology: A Problem-Oriented Approach*. 4th ed., pp 67–115. St Louis, MO: Elsevier Saunders.

Williams, D. L., Heath, M. F., and Wallis, C. (2004) "Prevalence of Canine Cataract: Preliminary Results of a Cross-Sectional Study." *Veterinary Ophthalmology*, 7(1): 29–35.

5

Hearing Loss

Brad Bates

Hearing loss is one of the most common clinical signs in our geriatric pets. Although there are other causes of hearing loss, age-related hearing loss, also known as presbycusis, is the most common cause of deafness in pets (Kay, 2015). Other known causes of hearing loss include ototoxic drugs and congenital deafness (Cunningham and Klein, 2007). This chapter includes a brief discussion of how noise is converted and interpreted into sound, causes of hearing loss, monitoring and testing geriatric pets for signs of hearing loss, and a discussion on the management techniques that can enhance the quality of life for a geriatric pet with hearing loss.

What is Sound?

Many animal species have a particularly acute sense of hearing, especially when compared with humans. Although hearing sensitivity of other species may be far beyond that in humans, the basic mechanisms of sound interpretation is similar among mammalian species. To hear a noise, sound waves must be transduced from the environment through the tympanic membranes (or ear drums) to the cochlea in the inner ear, where hair cell receptors are located. These hair cells mediate the conversion of sound waves into electrical activity, which is then propagated to the brain, where they are interpreted into what we perceive as sound (Cunningham and Klein, 2007). A full description of the physiology of sound interpretation is beyond the scope of this chapter.

Causes of Hearing Loss in Pets

Age-related hearing loss is the most common cause of deafness in pets. It typically begins with impaired ability to hear middle- to high-frequency sounds, and progresses to include the entire range of sound frequencies (Kay, 2015). As it develops, many pet owners mistakenly interpret their pet's partial hearing loss as a behavioral issue, similar to what some would consider "selective hearing." This is why many pet owners will not recognize hearing loss until it is quite advanced (Kay, 2015). In fact, deafness in animals

Treatment and Care of the Geriatric Veterinary Patient, First Edition. Edited by Mary Gardner and Dani McVety.
© 2017 John Wiley & Sons, Inc. Published 2017 by John Wiley & Sons, Inc.
Companion Website: www.wiley.com/go/gardner/geriatric

is usually only detected when there is bilateral hearing loss and when it is either completely or close to completely developed (Cunningham and Klein, 2007).

Deafness may be classified as either conductive, sensory, neural/nerve, central, or mixed hearing loss. Additionally, deafness can be characterized as congenital or acquired, with acquired deafness being related mostly to iatrogenic, traumatic, or degenerative changes (Cunningham and Klein, 2007; Scheifele *et al.*, 2012).

Conductive (or conduction) deafness is caused by the loss of normal sound transmission from the environment to the internal ear. Anything that affects sound propagation from the environment may be classified as a conductive hearing loss. These include otitis externa, otitis media, fracture of the middle ear ossicles, or ossicle degeneration, called otosclerosis, which leads to reduced ossicle vibration and impaired transduction of sound waves. Although otitis may be rather easy to diagnose, identification and diagnosis of ossicle damage in pets is often difficult (Scheifele *et al.*, 2012).

Sensory hearing loss occurs with any disruption of the normal cochlear structures. These can be congenital or acquired, with the most common causes being iatrogenic from ototoxic medications, excessive noise exposure, or presbycusis (Scheifele *et al.*, 2012).

Nerve or neural deafness is caused by dysfunction of the cochlear nerve fibers between the cochlea and the brainstem (Cunningham and Klein, 2007; Scheifele *et al.*, 2012). Conditions in people that can lead to damage of these nerve fibers include acoustic neuroma, acoustic neuritis, and multiple sclerosis (Scheifele *et al.*, 2012). Similar disease processes can be expected in pets, although diagnosis may be more limited than that in people. Owing to difficulties in specific diagnoses in pets, it is common to group sensory and neural causes into one group of conditions, known as sensorineural deafness (Scheifele *et al.*, 2012).

Central (or cortical) deafness is a decrease in auditory function in the absence of any loss of hearing sensitivity, and results from alterations in the brainstem or auditory cortex. These conditions are often underdiagnosed or misdiagnosed, even in humans. Given the difficulty with diagnosis, these conditions could very well be occurring in our pets but determining the cause would be unlikely on a routine basis (Scheifele *et al.*, 2012).

Congenital deafness in animals is usually a result of a congenital defect in the cochlea, a condition frequently associated with certain coat colorations (Cunningham and Klein, 2007). Congenital deafness has been noted particularly in pets with white, merle, or piebald coat colorations. Deafness has also been linked to certain breeds and breed characteristics, regardless of coat color. For example, dogs with heterochromia iridis, a condition where iris pigmentation is incomplete, have been shown to be predisposed to deafness (McDonnell, 2015). One source states that almost 25% of Dalmatians are born deaf in one ear and 8% are born deaf in both ears (Deaf Websites, 2013). Box 5.1 shows a list of breeds predisposed to congenital deafness. Deafness in these pets are usually caused by bilateral partial or complete absence of the cochlea. Less commonly, it is caused by absence of neural elements downstream from the cochlea (nerve deafness). Pets with congenital deafness can live normal lives, but may need extra attention especially in outside environments (Cunningham and Klein, 2007). Training for these pets will depend more on visual cues (see Management of Geriatric Pets with Hearing Loss below).

Box 5.1 Dog Breeds Predisposed to Congenital Deafness	
Akita	English Setter
American Pit Bull Terrier	Fox Terrier
American Staffordshire Terrier	Great Dane
Australian Heeler	Great Pyrenees
Australian Shepherd	Parson Russell Terrier
Beagle	Maltese
Border Collie	Miniature Poodle
Boston Terrier	Mongrel
Boxer	Old English Sheepdog
Bull Terrier	Papillion
Catahoula Leopard Dog	Pointer
Cocker Spaniel	Rhodesian Ridgeback
Collie	Scottish Terrier
Dalmatian	Sealyham Terrier
Dappled Dachshund	Shetland Sheepdog
Doberman Pincher	Walker Foxhound
Dogo Argentino	West Highland White Terrier
English Bulldog	
Source: McDonnell, 2015.	

Acquired deafness can be iatrogenic. For example, deafness may be induced by ototoxic medications, including certain antibiotics, diuretics and antineoplastic drugs (Cunningham and Klein. 2007). Common antibiotics that can cause ototoxicity include aminoglycosides, erythromycin, and polymyxin B. Loop diuretics can enhance the ototoxicity of certain drugs, especially aminoglycoside antibiotics. Ototoxic drugs cause deafness by binding to or damaging the hair cell receptors. The cells detecting high-frequency sounds are usually the first to be damaged by ototoxic drugs. Early detection of hearing damage is important, since some of this damage may be reversible (Pickrell *et al.*, 1993). Another less-discussed iatrogenic cause of hearing damage in pets, particularly in dogs, is hearing loss induced by excessive kennel noise. In some kennels, hearing protection devices may be required for workers by Occupational Health and Safety Administration (OSHA) guidelines (Scheifele and Clark, 2012), but the effect on pets in the kennels may be overlooked.

Monitoring Pets for Hearing Loss

As with many health conditions, behavioral changes are often the first sign of hearing loss in pets. Age-related hearing loss has a gradual onset, so recognition of changes in auditory function can be difficult. Some signs include sleeping or resting through sounds that would normally cause a response, a tendency to startle or snap with touch even after verbal cues were given, failure to respond to verbal cues, confusion with previously trained commands, an increase in time spent sleeping or resting, difficulty waking during sleep, disorientation and confusion, excessive barking or vocalization, changes in normal vocal sounds, and even agitation (Scheifele *et al.*, 2012).

Hearing loss is an important clinical sign that should be considered during examination of geriatric pets, as it can have a significant impact on the pet's quality of life and the bond between the pet and pet owner. During the examination, a veterinarian can test for signs of age-related hearing loss and evaluate the pet's ear canals for signs of disease. Diseases of the ear canal can include various growths (including some cancers), infections, allergic inflammation, and complications associated with foreign bodies that enter the ear canal. These diseases may contribute, predispose, or speed the development of deafness. Treatment of the ear canal diseases may restore some hearing that was impaired, and may also limit the continued progression of hearing loss (Kay, 2015). Hearing can be tested by using only auditory signals of different frequencies and positions in relation to the patient (for example, response to squeaking toys, clapping, snapping fingers, doorbells).

Advanced Screening for Hearing Loss

Congenital deafness has been found in more than 90 breeds, making hearing assessment an important screening test for breeds commonly affected. In addition, working and service dogs should be screened to ensure that they can appropriately respond to auditory cues (Scheifele and Clark. 2012). Pets diagnosed with hearing loss should be removed from breeding programs. In addition, removal of their parents should be considered, since they are likely to be carriers of genetic abnormalities that lead to deafness.

Advanced diagnostics to evaluate auditory function in dogs is possible. In humans, the auditory brainstem response is the primary screening test used to detect auditory abnormalities in infants. Similar to this test, the Brainstem Auditory Evoked Response (BAER) has been used in veterinary patients. BAER testing can be used on pets at five weeks and above (McDonnell, 2015). Two other electrophysiological tests have been evaluated in veterinary patients: Otoacoustic Emissions and the Auditory Steady State Response (ASSR; Scheifele and Clark, 2012).

The BAER test records neural activity generated in response to a controlled sound stimulus. This test evaluates each ear independently and can therefore be used to evaluate unilateral hearing loss. In humans, BAER combined with otoacoustic emissions leads to more accurate findings, and this can potentially be applied to veterinary patients in the future. The ASSR can be used to test hearing acuity (Scheifele and Clark, 2012). BAER testing is recognized by the Orthopedic Foundation for Animals (OFA), as the only acceptable testing modality to diagnose canine deafness. For this reason, BAER testing has been routinely used in veterinary patients to screen breeds commonly affected with congenital deafness and to evaluate working and service dogs. Otoacoustic emissions and ASSR are being examined as potential adjunctive tests for auditory function in pets (Scheifele and Clark, 2012).

Is There Treatment for Age-Related Hearing Loss?

Unfortunately, there are no standard strategies that have universally restored hearing in pets with age-related hearing loss. There are a few studies of middle-ear implants and hearing aid use in animals, but in general, care of pets with age-related hearing loss is focused on management techniques to improve communication, interaction, and quality of life for a pet with age-related hearing loss (Kay, 2015).

As stated above, therapies and management to prevent and treat concurrent issues, including ear canal infections, can limit development and progression of deafness in pets (Kay, 2015). Inherited deafness cannot be treated with treatments such as hearing aids or surgical treatment (McDonnell, 2015).

Management of Geriatric Pets with Hearing Loss

When a pet has hearing loss, management above and beyond routine care may be warranted. When deafness in a pet has been diagnosed, there are a few issues that should be considered. Veterinarians can discuss these issues and management techniques with their clients during a focused visit. An owner may notice that their pet is dealing with social and emotional effects that may be similar to those seen in people with hearing loss. The impact on the owner's interactions with their pet, how to optimize communication between the pet and owner, and consideration for safety issues arising from the pet's inability to hear the surrounding environment should all be discussed (Scheifele *et al.*, 2012). These efforts aim to improve communication and interaction between the pet and owner, and also to improve the quality of life for a pet with partial or complete hearing loss (Kay, 2015).

We should consider whether pets experience social and emotional changes similar to those seen in people with hearing loss. This has yet to be researched appropriately and fully answered. However, it is quite possible that some pets and certain members of a particular species may experience changes similar to (though not exactly the same as) our own. It is also possible that pet owners may place their own fears and anxieties about hearing loss onto our pets, and may anthropomorphize their feelings. Hearing loss in pets may have less of an impact than hearing loss in people, as many pets (especially domesticated dogs and cats) rely on their sense of smell more than their sense of hearing (Scheifele *et al.*, 2012). It is important to determine the depth of a pet owner's concerns and discuss which are truly applicable to their pets. Most importantly, a discussion of management techniques should take place.

We may not be able to assess the psychological changes and effects of hearing loss on pets as well as we can in people, but there are certain anxieties that are easy to identify in pets and common enough to warrant a discussion of general management techniques for these anxieties. For example, pets with hearing loss are often startled very easily, especially when resting. It is not uncommon for pets to experience enhanced generalized anxiety after hearing loss, and this may be related to the fear of being startled. Therefore, it is best to teach pet owners to approach a pet with hearing loss well within their field of vision. Before touching or interacting with a pet that is resting or sleeping, it is best to allow them to smell your hand first. Many pets will retain their sense of smell as they age. Using a familiar and well-liked scent may aid in awakening a deaf pet. When a pet does not awaken from smelling a nearby hand, gently touching a non-painful area of their body may be appropriate. It is important to be particularly aware of avoiding painful areas and the face. Caution should be taken when awakening a deaf pet or interacting with them after a period of rest. To avoid injuries, visitors and strangers should be prevented from interacting with a deaf pet until they have become familiar with the pet (Kay, 2015).

Since our pets rely on other senses (especially smell) more than people do, they may fall back on these senses when their hearing becomes diminished or absent. The psychological effects on pets with hearing loss may not therefore be as significant as the impact that hearing loss may have on the owner. Keeping this in mind, we should be aware that a pet's hearing loss may affect the human–animal bond. Owners may develop frustrations when communicating with a deaf pet, especially when that pet is highly trained and accustomed to many vocal commands (such as working and service dogs). Deafness in these pets may even lead to early retirement from their positions (Scheifele *et al.*, 2012).

Deaf pets should be leash-walked only, or supervised when they are allowed to be in a fenced yard. As a method of informing strangers about a pet's condition, it is recommended to use a collar, tag, and/or a clothing garment stating that the pet is deaf. This is especially helpful if a deaf pet gets loose from a leash or a yard and is found (Kay, 2015).

Deafness in pets, as well as the management ideas proposed in this chapter, should be discussed with all members of the family and all of the pet's caretakers. It is important to teach pet owners how to effectively communicate with their deaf pet. This is not only for safety reasons, but to also help maintain the human–animal bond. Training a pet to understand hand, arm, and body signals is an easy and effective technique to implement. Some pets, especially dogs, tend to learn these signals rather quickly. It may even be wise to educate pet owners early so that they can start to use verbal cues along with body and hand signals to train their pets prior to the onset of hearing loss. Many older pets can still be trained to learn new cues, but it is important to encourage pet owners to be diligent and consistent as they implement these new signals, tricks and cues. It is also important to use positive reinforcement and avoid negative punishment when training young or geriatric pets (Kay, 2015). Additionally, other cues that stimulate other senses can be implemented. Using an appealing scent to coax a pet or to get their attention is an easy technique and can be taught to all members of the family. Using a flashlight to get the attention of geriatric pets that still have eyesight is also effective. The light can even be used to guide their movement to where the owner wants the pet to walk. Some pets with hearing loss can actually still sense vibrations. Developing vibrations by stomping on the floor, hand clapping or knocking cans together can be used effectively to communicate with some deaf pets (Kay, 2015).

Quality of Life Assessment for Pets with Hearing Loss

Often hearing loss is shrugged off as something that is not "bad" and an ailment pets can "deal with". But hearing loss can certainly diminish quality of life for a geriatric pet, and may also affect the human–animal bond. Pet owners can become quite frustrated and disheartened if management techniques and training with nonverbal cues are not enough to maintain adequate communication and interaction between them and their pet. Not only will this affect a pet's quality of life, but it can also have profound effects on a pet owner's emotional bond with their pet.

It is important to support pet owners as much as possible and to discuss that some degree of failures with managing and training a deaf pet will occur. Like so many things, success is all about setting appropriate expectations, which should be discussed as early as possible. There are some benefits to hearing loss in some pets, particularly those prone to noise and storm phobias. The added interaction between the pet owner and pet can also heighten their relationship.

One could assume that hearing loss is not a painful ailment but it can lead to anxiety which is, to some humans, considered even worse than pain. Add hearing loss to other ailments that a geriatric pet is dealing with (cognitive dysfunction, decreased vision, and so on) and the compounding struggles often become too much for the pet and family. However, educating the family on best practices to manage hearing loss can be a huge benefit to families and the pet and most will live a relatively normal and happy life together for years.

References

Cunningham, J., and Klein, B. (2007) "Hearing." In *Textbook of Veterinary Physiology*. 4th ed., pp. 169–175. St Louis, MO: Elsevier Saunders.

Deaf Websites. (2013) A Guide to Deaf Dogs. Available from www.deafwebsites.com/ hearing-loss/deaf-dogs.html.

Kay, N. (2015) Eight Tips for Coping with Your Dog's Age-Related Hearing Loss. Pet Health Network. Available from http://www.pethealthnetwork.com/dog-health/dog-diseases-conditions-a-z/eight-tips-coping-your-dogs-age-related-hearing-loss.

McDonnell, J. (2015) Deafness (Hearing Loss) in Dogs. Pet Place. Available from www. petplace.com/article/dogs/diseases-conditions-of-dogs/symptoms/deafness-in-dogs.

Pickrell, J. A., Oehme, F. W., and Cash, W. C. (1993) "Ototoxicity in Dogs and Cats." *Seminars in Veterinary Medicine and Surgery (Small Animal)*, **8**(1): 42–49.

Scheifele, M. and Clark, J. G. (2012) "Electrodiagnostic Evaluation of Auditory Function in the Dog." *Veterinary Clinics of North America Small Animal Practice*, **42**(6): 1241–1257.

Scheifele, L., Clark, J. G., Scheifele, P. M. (2012) "Canine Hearing Loss Management." *Veterinary Clinics of North America Small Animal Practice*, **42**(6): 1225–1239.

6

Dentition and the Oral Cavity
Heidi B. Lobprise

Introduction

In many cases in a veterinary practice, the oral cavity does not get much attention until there is a problem: the oral odor is bad, the pet is not eating well, or there is obvious swelling or bleeding. Unfortunately, by the time signs are bad enough for an owner to notice, the disease process has been progressing unseen, inside the oral cavity. When this happens to our senior and geriatric patients, complete resolution of the problem can be very challenging, as full assessment and treatment typically requires general anesthesia.

When a pet stops eating, or is showing signs of discomfort, the oral cavity is certainly a primary focus for diagnosis. The practitioner must keep in mind that many conditions, from gastrointestinal to osteoarthritic changes, can result in a patient becoming anorectic, so all body systems should be taken into account. Returning the oral cavity to a comfortable function (for eating, drinking and grooming) is essential to the overall health and wellbeing of the patient, so all efforts should be made to keep the mouth pain free and working.

Conditions

Periodontal Disease

Periodontal disease is one of the most common problems in our pet population, particularly with older patients. It has been shown that the prevalence and severity of periodontal disease in dogs increase with the age of the pet (Harvey, 1994). This study also shows that periodontal disease has an inverse relationship to the size of the pet – the smaller the dog, the more advanced the periodontal disease. Factor in the "relative age" assessment – smaller dogs tend to live longer, and that combines to make dental disease an important factor in many of our smaller, aged dogs.

The biggest factor for the prevalence of periodontal disease in small dogs is the ratio of alveolar bone to tooth/root size: 2–3 mm of bone loss around a Great Dane canine

Treatment and Care of the Geriatric Veterinary Patient, First Edition. Edited by Mary Gardner and Dani McVety.
© 2017 John Wiley & Sons, Inc. Published 2017 by John Wiley & Sons, Inc.
Companion Website: www.wiley.com/go/gardner/geriatric

tooth is less significant than the same amount of bone loss around an incisor or premolar in a Chihuahua. Since the teeth are often crowded in small (and brachycephalic) dogs, there is even less bone surrounding the teeth, and a domino effect can happen as the infection progresses from tooth to tooth. In making treatment decisions, a smaller, less strategic tooth may be extracted to improve the access for treatment and health of an adjacent and more important tooth (lower canine or first molar).

Although periodontal disease is in fact preventable, few patients benefit from a lifetime of optimal dental care, so many are presented with advanced stages of the disease as mature or senior pets. Advanced periodontal infection can destroy significant tissues of attachment (gingiva, bone) around the tooth that extraction may be the only option. At times, the bone loss can be so severe that pathological fractures of the mandible may occur, often in the region of the first molar (Figure 6.1) Complete assessment with intraoral radiography is essential in all dental cases.

Dental disease is not just about the mouth and teeth, however. The presence of the infection of periodontal and oral disease adversely affects many of the body's systems, with studies showing the association of periodontal disease and histologic lesions in multiple organs (DeBowes *et al.*, 1996), and the systemic effects of this chronically infected 'wound' that is the oral cavity (Pavlica *et al.*, 2008). It has also been shown that the increasing severity of periodontal disease can be correlated to the increasing concentrations of inflammatory markers, which can be reduced with appropriate periodontal therapy (Rawlinson *et al.*, 2011).

It is not necessarily the risk of bacteremia coming in contact with that diseased heart valve or nephron that is the biggest concern for systemic consequences of untreated periodontal disease; rather, it is the chronic presence of infected tissues with the ongoing process of inflammation and the host response that can be so destructive to other body systems. Certainly, any patient with diabetes, renal disease, hepatic disease or cardiac disease would greatly benefit from having the oral infection brought under control.

The big challenge is determining when the risks of the anesthetic procedure might outweigh the benefits of appropriate dental care. In most cases, with adequate preoperative history, diagnostics and thorough physical examination, any underlying problems can be identified, and potentially alleviated sufficiently to stabilize the patient, minimizing

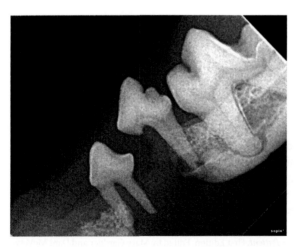

Figure 6.1 Severe periodontal bone loss of the mandible in an older dog has led to a pathological fracture.

Figure 6.2 Chronic osteitis/alveolitis in an older cat. The surrounding bone around the maxillary canines is expansile and enlarged and the teeth are super-erupted.

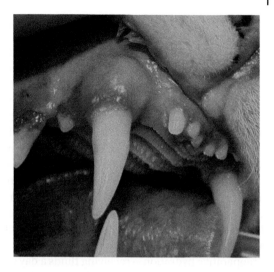

the pending risks. If a practitioner is uncomfortable with the prospect of anesthetizing, monitoring and maintaining an older patient through the recovery period, a referral should be offered to a veterinary dental specialist or to a facility with advanced anesthetic capabilities.

While all forms of periodontal disease can occur at nearly any age, there are a few specific conditions that are typically seen in senior patients. In older, smaller dogs, advanced bone loss due to periodontal disease may result in a mobile mandibular symphysis or even a pathological fracture of the mandible, often near the mandibular first molar. Cats may exhibit signs of chronic osteitis and alveolitis, where the maxillary canines (sometimes mandibular as well) seem to be super-erupted, and the surrounding bone is expansile and enlarged (Figure 6.2). If significant disease is present, these canine teeth can become mobile and uncomfortable.

There have been times when the oral disease becomes so uncomfortable that owners are willing to take even greater risks, being prepared for the possibility that the anesthetic event may be too much for their pet. It is much more likely, though, that the relief the pet is afforded through appropriate care will result in significant improvement, not just in the oral cavity, but in the entire health of the patient. Time and time again we hear, "He's like a new puppy!" While such miracles are great to experience, the ultimate benefit for the pet would be to have never have had to go through this disease, which is preventable for the most part.

Periodontal Disease Therapeutics

Conservative therapy of periodontal disease with antibiotics and pain medication may improve the oral condition of the patient and they will likely feel better, but as soon as the medication is finished, the level of disease will increase once again. Intermittent antibiotic therapy (pulse therapy) should be reserved only for those for whom an anesthetic procedure is not possible, both for the patient's sake and for appropriate antibiotic stewardship (American Veterinary Dental College, 2005). One function of prescribing the medication could be to show the pet owner that the infection and pain is truly affecting their pet, reinforcing the message that definitively treating the problem will be best for the pet.

Preparing the patient for the anesthetic event involves preoperative assessment and diagnostics, potentially including (but not limited to) complete blood work, urinalysis, thoracic radiographs and electrocardiogram (particularly for cardiac patients) and thorough examination. All medication and supplements should be reviewed carefully, as long-term use of fish oils can have an impact on clotting, so they should be stopped a week ahead of time. Most medications can be given the night before, while some cardiac medications can be administered for a morning dose the day of the procedure. Water can be made available to most senior patients until they leave for the clinic.

Specific conditions require special instructions, and a good resource for challenging anesthetic patients can be found at the Veterinary Anesthesia and Analgesia Support Group (www.vasg.org). Diabetics should receive one-half their typical morning dose of insulin, be fasted that morning, and have their blood glucose monitored before, during and after the procedure, with supplementation if needed. Renal patients benefit from preoperative hydration – receiving fluids a day or two ahead of time, as well as just prior to, and after, the procedure. Cardiac patients may benefit from a slower fluid administration, and preoperative oxygenation.

There are many analgesic and anesthetic protocols from which to choose, to tailor the regimen according to the patient's needs. A comprehensive analgesic protocol is essential with dental surgery, selecting preoperative agents, providing regional and local blocks, constant rate infusion and postoperative medication. Not only does this provided optimal comfort for the patient, but it also allows you to use decreased amounts of induction medication and inhalant anesthesia.

Intraoral radiography is absolutely essential when providing dental care for all of your patients, but even more so for your senior patients. The level of bone loss may be so advanced, making the jaw, particularly the mandible, fragile and susceptible to fracture during extraction. Reported cases of mandibular fracture during extraction without radiographs submitted to the AVMA Professional Liability Insurance Trust were 'indefensible' as compared with a standard of care (www.avmaplit.com).

The goal in providing dental care for senior patients is to remove the debris and source of infection as quickly as possible, minimizing anesthetic time, while closely monitoring the patient. Body temperature, blood pressure, heart rate and pulse quality should remain in a reasonable range, and if traditional methods of responding to decreases are not helpful (patient warming, decreasing inhalant anesthesia, increasing fluid rate), the patient should be recovered even before the procedure may be finished. Prepare ahead of time to have all materials, including emergency drugs, ready and close at hand. Do a quick assessment at the beginning of the procedure to identify the major problems and triage or rank them. Get the radiographs early to identify those problems and place the regional and local blocks in a timely manner. Removing the diseased teeth and the bulk of the plaque and calculus may be the primary goals rather than having meticulously cleaned crowns while leaving hidden disease under the gums.

As discussed earlier, some periodontal problems are found more often in aged pets. If the mandibular symphysis is mobile, it should be noted on the chart, and the extent of bone remaining around the canine teeth evaluated closely. Assess mobility of the individual canines by stabilizing the mandible on that side while putting gentle pressure on the canine. If the tooth is truly mobile, extraction may be necessary, but extreme care should be used to avoid further damage to the region. If bilateral mandibular canine extractions are needed, sometimes it is best to stage the treatment into two separate procedures, depending on the patient's stability. The rostral ends of the mandible will likely remain quite mobile, and effective chewing with the caudal teeth is lessened, but most patients manage nicely, though the tongue is likely to hang out on occasion.

Pathological fracture of the mandible at the first molar is more challenging to manage. Frequently, the bone loss is so significant that extraction of the first molar in the fracture site is necessary. There is seldom sufficient healthy bone to provide material to attempt interosseous wiring, and complicated bone grafting materials and mini-plate systems are not reasonable for these patients. For palliative care, it is sometime easiest to remove the remaining rostral portion of that side, with steps to ligate any vessels at the distal aspect of the fracture, splitting the symphysis to release that side, and excising gingiva and mucosa off the buccal and lingual aspects of the mandible to remove it. Simple suturing of the buccal mucosa to the sublingual tissue is often adequate, though a commisuroplasty (closing the upper to the lower lip at the corner) to provide additional support can be done. With bilateral fractures, removing a wedge of the lower lips/chin (cheiloplasty) to tighten the remaining tissue can provide a better cosmetic result.

Cats with chronic osteitis or alveolitis will often need the affected teeth to be extracted. Since the gingiva covering the expanded buccal bone gets very thin, it is often difficult to elevate a gingival flap without tearing the tissue. Since feline canines are fairly cylindrical, and most are already super-erupting or even mobile, it is easier to simply elevate the teeth without making a flap. Once the tooth is removed, the alveolus can be curetted and the inner edge of alveolar bone can be gently debrided sufficiently to release enough gingiva and palatal mucosa to allow a cruciate stitch to somewhat oppose the edges. The opposing teeth (mandibular canines) can be gently blunted with a white stone bur on a high-speed handpiece to minimize the trauma that these teeth can cause to the maxillary tissues post-extraction.

After any oral or dental treatment, patient aftercare is critical. Maintaining adequate hydration, nutritional support, and pain management is necessary to return the patient to normal function as quickly as possible. Supplemental fluids, nausea control, appetite stimulants, appropriate antibiotics, and pain management, and even feeding supplementation, may be needed. While most dental surgical patients do not require the placement of feeding tubes, softening the food for a few days to two weeks after surgery helps to protect the healing tissues. Some patients (cats) may not adjust to food changes, so if hard food is all they will eat, let them eat.

Oral Tumors

Tumors in older pets are fairly common, but tumors of the oral cavity can provide unique challenges. Since few pets are examined carefully on a regular basis, often tumors in the oral cavity can grow to a substantial size before they are detected. Inappetence, bleeding from the oral cavity and facial swelling may be the first signs noticed. In cats, cessation of grooming and an unkempt coat may be the first indications of a mass that is affecting the oral cavity or tongue. Unfortunately, outside a few more benign processes, many of the tumors in the oral cavity do not carry a good prognosis once they are large enough to cause the signs described above. In dogs, malignant melanocytic tumors, squamous cell carcinoma and fibrosarcomas are among the most common malignancies diagnosed. In cats, squamous cell carcinoma is by far the most common tumor found, with variations of location – gingival, sublingual and tonsillar.

Early detection of small tumors in the rostral portion of the oral cavity typically carry the best prognosis, as most patients will tolerate significant levels of mandibulectomy and maxillectomy. Full staging, including evaluation of lymph nodes and lungs, will provide information, with the histopathology and information about the presence of any tumor cells at the biopsy borders, to provide adequate treatment planning. More advanced tumors, whether by size or extent of metastasis, may be amenable to chemotherapy and radiation therapy options, but those choices can be difficult. Evaluation of the pet's quality of life should play an important part in those decisions.

Oral Pain

Many veterinary professionals do a reasonable job at providing adequate surgical pain management for their patients, and this is very important for any senior animal undergoing oral and dental treatment. Beyond the surgery time, however, pain management may be needed over the long term for the inflammation of periodontal disease, and even potential neuropathic pain. While initial treatment of periodontal disease focuses on removing the infection (surgically or with antibiotics), in human dentistry, a focus on the host's inflammatory response to periodontal pathogens is an important part of management. For those patients that may have to delay an anesthetic procedure, providing analgesic support can be helpful. There are also patients that may benefit from surgical procedures, and some that have chronic neuropathic pain associated with a chronic oral disease or inflammation. Pain modulators such as gabapentin may be needed to provide additional comfort. Further details on pain management in senior pets can be found in the Chapter 18. Providing sufficient care to allow the patient to eat comfortably is a primary goal of dental management.

End of Life decisions

Complete evaluation of a patient will include their ability to prehend, masticate and swallow sufficient nutrition to maintain life functions. Quality of life assessment extends this evaluation to include the patient's comfort in eating and grooming, and even its enthusiasm for and enjoyment of eating. When a patient cannot maintain a comfortable means of eating for extended periods, this may factor into the decision process for that individual.

Client Education

Client education is one of the most important components of supporting your patients' oral care, and the message must be a consistent one throughout the clinic team. Pet parent concerns about the cost and risks of anesthesia can be alleviated with discussion of the benefits of good oral health, and its impact on systemic health. This education should start with new puppies and kittens to minimize disease throughout life, but even with our senior pets, thorough examination and pre-anesthetic diagnostics, together with individualized anesthetic protocols and monitoring can make optimal oral care possible for nearly any patient.

Implementing home care instructions may be challenging for some patients, but should be encouraged in every case. Brushing on a daily basis with a soft bristled toothbrush and veterinary toothpaste is still the gold standard for care (try a toothpaste taste test at the two-week recheck), but often the care regimen should be customized for that particular patient–owner combination. If brushing is going to be too traumatic, then maybe an oral gel can be used, or dogs can be given an appropriate chewing device. Instruct the owner not to provide any chewing product that is hard and non-compressible: If you cannot bend it, or your thumbnail cannot depress the surface, it is likely to hard and rigid and can potentially break their teeth. Certain water additives may help, but they will not be as effective as mechanical means of removing the soft plaque before it hardens into tartar or calculus. One helpful guideline is a listing of products on the Veterinary Orasl Health Council website (www.vohc.org), which also includes information on periodontal disease for pet parents.

References

American Veterinary Dental College. (2005) *The Use of Antibiotics in Veterinary Dentistry.* (AVDC Position Statement). Meridien, ID: AVDC.

DeBowes, L. J., Mosier, D., Logan, E., Harvey, C. E., Lowry, S., and Richardson, D. C. (1996) "Association of Periodontal Disease and Histologic Lesions in Multiple Organs from 45 Dogs." *Journal of Veterinary Dentistry*, **13**(2): 57–60.

Harvey, C. E., Shofer, F. S., Laster, L. (1994) "Association of Age and Weight with Periodontal Disease in North American Dogs." *Journal of Veterinary Dentistry*, **11**(3): 94–105.

Pavlica, Z., Petelin, M., Juntes, P., Erzen, D., Crossley, D. A., and Skaleric, U. (2008) "Periodontal Disease Burden and Pathological Changes in Organs of Dogs." *Journal of Veterinary Dentistry*, **25**(2): 97–105.

Rawlinson, J. E., Goldstein, R. E., Reiter, A. M., Attwater, D. Z., and Harvey, C. E. (2011) "Association of Periodontal Disease with Systemic Health Indices in Dogs and the Systemic Response to Treatment of Periodontal Disease." *Journal of the American Veterinary Medical Association*, **238**(5): 601–609.

7

The Nose and Smelling

Faith Banks

"The nose knows." This may be very true in young cats and dogs, but as they age their ability to sniff and smell the world around them may not be up to snuff. Very little is known about olfactory dysfunction in aging people, and even less is known about it in aging cats and dogs.

The sense of smell, known as olfaction, is a very important sense for our pets. Evidence shows that cats have 80 million smell receptors and dogs have 300 million. Comparatively, humans have been shown to have a mere five million smell receptors in their noses (Trumps, 2015).

The external and internal surfaces of the nose have many scent receptors. When dogs sniff the air, they are sending the inhaled scents deep into the nasal cavities where the chemical scent gets trapped within mucus (Kidd, 2004). The moistness of the nose aids in trapping the smell to allow a pet to breakdown and subsequently interpret the odor. This is the theory behind a healthy dog having a wet nose – the better to smell you with, my dear. Dry noses can decrease their ability to hold a scent and then decipher it, so dogs may lick their nose to moisten it and thus improve their scenting ability.

In the nasal cavity are sensory cells with associated projections of cilia. Each of these cilia contains many scent receptors. When a scent is captured into these scent receptors, it is processed by the sensory cells, then a signal travels through axons to deliver the messages through the ethmoid bone (the caudal part of the nose) directly to the large olfactory bulb of the brain. When scent signals reach the olfactory bulb, they are transported to the frontal cortex for analysis and then to other centers of the brain for further interpretation (Kidd, 2004). It is theorized that one-third of the dog's brain is involved with scenting and a dog's sense of smell is up to 100,000 times greater than that in humans (Kidd, 2004).

Decline of Smell

Little is known about the actual decline of smell in geriatric dogs, but studies in humans have shown disturbances of olfaction are quite common (Figure 7.1). Prevalence rates increase to 13.9% in individuals older than 65 years, to over 50%

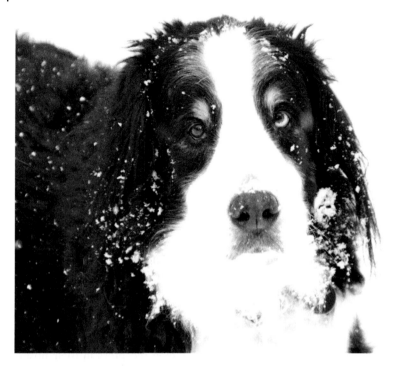

Figure 7.1 Geriatric patient Smudge.

in people between 65 and 80 years, and up to 80% in those above 80 years of age, respectively (Attems *et al.*, 2015).

As pets age, there is no specific disorder that affects their ability to smell. However, the cells within nerve and brain tissue are vulnerable to the effects of oxidative damage. They can undergo changes that cause a patient's sense of smell to decrease or completely diminish (Roberts, 2015). Loss of nerve endings in a pet's nose will also cause a decrease in the production of mucus, which normally helps to trap odors. Less mucus means the odors will not remain long enough for the pet to decipher the smell.

A decrease in a pet's sense of smell may be partial (hyposmia) or complete (anosmia) and can lead to a decreased appetite, malnutrition or weight loss, as smell and taste are both involved with "tasting" food. Currently, there is no gold standard test to diagnose deterioration in a pet's sense of smell. Changes in their perception of flavor is actually more a result of changes within the nose, rather than a decrease in taste bud number or function (although this may also play a part). Many people rely on their pet's appetite as a marker of their general health (Figure 7.2). A decreased appetite may give the owner an impression that their pet is not well, but it may simply be because food is no longer as palatable as it was in their youth. A food's decreased aroma, as interpreted by the geriatric pet, will require additives or tasty morsels to stimulate the pet's interest and thus their overall appetite. Hand feeding and warming up food (which helps to vaporize the aroma) may also increase a pet's interest in eating, and is a simple management recommendation that should be mentioned to pet owners.

Figure 7.2 Geriatric patient Serissa, whose pigmentation change caused more alarm to the owner than her decreased ability to smell.

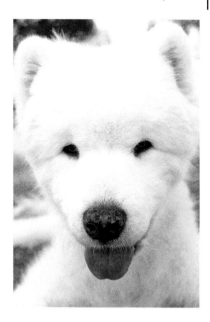

Contributory Factors

There are many contributing factors that can lead to olfactory deterioration. It is seen in humans with Alzheimer's disease, so it is likely that pets with cognitive dysfunction syndrome may also experience similar changes. Irritants causing ongoing allergic sinusitis or rhinitis may occur, with seasonal changes being observed. Other environmental irritants, such as cigarette smoke, dust, mold, and abnormal odors, may have a negative cumulative effect on nasal health. Viral rhinitis or secondary bacterial infections will alter the mucus within the nasal passages, thus negatively impacting a pet's sense of smell. The most common causes of acute rhinitis or sinusitis in dogs are canine distemper, adenovirus types 1 and 2, and parainfluenza (Kidd, 2004).

Other olfactory conditions seen with older pets may be related to dental disease, foreign bodies, or fungal infections. The nose's texture or sores on the nose may be a sign of underlying disease. Nasal hyperkeratosis is a disorder commonly seen in older dogs or certain breeds (Cocker Spaniel, Labrador Retriever) where the nose takes on a dry, callus-like appearance due to excess production of keratin (Mahaney, 2013). These changes to the nasal planum may not lead to a significant reduction in olfaction, but they could be a contributing factor. Certain breeds with stenotic nares may also have decreased ability to smell, owing to the structural anatomy of their nose.

The most common condition seen in geriatric pets involving the nose and smelling is neoplasia. Owners may first see nasal discharge, epistaxis, noisy breathing, or even changes in the physical appearance of their pet's face. The most commonly observed form of cancer in the nasal cavity in geriatric dogs is nasal adenocarcinoma (Roberts, 2015), while the most common form of nasal planum tumor is the mast cell tumor (Figure 7.3). In cats, squamous cell carcinoma is the most common type, and is usually induced from exposure to the sun (Geiger, 2014). Diagnosis is made through x-rays or computed tomography, biopsy, and histopathology of the affected nasal tissue. Currently,

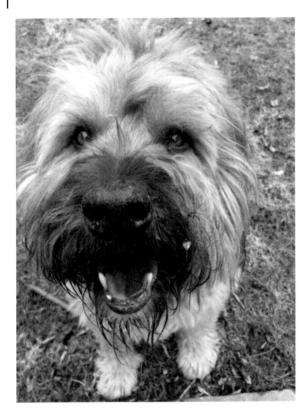

Figure 7.3 Chase, 12 years old, has an aggressive nasal tumour and subsequent epistaxis.

the best treatment for dogs with nasal adenocarcinoma is radiation therapy. Treatment for cats with nasal squamous cell carcinoma may involve surgery, radiation therapy, cryosurgery, photodynamic therapy, intralesional chemotherapy, or immunotherapy, depending on the size and invasiveness of the lesion. The Veterinary Society of Surgical Oncology (2011) has an informative website with treatment recommendations based on the location of different types of tumors.

A decrease in a pet's ability to smell does not initially seem to be an issue of concern for caregivers of geriatric pets. However, if their sense of smell decreases, the pet may lose the ability to "taste" food, as taste is associated with the nose. This will cause a decrease in appetite, which may be a concern for caregivers. Veterinarians often recommend adding foods/treats that are more palatable, but at the same time, these food/treats may also be more aromatic, thus increasing their appeal. If an underlying issue is present (tumor, infection, inflammation, other), addressing and ameliorating the problem would be the only way to improve the pet's decreased olfactory ability.

Therapy

Age-related smelling decline cannot be reversed and does not require specific therapy, especially if a pet is still eating and interested in food. Nasal tumors with subsequent decreased smelling ability would be the reason a pet may be euthanized for olfactory reasons, but this is due to the tumor and not its effect on olfaction.

Currently, there are no known therapies to increase a diminishing sense of smell for an aged pet. Managing the underlying issue (related to neoplasia or infection), or palliating the outcome (decreased appetite or interest in food) are the only options available. There is no direct way to increase a pet's ability to smell. However, knowing that this is a common issue with aging pets should alert the clinician to monitor geriatrics for a waning appetite or weight loss and to make changes in the diet by increasing the aroma of a food and its palatability to stimulate interest and appetite.

References

Attems, J., Walker, L., and Jellinger, K. A. (2015) "Olfaction and Aging: A Mini-Review." *Gerontology*, **61**(6): 485–490.

Geiger, T. (2014) "Nasal Planum Neoplasia." Veterinary Information Network. Available at http//:www.vin.com/Members/Associate/Associate.plx?from=GetDzInfo&DiseaseId=1057.

Kidd, R. (2004) "The Canine Sense of Smell, Getting to the Source of the Dog's Ability to Smell." *The Whole Dog Journal*, November. Available at http://www.whole-dog-journal.com/issues/7_11/features/Canine-Sense-of-Smell_15668-1.html.

Mahaney, P. (2016) "What your Dog's Nose Can Tell You." Animal Wellness Magazine. Available at http://animalwellnessmagazine.com/what-her-nose-can-tell-you.

Roberts, B. (2015) "The Effects of Age on a Senior Dog's Eyes, Ears and Nose." petcha.com. Available at http://www.petcha.com/the-effects-of-age-on-a-senior-dogs-eyes-ears-and-nose.

Trumps, V. (2015) "Who Has a Stronger Sense of Smell, Cats or Dogs?" Pet360. Available from: http://www.pet360.com/dog/lifestyle/who-has-a-stronger-sense-of-smell-cats-or-dogs.

Veterinary Society of Surgical Oncology (2011) Welcome to the Veterinary Society of Surgical Oncology (VSSO). Available at www.vsso.org.

8

Cognitive Dysfunction and Related Sleep Disturbances
Dawnetta Woodruff

Introduction and Background

Pathology within the brain can lead to a whole host of disorders, each with its own set of diagnostic challenges and appropriate treatments. In this chapter, we focus on cognitive dysfunction and sleep disturbances that are common in geriatric pets. When pathology in the brain leads to changes in mental function and cognitive ability, a pet's entire demeanor is often affected. While subtle at first, significant memory deficits and personality changes tend to be progressive in nature. The development of such disease leads to a gradual but considerable decline in a pet's overall quality of life. This chapter addresses the causes of cognitive dysfunction, the best diagnostic approaches, and the numerous treatment options that are available to increase and prolong the quality of life of the geriatric patient and their caretakers.

Modern veterinary medicine has noted a change within the companion animal population. More and more families have pets that fall into the categories of "senior" or "geriatric". Additionally, "advanced age [in the pet population] is frequently associated with severe behavioral and cognitive deficits" (Head and Zicker, 2004). The symptoms of cognitive dysfunction syndrome are quite prevalent in the aging pet population, and cause concern for both veterinarians and their clients. A 2001 study evaluated 180 dogs with no identifiable health problems. In the 11–12 years group, 28% of owners reported one category of cognitive dysfunction and 10% reported two or more categories. In dogs between 15 and 16 years of age, the numbers rose to 68% and 36%, respectively (Nielson et al., 2001). Cognitive disorders are also a concern for our feline patients. A 2010 study of 154 cats age 11 years and over showed that 35% were diagnosed with possible cognitive dysfunction syndrome, and this value was found to increase with age. While 28% of cats age 11–15 years were affected, 50% of cats older than 15 years were showing clinical signs (Landsberg et al., 2010).

One problem with the diagnosis and treatment of cognitive dysfunction is that symptoms are initially subtle and can be written off as the pet "just getting old." Pet owners may not bring these early or mild symptoms to their veterinarian's attention. Nevertheless, the symptoms may still be creating problems at home for both the pet and

Treatment and Care of the Geriatric Veterinary Patient, First Edition. Edited by Mary Gardner and Dani McVety.
© 2017 John Wiley & Sons, Inc. Published 2017 by John Wiley & Sons, Inc.
Companion Website: www.wiley.com/go/gardner/geriatric

their human family. With time, as symptoms progress, the problems affect quality of life and begin to break down the strength of the human–animal bond. Eventually, the symptoms become so intrusive that everyday activities like eating and elimination are no longer happening without the owner's intervention. At this point, many people will bring their pet in to the veterinarian's office specifically for cognitive concerns. However, when the disease has progressed to an advanced stage and the human–animal bond has already been broken, therapy is typically minimally effective at returning the pet to a reasonable quality of life, and euthanasia is often considered. For this reason, it is imperative that the entire veterinary team become proactive in questioning owners and recommending appropriate therapeutic options early in the disease, when therapy has the highest likelihood of a positive outcome.

Common Symptoms of Cognitive Dysfunction

Symptoms of cognitive dysfunction fall into several broad categories. Pets may show symptoms in any or all of the categories, with the number and severity of symptoms generally increasing with age and disease progression (Figure 8.1a, b). When categorizing these symptoms, the acronym "DISHA" is helpful, and can serve as a guideline when talking with clients to determine if cognitive dysfunction is present. DISHA stands for disorientation, interactions, sleep-wake cycle disturbances, house-soiling, and activity-level alterations (Table 8.1).

When talking with clients during senior wellness visits, it is imperative for the veterinary team to mention a few examples of cognitive dysfunction symptoms. Simply asking clients if their pet has any signs of dementia may not be adequate. Some clients are familiar with dementia and Alzheimer's disease in humans, but may not relate the symptoms their pet is experiencing to the disease they are familiar with. Other clients may have no personal experience, and thus no framework in which to evaluate their pet's mental status. Figures 8.2 and 8.3 illustrate the most common owner reported behavior symptoms in canines and felines, respectively (Landsberg *et al.*, 2012). Often, clients do not recognize

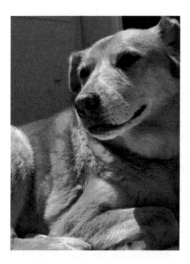

Figure 8.1A Nevada, a 13-year-old Labrador mix with cognition issues, having a moment of relaxation.

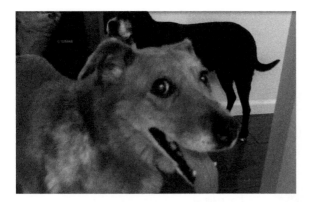

Figure 8.1B Nevada panting and pacing – owners report that 75% of her waking day is in this state; eyes wide, ears back, panting, drooling and pacing into and out of every room.

Table 8.1 The DISHA acronym (Landsberg *et al.*, 2010, 2012).

Initial	Stands for	Explanation
D	Disorientation	Confusion, wandering from room to room, abnormal vocalizations (sometimes present during the daytime, but especially evident at night), pacing, appearing lost in the normal environment, not responding to their own name, getting "stuck" with their head in a corner, staring vacantly into space.
I	Interactions with people or other pets	Lack of interest in family, failure to recognize family members, hiding or sleeping in unusual places, change in playfulness with housemates, aggression towards human family members, fighting with housemates, becoming clingy or aloof (as a change from previous behaviors).
S	Sleep–wake cycle disturbances	Sleeping all day and awake all night, pacing at night, unable to sleep, restless during normal sleep times.
H	House soiling, loss of house or litter box training	Urine and/or stool found in the home (outside the litter box for cats), inability to hold urine/stool while owners are away, urination or defecation while standing in front of family members, urination/ defecation while seemingly unaware of the process.
A	Activity level alterations	Constant pacing (often associated with panting), refusal to engage in enjoyable activities (walks, playtime, brushing, etc.), no longer grooming themselves, not responding to well-known commands, loss of interest in toys.

these symptoms as early signs of cognitive disease until it is pointed out, or until the symptoms significantly worsen. To make this discussion easier, a "cognitive wellness checklist" can be used during senior wellness visits (Figure 8.4). The client may complete the checklist and then the results should be reviewed together with their veterinary team. Based on the family's answers and the clinician's review, a treatment plan can be developed before symptoms worsen to the point of being unresponsive to therapy. This allows the best chance for therapeutic success and lengthens the time during which the pet may enjoy good quality days with their family. Veterinary teams are encouraged to copy

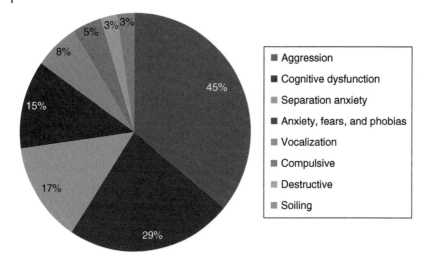

Figure 8.2 Prevalence of owner-reported signs in senior dogs. Fears and phobias include generalized anxiety; compulsive includes repetitive and stereotypic behavior; cognitive dysfunction include disorientation, wandering, waking and anxious at night. Behavior signs were combined from three studies: a Spanish study of 270 dogs older than age 7 years presenting with behavior problems, 103 dogs referred to a veterinary behaviorist, and a search of the Veterinary Information Network of 50 dogs aged 9–17 years.

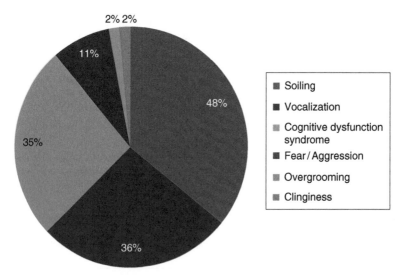

Figure 8.3 Prevalence of owner-reported signs in senior cats. Soiling includes marking; cognitive dysfunction includes disorientation, wandering and night waking; and fear/aggression includes fear and hiding. Behavior signs were combined from a Veterinary Information Network data search of 100 cats aged 12–22 years and 83 cats from three different behavior referral practices.

Figure 8.4 for their own patient assessments, but there are also several other behavioral questionnaires and scoring methods available online and in the literature (Dog Dementia, 2016; PetSci, 2016; Salvin *et al.*, 2010). One such scoring method (the Canine Cognitive Dysfunction Rating scale) was evaluated in a 2010 study, which analyzed its efficacy in correctly diagnosing canine cognitive disease (Salvin *et al.*, 2010). This evaluation of 27 behaviors was found to be a useful tool in research and perhaps in a clinical setting as well.

Cognitive Wellness Checklist (For Canines & Felines)

Client Name		Date	
Patient Name		Patient Age	

Symptom Category	Symptom Name/Description	Happens Daily	Happens Weekly	Happens Monthly
Disorientation	Confusion			
	Wandering room to room			
	Abnormal vocalizations(day or night)			
	Pacing/appearing lost			
	Staring absently into space			
	Standing "stuck" in a corner			
Interactions	Disinterest in greeting family members			
	Does not recognize family			
	Hiding/sleeping in unusual places			
	Does not play with housemates			
	Aggression/fighting with housemates			
	Acting clingy or aloof			
Sleep Issues	Sleeping more than awake during day			
	Awake at night			
	Pacing at night			
	Restless during sleep hours			
House Soiling	Urine found in home			
	Feces found in home			
	Urination in front of owner			
	Defecation in front of owner			
	Urinating while unaware			
	Defecating while unaware			
Activity Alterations	Lack of interest in play			
	Lack of interest in grooming			
	Lack of interest in walks			
	Loss of trained commands			
	Loss of interest in toys			

Special Concerns:

Figure 8.4 Cognitive wellness checklist for canines and felines.

The most important point in discussing symptoms of canine cognitive disease is to open an early dialogue with owners. As mentioned previously, clients often notice initial signs but pass them off as the patient "just getting old." They may not be aware that the symptoms are related to one another, or they may not feel that there is anything that can be done. This may allow the disease to advance into its end stages before the family feels desperate and begins looking into therapeutic options. At that time, they either realize it is too late, or they begin therapy which inevitably fails because of the advanced nature of the disease. It is a case of "too little too late," which can worsen client grief and feelings of guilt. The family often assumes that if they had known of the therapeutic options earlier, they could have given their pet more good days, or a longer, better-quality life. By opening the veterinarian–client dialogue early in the course of the disease, we can not only increase patient comfort and quality of life but also decrease the family's long-term feelings of guilt, thus speeding their healing and assisting with the grieving process.

Development and Pathophysiology

In order to better diagnose and treat cognitive dysfunction, it is important to discuss our current understanding of the pathophysiology of the disease process. The disease shares many similarities with human Alzheimer's Disease and is a result of age-related physiological and chemical changes within the brain. With the passage of time, the aging canine brain experiences neuronal loss and progressive atrophy, leading to neuro-degenerative changes that include (Araujo *et al.*, 2005; Head *et al.*, 2008; Landsberg *et al.*, 2011; DePorter, 2014):

- reduction in brain mass (and decrease in frontal volume)
- increased ventricular size
- cortical atrophy
- meningeal calcification
- demyelinization
- acetylcholinesterase reduction
- reduction in Purkinje cells
- increased lipofuscin and apoptic bodies
- neuroaxonal degeneration
- reduction in neurons
- increased accumulation of diffuse beta-amyloid plaques with perivascular infiltrates (similar to those seen in the brains of humans with Alzheimer's disease)
- depletion of catecholamines and an increase in monoamine oxidase B activity, resulting in a decline in the cholinergic system
- decrease in dopamine within the brain and presence of oxidative stressors
- perivascular changes including microhemorrhage.

The feline brain undergoes similar changes (although not as well studied or defined) that include: (Landsberg *et al.*, 2010, 2011):

- neuronal loss
- decrease in number of dendrites in Purkinje cells
- cerebral atrophy
- widening of the sulci
- increased ventricular size
- perivascular changes including microhemorrhage

- decrease in dopamine within the brain and presence of oxidative stressors
- compromised blood flow and hypoxia secondary to factors such as hypertension and cardiac disease.

Numerous studies show a correlation between the presence of morphologic aging changes and the presence of cognitive dysfunction symptoms (Head *et al.*, 2008). The existence of beta-amyloid plaques, in particular, receives a significant amount of attention and research focus. This is because the presence of proteinaceous plaques is linked to the development of Alzheimer's disease in humans, and the primary component of these plaques (the beta-amyloid peptide) has an identical amino acid sequence in dogs and in humans (Head *et al.*, 2008). "Beginning around age 8, the formation and maturation of diffuse beta-amyloid deposits are observed by immunostaining in all layers of canine cortical gray matter in a characteristic four-stage distribution" (Bosch *et al.*, 2015). The presence and severity of these plaques, as well as their location within the brain, has a distinct correlation with the presence and severity of the symptoms of cognitive dysfunction. "Beta-amyloid plaques in the cranial part of the parietal lobe correlated with behavioral changes in aged companion animals related to appetite, drinking, incontinence, day and night rhythm, social behavior (e.g., interaction with owners and other pets, personality), orientation, perception and memory" (Head *et al.*, 2008). Additional research in this area shows promise for increasing our understanding of the disease, as well as the potential for developing more effective therapies.

While beta-amyloid plaques are undoubtedly important, they do not fully explain cognitive dysfunction syndrome in and of themselves. Other neurochemical factors (such as oxidative damages) are present and play an important role in the development of cognitive dysfunction (Opii *et al.*, 2008). The young brain has multiple safeguards in place, protecting it from free radicals and oxidative damage. With age, however, these safeguards decline or become less effective (Head *et al.*, 2008). Superoxide dismutase is one example of this type of protective enzyme. It is present in the normal, healthy brain, and by converting reactive superoxide ions to hydrogen peroxide, it decreases the presence of damaging free radicals. However, concentrations of superoxide dismutase decline within the aged canine brain, presumably leaving the brain of geriatric pets more vulnerable to damage from free radicals. "Evidence of increased oxidative damage to DNA or RNA in the aged canine brain has been reported [and that damage] may also be associated with behavioral decline. Rofina and collaborators found that increased oxidative end products in aged canine brain correlate with severity of behavior changes attributable to cognitive dysfunction" (Head *et al.*, 2008). Oxidative damage leads to demyelination and the production of cytokines, which may in turn play a role in the production of beta-amyloid proteins and plaques (Head *et al.*, 2008). It therefore stands to reason that preventing or reducing oxidative damage within the brain could lead to a slowing of the progression of cognitive dysfunction syndrome.

Similar to Alzheimer's disease in humans, we recognize that the development of cognitive dysfunction syndrome in our pets is multifactorial. It is suspected that some animals are genetically predisposed to developing cognitive dysfunction, but environmental and nutritional factors also play a role. The combination of factors causes a breakdown in the brain's ability to function normally and leads to the development of clinical signs of cognitive dysfunction syndrome. We are beginning to better understand the nature of the disease, but we do not fully recognize why some dogs are burdened with cognitive disease early in life while others progress to an elderly age with minimal symptom development. As research continues, we hope to gain a better understanding of not only the disease process itself, but also the predisposing factors. This may eventually lead us to a cure or even a prevention for cognitive dysfunction.

Differential Diagnoses

Cognitive disorders produce many symptoms that are easily overlooked early in the course of the disease. The symptoms frequently overlap with symptoms of other diseases that are also common in the geriatric population. Additionally, there is no definitive diagnosis for cognitive dysfunction syndrome. For these reasons, we realize that the syndrome is underdiagnosed and under-reported. It is imperative for veterinary professionals (doctors, technicians, and support staff) to make an intentional effort to recognize cognitive disorders in their patients. Obtaining a thorough history is the first step in this process. Understanding which symptoms presented first can be vital in determining if the symptoms are a result of a medical or a cognitive disorder. Often, a clinician will strongly suspect cognitive dysfunction based on the given history. However, cognitive dysfunction syndrome is a diagnosis of exclusion. It is therefore necessary to perform medical diagnostics to rule out other potential health concerns before confirming the diagnosis. These diagnostics vary from patient to patient, depending on the observed symptoms, the patient's pertinent history, and the client's budget. In general, they may include a chemistry panel (including electrolytes), thyroid testing, a urinalysis and/or a urine culture, possible imaging of the bladder (radiographs and/or ultrasound), a neurologic exam, and a workup for arthritis and pain (thorough physical exam, orthopedic exam, radiographs, etc.). A clinician should be thorough, but judicious, when determining which testing is necessary for any given patient. When test results become available, they may reveal the presence of a disease or multiple disease processes that require their own medical or surgical intervention. Medical disorders that can mimic the symptoms of cognitive disorders are numerous. Similar symptoms may be the result of sensory dysfunction (loss of sight, hearing, smell), urinary tract disease (urinary tract infection, bladder stones, bladder neoplasia), generalized pain (neuropathy, osteoarthritis), endocrine disorders (hyper or hypothyroidism, hyper- or hypoadrenocorticism, pituitary disease, diabetes, insulinoma), or neurologic disorders (primary or secondary intracranial tumors, seizure disorders), and so on. The symptoms of these diseases, which may mimic or overlap with the symptoms of cognitive dysfunction syndrome, are listed in Table 8.2.

When testing is performed and other diseases have been appropriately treated, symptoms may still be present which indicate the presence of cognitive dysfunction syndrome. At this time, or when testing reveals no other diseases that can account for the cognitive changes being observed, cognitive dysfunction syndrome is diagnosed by exclusion. While this is method of diagnosis is most common, response-to-therapy is another approach that can be elected based on patient need, owner finances, and the urgency of beginning therapy. This method skips some (or all) of the testing listed above. Rather, it involves arriving at a diagnosis based upon the response to a therapeutic trial. While a diagnosis of exclusion is medically desired, it is sometimes more reasonable to focus financial resources on therapy, rather than on diagnostic testing.

Table 8.2 Symptoms of diseases that mimic or overlap with symptoms of cognitive dysfunction syndrome (modified from Landsberg *et al.*, 2011).

Medical condition	Presentation	Examples of behavioral signs
Neurologic	Central (intra- or extracranial), particularly if affecting forebrain, limbic/temporal, and hypothalamic; rapid eye movement sleep disorders	Altered awareness, response to stimuli, loss of learned behaviors, house soiling, disorientation, confusion, altered activity levels, temporal disorientation, vocalization, soiling, change in temperament (fear, anxiety), altered appetite, altered sleep cycles, interrupted sleep
Partial seizures	Temporal lobe epilepsy	Repetitive behaviors, self-traumatic disorders, chomping, staring, alterations in temperament (eg intermittent states of fear or aggression), tremors, shaking, interrupted sleep
Sensory dysfunction	Loss of sight, hearing, smell, or a combination of the senses	Altered response to stimuli, confusion, disorientation, irritability/aggression, vocalization, house soiling, altered sleep cycles
Endocrine	Hyper- or hypothyroid, hyper- or hypoadrenocorticism, insulinoma, diabetes, testicular or adrenal cancers	Altered emotional state, irritability/aggression, lethargy, decreased response to stimuli, anxiety, house soiling/marking, night waking, decreased or increased activity, altered appetite, mounting
Metabolic disorders	Hepatic, renal	Signs associated with organ affected: anxiety, irritability, aggression, altered sleep, house soiling, mental dullness, decreased activity, restlessness, increased sleep, confusion

In such cases, it is important to counsel owners that we may have missed another (possibly treatable) disease, and diagnostics may still be indicated in the future if the pet is not responding appropriately to therapy for cognitive dysfunction syndrome. If the owners understand the risks of a response-to-therapy approach, it can be an effective avenue of diagnosis and treatment.

In a research setting, there are multiple neuropsychologic learning tests that provide a more objective measure of a dog's cognitive function. These tests include the open field test, curiosity test, spontaneous activity test, food searching task, problem solving task, various learning tests, and various memory tests (Rosado *et al.*, 2012; Landsberg *et al.*, 2011, 2012; Gonzalez-Martinez *et al.*, 2013). They certainly have significant value in our quest to better understand and identify the disease. According to Gary Landsberg, DVM, MRCVS, "Collectively, these tests have provided valuable new insights into the diagnosis and treatment of cognitive dysfunction in dogs. For example, the typical age of onset for clinical cases is usually reported at 11 years of age, or greater, while laboratory tests have documented cognitive decline from as early as 7 years"… This is similar to neurodegenerative diseases in humans, such as Alzheimer's disease, where impairments in patients undergoing regular cognitive testing can be detected long before clinical signs appear in the day-to-day environment. Laboratory testing also provides an objective measure for controlled studies that can predict the effect of therapeutic intervention in the treatment of cognitive dysfunction in pet dogs" (Landsberg *et al.*, 2005). However, these tests are labor intensive and it is questionable whether they can be practically applied in clinical practice. In the future, we hope to have advances in the field of cognitive disorders that could provide a definitive method of diagnosis. In the meantime, using a combination of client questionnaires, clinical impression, diagnosis of exclusion, and response-to-therapy approaches is most clinically relevant.

Therapeutic Options

Once we determine that it is time to treat a patient for cognitive dysfunction syndrome, we have many therapeutic options. Unfortunately, treatment is not straightforward nor simple. It requires an abundance of patience and dedication. However, it can be a worthwhile endeavor that provides positive results in many cases. An excellent comment that can be applied to patients with cognitive dysfunction syndrome comes from Dr Marsha Reich, a diplomate of the American College of Veterinary Behavior:

> Just because he's getting old doesn't mean that we just stand on the sidelines and let him get old. There are things we can do to intervene and improve the [pet's] ability to function and improve its quality of life.
>
> (Neutricks, 2017).

Treatment for cognitive dysfunction syndrome is not a curative process. Rather, the goal is to minimize the impact of the disease on the pet's daily activities, thus improving their quality of life. The treatment process can be a significant challenge both for the family and for the veterinary team because there is no one approach or set of therapies that will be successful in all cases. Rather, a variety of therapeutic approaches, medical treatments, and nutritional supplements should be used. It is up to the client and the veterinary team to determine how many and which of these options to implement. This decision should always include a discussion with the pet's family regarding their financial and emotional ability to execute such treatments and therapies.

Treatment options fall into three major categories: traditional medical therapies, alternative medical therapies, and environmental management. While we cannot provide an exhaustive list of all available options, we discuss specific examples of each of these in more depth.

Traditional Medical Therapies

Selegiline
At the time of publication, selegiline is the only pharmaceutical in the United States that is approved by the Food and Drug Administration for use in slowing the progression of canine cognitive dysfunction. It is a selective and irreversible inhibitor of monoamine oxidase B that is used in human medicine to treat Alzheimer's disease, as well as Parkinson's disease and Cushing's disease. According to the manufacturer, the drug works at the hypothalamic–pituitary level to normalize dopamine levels (Zoetis Inc., 2017). It is not fully understood how this produces a clinical improvement in dogs with cognitive dysfunction syndrome, but "enhancement of dopamine and perhaps other catecholamines in the cortex and hippocampus is presumed to be an important factor"

(Landsberg, 2005). In general, selegiline can be quite helpful if started early, but seems to be less effective when the disease is already at a more advanced stage. For canines, selegiline is dosed at 0.5–1.0 mg/kg once daily, typically in the morning. If, after 30 days, the improvement is not adequate, the dose can be increased to the next tablet size for an additional 30 days. The American Association of Feline Practitioners also supports the off-label use of this medication for cats at a dose of 0.25–1.0 mg/kg once daily (Herron, 2012). Additional dosing information and drug interaction warnings can be found on the product label.

Anxiolytic Drugs

Anxiolytic drugs (such as alprazolam, amitriptyline, clomipramine, fluoxetine and trazodone) may be necessary for the treatment of anxious behaviors associated with cognitive dysfunction syndrome. If the patient is receiving selegiline, caution should be used when considering these medications, as some may interact with monoamine oxidase inhibitors. When anxiolytic drugs are indicated, there are many options, and finding the best drug may be a process of trial and error. Clinicians should discuss this with clients when prescribing the first medication for anxiety. Clients should be informed that while they may see some results immediately, most anxiolytic drugs have an additive effect over time. It is important to encourage clients that they must commit to the medication trial long enough (often for a period of two to six weeks) to gauge its full efficacy. They should also be aware that, after such a time, if the response is not adequate a dosing change, medication change, or the addition of another medication may be required to achieve the desired results. The process of finding the right medication(s) for anxiety can be frustrating. However, if veterinarians help clients go into the process with realistic expectations, they are more likely to persevere until they find something that works for their pet.

Benzodiazepines

Benzodiazepines may be useful as adjunctive therapy for restlessness and nighttime waking. According to the Ohio State University, oxazepam may be the safest choice for geriatric pets (who often have concurrent liver disease) because it does not have active liver metabolites. For canines and felines, it can be dosed at 0.04–0.5 mg/kg and given at bedtime (note that this dosage is lower than published doses used for treating fears and phobias). The recommendation is to start low and titrate the dosage upward on an as-needed basis. Another liver-sparing alternative is lorazepam, given to canines at 0.1–0.5 mg/kg, also at bedtime. For cats, it is suggested to start at one-quarter or one-half of a 0.5 mg tablet (0.125–0.25 mg per cat) and titrate upwards if necessary (Herron, 2012).

Immunotherapy

Immunotherapy is an emerging area of study in the battle against cognitive dysfunction syndrome, Alzheimer's disease, and associated cognitive decline. Researchers are investigating an active vaccine that can modify the presence of the beta-amyloid plaques within the brain. A study published in 2015 shows that anti-beta-amyloid immunotherapy does modify the shape and density of the beta-amyloid plaques. The same authors had previously shown that the vaccine led to "a very rapid cognitive improvement in all treated CDS dogs, with no evident side effects" (Bosch *et al.*, 2015).

The details are beyond the scope of this text, but their potential as a future treatment option appears promising.

Alternative Medical Therapies (including Nutritional and Supplemental Support)

Acupuncture

According to the Healthcare Medicine Institute (2014), research is beginning to provide evidence that acupuncture is beneficial in humans with Alzheimer's disease. It may increase acetylcholinesterase reactivity in the hippocampus, and it may also increase the activity of antioxidants such as superoxide dismutase (Leung *et al.*, 2013). More research is needed (in human and animal models) to fully understand the benefits of acupuncture for cognitive dysfunction. For more information regarding appropriate acupuncture therapy for cognitive dysfunction syndrome, it is recommended to consult with a certified veterinary acupuncturist in your area.

L-Theanine

While not a treatment for CDS directly, L-theanine (Anxitane®) is a product made from green tea leaves which can be beneficial in treating the associated anxiety. According to product literature, an open field trial showed a 62.1% reduction in the observed signs of anxiety within a 30-day period. It will likely not be adequate in and of itself to relieve a CDS patient's anxiety, but it can augment the results from other treatments and behavior modification techniques (Virbac US, 2017).

Special Diets

Brain Aging Care B/D™ Hills® Prescription Diet® Hills® Pet Nutrition is reported to work because it includes high levels of omega-3 fatty acids. This diet has excellent reviews and empirical evidence for its efficacy. Clinical studies also back up the idea that a diet rich in antioxidants and mitochondrial enzymatic cofactors can help minimize the effects of cognitive decline (Head, 2009; Head *et al.*, 2008). One study showed that "age-associated decline was reduced in the animals fed the enriched food, particularly on the more difficult tasks. These results indicate that maintenance on foods fortified with complex mixtures of antioxidants can partially counteract the deleterious effects of aging on cognition" (Milgram *et al.*, 2002).

Bright Mind™ diet by Purina® Pro Plan® is a proprietary diet blend that is rich in arginine (an essential amino acid), antioxidants (including vitamins E and C), docosahexaenoic acid and eicosapentaenoic acid (from fish oil), and B vitamins (including folic acid and pyridoxine). According to the manufacturer, the food's unique formula focuses on providing medium-chain triglycerides from "enhanced botanical oils like palm kernel oil and coconut oil" as fuel that the aging canine brain can use as an effective energy source. One study showed that feeding this diet "significantly improved performance on several cognitive tasks" (Landsberg *et al.*, 2012). This diet also has excellent reviews and empirical evidence for its efficacy (Purina Pro Plan, n.d.).

Gamma-Aminobutyric Acid

Gamma-aminobutyric acid (GABA) has been used in humans for its beneficial effects on patients suffering from severe psychiatric disorders. A 2005 study evaluated canine patients who received GABA at a dose of 30 mg/kg once daily for two weeks (Inagawa *et al.*, 2005). Patients' owners reported a perceived improvement in CDS signs in the areas of frequent whining and barking at night, whines and barks when left alone, continual sleep during day and night, walking around without particular intention, and rough respiration. Overall statistical data are lacking, but the Inagawa study "strongly suggests ... that GABA administration has beneficial effects [and improves] the quality of life of aged dogs" (Inagawa *et al.*, 2005).

Gingko
A clinical trial in Europe showed a "reduction of behavioral disturbances" when geriatric canines received Ginkgo biloba (Robinson, 2009). Said to improve blood flow to the brain and act as an antioxidant, Gingko could be used alone, but is often found in combination products (such as Senilife®, as noted below).

Melatonin
Melatonin is specifically for the sleep disturbances associated with CDS. A single dose of 0.1 mg/kg (alternatively, 1–9 mg per dog, or 1.5–6 mg per cat, depending on size) is best given approximately 30 minutes before bedtime, and works more effectively with a predictable bedtime routine. Use with caution with benzodiazepines, as melatonin may potentiate their effects (Landsberg *et al.*, 2011).

Apoaequorin
Neutricks food supplement (canine and feline versions available) contains apoaequorin, a substance derived from jellyfish. Apoaequorin is a protein that binds calcium and has a neuroprotective effect on the brain. Studies show that its use improves ability to perform learning and attention tasks compared with both a placebo and selegiline (Landsberg *et al.*, 2012; Neutricks, 2017).

Antioxidants and Plant Extracts
Supplements that include omega-3 fatty acids, such as Platinum Performance®, a blend of 55 ingredients, may help to support cognitive function. According to the manufacturer, dogs fed their normal food with the addition of the Platinum Performance supplement learned tasks more quickly while also improving their recall ability (Platinum Performance, 2017).

Resveratrol is a plant polyphenol, which is thought to act like an antioxidant. It can be used alone, or in combination products such as Senilife (see below) and Actistatin® (which may also be helpful for improving joint health and patient comfort).

S-Adenosyl-L-Methionine
S-adenosyl-L-methionine (SAMe) is made naturally in the body from methionine, and can also be synthesized. SAMe is involved in the formation, activation, or breakdown of other chemicals in the body, including hormones, proteins, phospholipids, and certain drugs. In one double blinded, placebo-controlled study, test subjects were given SAMe as their only treatment (no behavioral therapy was allowed). Results showed that dogs receiving SAMe had a significant increase in activity levels (41.7% compared with 2.6% after 4 weeks, $P < .0003$; 57.1% compared with 9.0% after 8 weeks, $P < .003$) and cognitive awareness (33.3% compared with 17.9% after 4 weeks, $P < .05$; 59.5% compared with 21.4% after 8 weeks, $P < .01$) as controlled with test subjects who received the placebo.

e is marketed for canines as Denosyl®. Dosing can be based on Denosyl product labels, or figured at 18 mg/kg and rounding to the nearest tablet size (Reme *et al.*, 2008).

Senilife
Senilife is a blend of phosphatidylserine, pyridoxine, Ginkgo biloba extract, resveratrol, and D-alpha-tocopherol (canine and feline versions available). According to the manufacturer, "the components of Senilife work synergistically and have a specific neuroprotective action to help combat your dog from the brain-aging-related behavior signs often seen in senior pets" (Ceva Animal Health, 2015). A Canadian study also showed that Senilife improved short-term memory performance compared with administration of a placebo (Araujo *et al.*, 2008). Another study also showed that "dogs on Senilife showed a marked improvement of CDS related signs, even if the dogs failed to show a complete remission of symptoms" (Osella et al., 2007). Dosing is according to product label.

Alpha-casozepine
While not a treatment for CDS directly, alpha-casozepine (Zylkene®) is a product made from milk proteins that can be beneficial in treating the associated anxiety. Its structure is similar to that of GABA and one blinded trial showed that its efficacy was equal to that of selegiline (Beata *et al.*, 2007). It will likely not be adequate in and of itself to control anxiety, but it can augment the results from other treatments and behavior modification techniques (Vetoquinol USA, n.d.).

Environmental Management and Occupational Therapies

Home Environment
It is important to make a CDS patient's living quarters as low stress as possible. This will decrease anxiety levels and increase overall quality of life, and the process is quite simple. Remind clients not to rearrange furniture or purchase new items (if possible). If patients are prone to wandering, closing doors or placing baby gates in doors and stairways is a simple way to ensure that they do not injure themselves during their wandering. For cats and small dogs, the addition of stairs may be helpful to reach favorite places (like the bed or a windowsill). If cats are not jumping well, it may be advisable to remove tall cat trees and other climbing objects (Figure 8.5). It is important to place food and water dishes (and litter boxes) in an easily accessible area. If the pet's food and water dishes have always been in the same place, take care not to move them, as this may be confusing to a patient with CDS. Consistency is the top priority, with ease of access being a close second.

Consistent Daily Routine
With people with dementia and Alzheimer's disease, a consistent daily routine brings a bit of stability in the midst of a world that may feel like it is falling down around them. Knowing what is going to happen throughout the day and having the ability to anticipate what will happen next can bring calm in the midst of internal chaos. This seems to be true for our pet patients with CDS as well. A predictable time for feedings, treats, walks, and play sessions can act as an anchor. It is not always possible, but humans having a predicable "home and away" schedule can also be helpful to pets with cognitive disorders. The predictability of a routine gives them the ability to better cope with other things that may surprise them throughout the day.

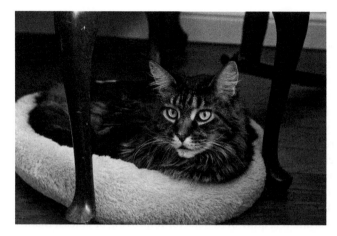

Figure 8.5 Beds placed on the ground in "safe" spots for the pet to sleep on.

Exercise

Consistent, gentle exercise (tailored for each patient's ability level) is good for geriatric pets in many ways. It improves mobility, helps to maintain muscle strength, and contributes to mental stimulation. Exercise releases endorphins which may also act to calm the pet and decrease anxiety that often accompanies CDS. Pets may still do the activities they loved in the past, with care given to shorten the duration and intensity of the exercise sessions. Gentle walks, limited games of fetch, and swimming for short periods of time are all excellent outdoor activities to recommend. Indoors, a pet may enjoy yoga, games of hide-and-seek, range of motion exercises, or even massage (from the owner or a professional). Encourage pet owners to find an exercise routine that fits their schedule and is enjoyable for both the pet and their human family members.

Love

This recommendation may seem to be a bit tongue-in-cheek, but it is important to consider and worth recommending love to clients. Oftentimes, the daily tasks and duties involved in geriatric nursing care can become burdensome and stressful. Patients with dementia do not always cooperate well with bathing, grooming, and the administration of medications. For this reason, a caretaker can easily become frustrated with their pet, or slip into the responsibility of being their pet's nurse and leave the role of loving family member behind. According to Gary Landsberg, DVM, MRCVS, "Interactions that support the human–animal bond are especially critical in pets that are aging and ill because owners need to be responsive and sensitive to their pet's subtle changes in behavior as indicators of pain, welfare, and quality of life. Positive and pleasant shared experiences provide caregivers a sense of accomplishment rather than anguish about their pet's illness" (Landsberg *et al.*, 2011). For these reasons, it is worthwhile to "prescribe" 15–20 minutes of intentional love and affection each day. This should be a time where family members focus on simply enjoying time with their beloved companion, rather than attending to their daily needs. It is a simple prescription, but can go a long way towards maintaining the connection between a pet and their people!

Mental Stimulation

Asking patients to figure out a new concept or perform a task can be an excellent tool in the fight against the progression of CDS (Cory, 2013). Short, scheduled sessions of mental stimulation encourages healthy brain activity, reduces neuron loss, and may greatly improve a pet's overall quality of life (Siwak-Tapp *et al.*, 2008). If pets are still physically able to go on walks, encourage owners to take a new route where their dog can enjoy new sights and smells. Have them purchase novel toys that encourage sensory stimulation, "brain teaser" toys that reward their pet with food when they have figured out the puzzle (examples are available online at www.dogdementia.com), and place favorite toys on a rotation schedule so that a "new" favorite toy is available every few days. Remind clients to spend time strengthening their pet's training. The concept of "sit," or "down," or "shake" may not be new, but spending a few minutes each day reinforcing these concepts can be helpful. And contrary to the popular old saying, you *can* teach an old dog new tricks, and it is quite beneficial for improving or at least maintaining their cognitive function.

Sleep Disturbances

Nighttime waking is one of the most common complaints that triggers an owner to schedule a veterinary exam for their geriatric pet. When a pet is sleeping all day and agitated and noisy all night, the resulting lack of rest has a significant deleterious effect on the patient and his or her human caretaker's general wellbeing. The patient may be dealing exclusively with CDS and its resultant sleep–wake cycle disturbances, or (more commonly), the pet's disruption of normal sleep patterns is the result of multiple medical and behavioral issues that all contribute to interrupted sleep. As discussed earlier in the chapter, it is often difficult to fully differentiate between these disorders and their overlapping symptoms. The pet may be experiencing anxiety or phobias that worsen at night, or they may have a need for nighttime elimination related to polyuria/ polydipsia. Regardless of its cause(s), a lack of restful sleep can quickly wear down even the most tolerant person. When a patient and their family are chronically not sleeping well, euthanasia is much more likely to become a consideration. Therefore, it is essential to regard management of this symptom as a vital component of geriatric care.

As with everything related to CDS, therapy for sleep-disturbances is not simple or "one size fits all". Rather, a multimodal approach must be taken. When possible, all medical causes should be considered and treated (especially those related to elimination issues). As previously mentioned, melatonin may be beneficial as a first line of therapy for enhancing nighttime sleep. It should not be redosed at other times of the day when trying to reestablish nighttime sleeping patterns (Landsberg *et al.*, 2011). Other aforementioned therapies (such as exercise, mental stimulation, and a consistent daily routine) can also have favorable results with regards to nighttime waking. However, these therapies are not usually adequate in and of themselves. The addition of a predictable nighttime routine and a relaxing, comfortable place to sleep can also be helpful. Much like a newborn baby, geriatric pets benefit from signals that nighttime is approaching and it is time to get ready for sleep. Always taking the pet to the same place, lowering the lights, turning off electronics, and even using pheromone sprays or collars (such as Feliway and Adaptil) at bed time can help a pet fall asleep (DePorter, 2014). Some pets benefit from having their activity restricted at night by way of baby gates in doorways or by encouraging them to sleep in a crate (especially if they were crate trained early in life). Ambient temperature should be comfortable for the pet's needs (not too hot or too cool), and in some cases a heated bed should be used to support healthy sleep patterns by soothing a pet's muscles and joints. For CDS patients that are still having a difficult time falling asleep, it is often necessary to give anxiolytic drugs and/or benzodiazepines to provide necessary rest to both the patient and their caretakers (see Therapeutic Options earlier in this chapter for additional detail).

For pets that easily fall asleep but then wake during the night, it is important to ensure that the patient is not waking due to pain. If this is suspected, adjusting the doses or adding stronger pain medication may be required. A trial of gabapentin, or the use of combination products such as acetaminophen with codeine (for canines only, administered before bed) can also be helpful in providing pain relief and nighttime sedation (See Chapter 18).

As a final note regarding sleep–wake disturbances, it is essential to advise families that there should be no scolding or punishment for night waking. For a pet that is already confused and disoriented, punishment will only further add to their anxiety. Family members should be encouraged to care for their pet's needs, provide reassurance when the pet is anxious, and help their pet settle back into the appropriate place for sleep. However, other positive reinforcements (walks, feeding, turning lights on and watching television, and so on) should be avoided since they could encourage the undesired behavior.

End of Life Considerations

In summary, caring for an aging pet requires a significant investment of time, monetary resources, mental fortitude, and often physical strength. The pet likely needs an abundance of patience, love and nursing care that can be difficult to provide. Oftentimes, there is one person within the family structure that bears the weight of the responsibility for those needs. Managing an ailing pet's medication schedule, providing bathing and nursing care, and finding time for exercise, therapy, and enrichment activities are tasks that can quickly become overwhelming. As the primary caregiver strives to balance their pet's increasing needs with their family responsibilities, work, and other daily tasks, they are frequently burdened with an enormous amount of guilt as the various emotional, physical, and monetary budgets wear thin. This is especially true with cognitive disorders. The family frequently feels as though they are "giving up" on their beloved pet. However, the numerous physical, mental, and emotional stresses (for both the pet and the caregivers) that come along with CDS can break the human–animal bond and rob the pet of its ability to enjoy his or her days. The consideration of euthanasia is not a "last resort" or a selfish decision on the part of the caretakers, but rather a merciful and kind choice that focuses on the pet's quality of life. It is worthwhile to remind clients that the decision for end-of-life care is giving their pet a much needed escape from a confused and anxious reality that they can no longer cope with. They are truly providing their pet with the gift of no more bad days, and are shortening the length of their final struggle – and that is a beautiful (albeit incredibly difficult) decision.

References

Araujo, J., Studzinski, C., Milgram, M. (2005) "Further Evidence for the Cholinergic Hypothesis of Aging and Dementia from the Canine Model of Aging." *Progressive Neuropsychopharmacol Biol Psychiatry*, **29**(3): 411–422.

Araujo, J., Landsberg, G., Milgram, N., Miolo, A. (2008) "Improvement of Short-Term Memory Performance in Aged Beagles by a Neutraceutical Supplement Containing Phosphatidylserine, Ginkgo Biloba, Vitamin E, and Pyridoxine." *Canadian Veterinary Journal*, **49**(4): 379–385.

Beata, C., Beaumont-Graff, E., Diaz, C., Marion, M., Massal, N., Marlois, N., Mueller, G., Lefranc, C. (2007) "Effects of Alpha-Casozepine (Zylkene) Versus Seligiline Hydrochloride (Selgian, Anipryl) on Anxiety Disorders in Dogs." *Journal of Veterinary Behavior*, **2**: 175–183.

Bosch, M., Pugliese, M., Andrade, C., Gimeno-Bayon, J., Mahy, N., Rodriguez, M. (2015) "Amyloid-Beta Immunotherapy Reduces Amyloid Plaques and Astroglial Reaction in Aged Domestic Dogs." *Neurodegenerative Diseases*, **15**: 24–37.

Ceva Animal Health. (2015) Introducing Senilife: Helping Older Dogs Get Back to Life. Available at www.senilife.com.

Cory, J. (2013) Identification and management of cognitive decline in companion animals and the comparisons with Alzheimer disease: A review. *Journal of Veterinary Behavior* **8**(4), 291–301

DePorter, T. (2014) "Cognitive Dysfunction Syndrome." *Michigan Veterinary Medical Association Conference Proceedings*. Available at http://c.ymcdn.com/sites/www.michvma.org/resource/resmgr/mvc_proceedings_2014/deporter_03.pdf.

Dog Dementia. (2016) Canine Cognitive Dysfunction Checklist. Dog Dementia: Help and Support. Available at http://dogdementia.com.

Gonzalez-Martinea, A., Rosado, B., Pesini, P., Garcia-Belenguer, S., Palacio, J., Villegas, A., Suarez, M-L., Santamarina, G., Sarasa, M. (2013) "Effect of Age and Severity of Cognitive Dysfunction on Two Simple Tasks in Pet Dogs." *Veterinary Journal*, **198**: 176–181.

Head, E. (2009) Oxidative Damage and Cognitive Dysfunction: Antioxidant Treatments to Promote Healthy Brain Aging. *Neurochemical Research* **34**(4), 670–678

Head, E., and Zicker, S. (2004) "Nutraceuticals, Aging and Cognitive Dysfunction." *Veterinary Clinics of Small Animals*, **34**: 217–228.

Head, E., Rofina, J., Zicker, S. (2008) "Oxidative Stress, Aging, and Central Nervous System Disease in the Canine model of Human Brain Aging." *Veterinary Clinics of North America Small Animal Practice*, **38**: 167–178.

Healthcare Medicine Institute (2014) Acupuncture Continuing Education. Acupuncture Rejuvenates Alzheimer's Disease Patients (News Article). Available at http://www.healthcmi.com/Acupuncture-Continuing-Education-News/1403-acupuncture-rejuvenates-alzheimer-s-disease-patients.

Herron, M. (2012) "Behavior Changes in the Aging Pet: An Overview of Common Problems – Part 2." *Ohio State University College of Veterinary Medicine Behavior News*, **5**: 1–3.

Inagawa, K., Seki, S., Bannai, M., Takeuchi, Y., Mori, Y., Takahashi, M. (2005) "Alleviative Effects of Gama-Aminobutyric Acid (GABA) on Behavioral Abnormalities in Aged Dogs." *Journal of Veterinary Medical Science*, **67**(10): 1063–1066.

Landsberg, G. (2005) "Therapeutic Agents for the Treatment of Cognitive Dysfunction Syndrome in Senior Dogs." *Progress in Neuropsychopharmacology and Biological Psychiatry*, **29**: 471–479.

Landsberg, G., Denenberg, S., Araujo, J. (2010) "Cognitive Dysfunction in Cats: A Syndrome We Used to Dismiss as 'Old Age.'" *Journal of Feline Medicine and Surgery*, **12**: 837–848.

Landsberg, G, DePorter, T., Araujo, J. (2011) "Clinical Signs and Management of Anxiety, Sleeplessness, and Cognitive Dysfunction in the Senior Pet." *Veterinary Clinics of North America Small Animal Practice*, **41**: 565–590.

Landsberg, G., Nichol, J., Araujo, J. (2012) "Cognitive Dysfunction Syndrome: A Disease of Canine and Feline Brain Aging." *Veterinary Clinics of North America: Small Animal Practice* **42**: 749–768.

Leung, M., Yip, K., Lam, C., Lam, K., Lau, W., Yu, W., Leung, A., So, K. (2013) "Acupuncture Improves Cognitive Function: A Systematic Review." *Neural Regeneration Research*, **8**(18): 1673–1684.

Milgram, N., Zicker, S., Head, E., Muggenburg, B., Murphey, H., Ikeda-Douglas, C., Cotman, C. (2002) "Dietary Enrichment Counteracts Age-Associated Cognitive Dysfunction in Canines." *Neurobiology of Aging*, **23**: 737–745.

Neilson, J., Hart, B., Cliff, K., Ruehl, W. (2001) "Prevalence of Behavioral Changes Associated with Age-Related Cognitive Impairment in Dogs." *Journal of the American Veterinary Medical Association*, **218**(11): 1787–1791.

Neutricks. (2017) Frequently Asked Questions About Neutricks. Available at http:// neutricks.com/frequently-asked-questions-neutricks.

Opii, W., Joshi, G., Head, E., Milgram, N., Muggenburg, B., Klein, J., Pierce, W., Cotman, C. Butterfield, D. (2008) "Proteomic Identification of Brain Proteins in the Canine Model of Human Aging Following a Long-Term Treatment with Antioxidants and a Program of Behavioral Enrichment: Relevance to Alzheimer's Disease." *Neurobiology of Aging*, **29**(1): 51–70.

Osella, M., Re, G., Odore, R., Girardi, C., Badino, P., Barbero, R., Bergamasco, L. (2007) Canine Cognitive Dysfunction Syndrome: Prevalence, Clinical Signs and Treatment with a Neuroprotective Nutraceutical. *Applied Animal Behaviour Science* **105**(4), 297–310.

PetSci (2016) Canine Cognitive Dysfunction Questionnaire. Available at http://petsci.co. uk/canine-cognitive-dysfunction-questionnaire.

Platinum Performance. (2017) Support for Cognitive Function Conditions. Supplements for Cognitive and Antioxidant Support Available at http://www.platinumperformance. com/dogs-cats/dog-cat-conditions/dog-cognitive-health.

Purina Pro Plan. (n.d.) The Bright Mind™ Effect: Nutrition for Cognitive Health. Available at https://www.proplan.com/dogs/platforms/bright-mind-effect#dognitionbrightmind.

Reme, C., Dramard, V., Kern, L., Hofmans, J., Halsberghe, C., Mombiela, D. (2008) "Effect of S-Adenosylmethionine Tablets on the Reduction of Age-Related Mental Decline in Dogs: A Double-Blinded, Placebo-Controlled Trial." *Veterinary Therapeutics: Research in Applied Veterinary Medicine*, **9**(2): 69–82.

Robinson, N. (2009) "Supplements Can Ease CDS." *Veterinary Practice News*, April. Available at http://www.veterinarypracticenews.com/April-2009/Supplements-Can-Ease-CDS.

Rosado, B., Gonzalez-Martinea, A., Pesini, P., Garcia-Belenguer, S., Palacio, J., Villegas, A., Suarez, M-L., Santamarina, G., Sarasa, M. (2012) "Effect of Age and Severity of

Cognitive Dysfunction on Two Spontaneous Activity in Pet Dogs – Part 1: Locomotor and Exploratory Behavior." *Veterinary Journal*, **194**: 189–195.

Salvin, H., McGreevy, P., Sachdev, P., Valenzuela, M. (2011) "The Canine Cognitive Dysfunction Rating Scale (CCDR): A Data-Driven and Ecologically Relevant Assessment Tool." *Veterinary Journal*, **188**(3): 331–336.

Siwak-Tapp, C., Head, E., Muggenburg, B., Milgram, N., Cotman, C. (2008) "Region Specific Neuron Loss in the Aged Canine Hippocampus is Reduced by Enrichment." *Neurobiology of Aging*, **29**(1): 39–50.

Vetoquinol USA. (n.d.) Zylkene®. Available at http://www.vetoquinolusa.com/content/zylkene.

Virbac US. (2016) Anxitane® L-Theanine Chewable Tablets. Available at http://www.virbacvet.com/products/detail/anxitane-l-theanine-chewable-tablets.

Zoetis Inc. (2017) Anipryl Product Information. Available at https://www.zoetisus.com/products/anipryl.aspx.

9

Smelly Old Dog: Addressing the Dermatological Concerns of Our Geriatric Patients

Melanie Hasson Cohen

The Skin and the Changes

"Age is not a disease" is a phrase that is often thrown around and it is entirely true. Medical examiners will not write "old age" on death certificates. They indicate the terminal outcome of the body's dysregulation, or its inability to repair the perfect storm that set off a series of failures and ultimate demise. Often taken for granted but completely essential, skin plays an integral role as the barrier and protector to the outside world, as well as to a lifetime of physical, chemical and pathogenic insults. It allows us to sense and perceive our environment. It is essential in temperature regulation, immunosurveillance, and electrolyte regulation, and it assists with vitamin E production (Baker, 1967).

While there are no skin diseases found exclusively in older animals, senility tends to predispose dogs and cats to a multitude of skin pathologies (Goldston, 1989). With aging, the skin's immune system shows a decline in its adaptive capability or a dysregulation of the immune system (Cooley *et al.*, 2001). Cutaneous specific and non-specific manifestations of internal disease become more common, and structural changes of the skin will lead to higher incidences of infections and tumors (Goldston, 1989).

The most pronounced dysregulation is seen in T cells, which leads to both an increase in viral and intracellular pathogens as well as neoplastic diseases (Moore *et al.*, 1998). This T-cell dysregulation will lead to a decreased T-cell mediated immunity cell function, which is the ability of T cells to proliferate (Moore *et al.*, 1998). It also leads to their production of interleukin-2 (IL-2). The frequency and intensity of dysregularity has been shown to consistently increase with advancing age (Cooley et al., 2001). These changes will limit the patient's ability to develop an adequate response to presenting antigens by decreased production of antibodies (mediated via B cells) in both primary and secondary antibody responses (Cooley et al., 2001). This has been demonstrated in vivo with the inability of aged human and laboratory animals to develop an appropriate delayed-type hypersensitivity (DTH) skin response (Moore *et al.*, 1998). In addition, there is an age-associated increase in prostaglandin E_2 (PGE_2), which in turn can contribute to a reduction of antibody, DTH, IL-2 production as well as lymphocyte proliferation and ability to respond (Moore *et al.*, 1998).

Treatment and Care of the Geriatric Veterinary Patient, First Edition. Edited by Mary Gardner and Dani McVety.
© 2017 John Wiley & Sons, Inc. Published 2017 by John Wiley & Sons, Inc.
Companion Website: www.wiley.com/go/gardner/geriatric

Although there has been extensive research on human aging and changes of the skin, unsurprisingly there is very little written concerning skin gerontology of our cats and dogs. This may be due to a lack of a booming cosmetic anti-aging industry for our domestic animals. Our geriatric patients will commonly present with seborrhea, dry, dull and sparse hair coats due to follicular atrophy, as well as decreased quantity and altered quality of sebum production, making it more waxy (Davies, 1996). The skin will thicken and become less pliable with age, owing to a decrease in elastin. In addition, nasal planum and footpads will become hyperkeratinized and nails will often be long and brittle as they lose their water content and become malshaped (Moiser, 1989). Many patients may develop brown pigmented areas on their integument. The pigment lipofuscin, also known as the "wear and tear" pigment, is deposited in many other body tissues (neurons, cardiac and skeletal myocytes and integument; Moiser, 1987). With age, lipofuscin may be deposited in the dog at a rate fives times as fast as that seen in humans. Lipofuscin is the end result of autophagocytosis of cell constituents that results in a yellow-brown pigment or "age spots" which cannot removed by further lysosomal degradation (Moiser, 1987).

Alterations in hair color and condition are often the first and most predominant changes our clients will notice and associate with the aging condition of their pets (American Humane Association, 1994). Hair will grow gray and then white as the natural lifecycle of pigment cells reaches its end and the stem cells responsible for migrating to the surface to replace them become delayed and then absent (Baker, 1967). Often this starts around the muzzle and eyes but in some cases it may become widespread. Figure 9.1 shows a Pug pictured at 12 weeks, and again 10 years later, exhibiting typical age related dermatological changes including, graying, hyperkeratosis of nasal planum and pigmentary keratosis. Many factors may influence the loss and quality of hair. In general, the hair is controlled, but not limited by, the photoperiod, ambient temperature and nutritional status (Moiser, 1989). Anagen (hair growth) will be stimulated by

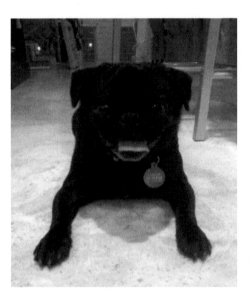 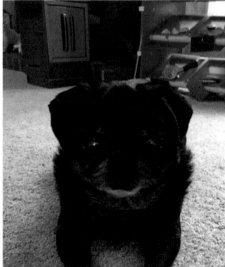

Figure 9.1 Twelve-week old Pug (left) and same dog at 10 years old (right).

thyroid hormones and inhibited by excess of glucocorticoids and estrogen. Hair is predominantly protein, and thus with malnutrition or protein losing enteropathies or nephropathies there will be a profound effect on the quality of the hair shaft which leads to a dull, brittle and thin hair coat (Fortney, 2004). With advanced disease, the anagen phases may be shortened resulting in hairs that are in telogen and thus more likely to be lost. In cases of severe illness, a condition of "telogen defluxion" may result, whereby hairs will synchronously enter telogen and shed simultaneously (Moiser, 1987).

The Patient: The Gold Standard and the Reality

Whether the patient is presented for a routine geriatric exam, or because the guardian has noted a specific dermatological abnormality, a thorough dermatological history can often provide as much information as the physical exam, and thus guide the need for further ancillary testing. Endocrinopathies, neoplastic and paraneoplastic conditions, and atopies are often seen with increased frequency in older patients and may need to be ruled out (Davies, 1996; Goldston, 1989).

As veterinarians, most of us were trained to recognize and categorize a list of symptoms into presenting complaints, then assign them differential diagnoses, as we systematically rule out or diagnose and identify problems we can fix. In general, these "problems" will be placed in a list of essential and nonessential concerns that form an informal hierarchy or priority list. Our priorities or concerns may change depending on the presence of concurrent disease and with the age of the patient. Although never formally part of my veterinary education, I recognized this subconscious pathway of problem solving when I visited Meg, a gorgeous Golden Retriever and her adoring guardians. At our initial consult, Meg was already in the throws of advanced renal failure. Her guardians were well versed in symptomatic and supportive therapies and were administering subcutaneous fluids daily and had a mini pharmacy of medications to keep her comfortable and eating well. During our visit, I noted her flaky skin, hair that was placating off in clumps and areas of alopecia along her dorsum. Meg was not pruritic, nor did she show any discomfort or signs of secondary infection. Her changes were associated with her current protein-losing nephropathy and persistent catabolic state. We were already optimizing her nutritional intake and addressing her nausea. I left our consult noting her dermatological changes as consequential but not a priority. There was a plentitude of therapies I could have suggested to address her seborrhea and hair loss, a wonderful array of patch jobs and maintenance attempts. But what would be the overall purpose? The patient had no discomfort. The anomalies were a cosmetic reminder of the bigger picture, her impending mortality that we could slow but not stop.

Reflecting back to the rhythm of general practice, I remember how many of my "sick visits" were dermatological in nature and the issue of dry, flaky skin and hair loss would have been listed as the highest priority and primary concern.

There is no secret formula or algorithm that I am aware of that tells us when to pursue further diagnostics and treat for primary or secondary conditions. The variables in the decision to investigate and treat are great, and the reality involves not just the patient presenting complaints but more the concerns and expectations of the guardian, as well as their financial limitations. The decision not to pursue diagnostics and symptomatic treatment with Meg was simple. At what point would I be crossing the line of actively inflicting harm on my patient versus confronting the idea of mortality with her guardians?

A close colleague of mine was presented with an entirely different scenario. Dax, a 9-year-old Box-a-Shar had a history of chronic allergies. He was self-mutilating deep lesions into his skin unless he remained in an e-collar 24 hours a day. His skin had been diminished to an alopecic sea of lichenification, hyperpigmentation with islands of ulcerations and deep pyoderma. Dax was miserably uncomfortable, at first spending many hours pacing and rubbing against both the furniture and his family, leaving a trail of yeasty film on everything he passed. Their discussion of his medical history revealed symptoms that had started seasonally some five years before and were treated with the flavor of the month, a steroid shot. Soon, the once or twice annual occurrence was every six weeks during the summer season, and then progressed to year-round intense pruritus. Dax had been through food trails and a slew of immunosuppressive drugs, antifungals and antibiotics. He had remained on parasiticides every three weeks and had a cabinet of mostly empty prescription shampoos and topical preparations that could fill a retail display at any respectable salon. My colleague was left with the reality that a patient had a long history of probable atopy that had failed to be controlled through the conventional therapies and was utterly miserable and cornered in the only part of the house that was easy to clean. The questions and hypotheses were endless. Would he have been successfully managed under the guidance of a boarded dermatologist, or perhaps have had relief under the simultaneous care of traditional eastern medicine and acupuncture? Perhaps. Dax was now one-third of his former weight; his quality of life had been diminished to a mere existence.

Shortly after my colleague shared her story of Dax, I met Bandit. Bandit was a German Shepherd that had dermatological changes associated with concurrent disease that was leading to poor quality of life. Bandit was a large stocky and regal boy with multi-decade champion bloodlines. His guardians were a veterinarian's dream of perfect compliance and the financial resources to perform and visit any specialist. As a result, Bandit was one of the few patients I have encountered that had a confirmed diagnosis of degenerative myelopathy. When I met Bandit, he was a shell of his former self, but remained stoic and was a complete gentleman. He was in late stage degenerative myelopathy and had flaccid paraparesis, urinary and fecal incontinence, and widespread muscle atrophy. Bandit had a painful case of pododermatitis, urine scalding of ventral and inguinal areas of his abdomen, multiple abrasions from dragging on lateral and dorsal aspects of both tarsi and decubital ulcers over his coxofemoral and scapula–humeral joints. Bandit's guardians were fully informed on the poor prognosis and debilitating progression the disease would take, but they felt uncertain of the path ahead. Although we went over the details, descriptions and options at length, some of the descriptions only fueled additional fears and concerns, necessitating important and hard questions. I had to determine their wishes concerning Bandit's health and wellbeing and how those preferences fit in with reality. I then selected which options were most likely to achieve these priorities.

Bandit's dermatological conditions were placed on the top of the priority list, as their progression would most certainly be responsible for the timing of compassionate euthanasia. Treatment would need to be directed at addressing current infection and instituting appropriate husbandry measures to limit exacerbation of these conditions. Topical and broad-spectrum oral antibiotics were initiated, and the larger wounds were cleaned

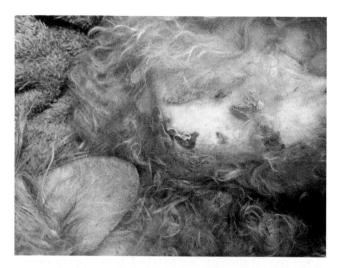

Figure 9.2 Decubital ulcers in a 16-year-old Poodle (post mortem).

and bandaged with donut-shaped bandage to alleviate pressure on the areas (Figure 9.2). A sanitary clip was performed to improve the ability to keep him dry and clean. Bandit's bedding was changed to an absorbent material over a well-cushioned crib mattress that was waterproof, to wick away moisture and prevent further urine scalding. A combination of talc-free baby powder and A&D ointment was used to create a barrier against moisture. Appropriate pain management measures were started and he was fitted for protective and waterproof boots to be used only when he was ambulatory with the assistance of his correctly fitted sling. We addressed his current pododermatitis with appropriate foot soaks and antifungals. Although intermittent bladder catheterization and manual expression were discussed, they were not within the comfort level of his guardians and if they became a necessity, were recognized as extreme and invasive measures to the family.

While Bandit readily accepted help and nursing care at first, he did not take to his cart and became a ball of anxiety. He refused to interact with his family, eat or even play ball, a pastime he had especially enjoyed. His family understood that there would be a limited time before he would have tetraplegia. Although a cart was available, it was not appropriate for Bandit, then or ever. While Bandit's dermatitis and pyoderma began to resolve, his anxiety built and he grew to resent the repeated cleaning and application of protective measures. It was a point of harsh realization that although the pot of physical and financial resources was full, the emotional tolls were high and treatment was beginning to inflict harm on both patient and guardian. Bandit was compassionately euthanized before he could progress to stage IV.

When We Need to Address "The Elephant"

I have only come across two people who admitted that their pet's appearance was their primary concern, both apologizing profusely for saying it out loud. I explained to them that these changes were associated with underlying pathologies. The damage was done, the guilt was present, and now the pieces of the human–animal bond needed to be salvaged. Although very few boldly stated their cosmetic concerns, a large number of the families I have encountered have expressed guilt concerning their altered relationships with their pets. As a species, we are very focused on the physical, bombarded daily with images of youth and perfection.

There is a perpetual "elephant in the room". No one wants to acknowledge it, and risk coming across as superficial, but it is there staring at them everyday and it is slowly breaking down the human–animal bond. Avoidance of such a subject can often lead to avoidance of the pet, as the family tries to keep the guilt at bay, and this break in relationship is a point of failure.

A mentor of mine shared a story of a hospice consultation. The patient, Bailey, was a typically loveable Golden Retriever. She had been an integral part of the family for more than 14 years. She was the couple's first adoption, the first big responsibility and their introduction to parenthood. Fourteen years later, the couple had three kids, two well into their teens, and a full schedule of school and extracurricular activities. The mother was struggling with guilt. It took her several attempts just to schedule the appointment. After she grew more comfortable and at ease, she explained the notion of someone coming into her house and seeing Bailey's state and fracturing her happy family façade had been causing sleepless nights. My mentor recounted the day of her initial consult. She was warmly greeted by each family member, then led to the back of the house into a comfortably converted sunroom they had made Bailey's assigned living quarters.

Bailey was thrilled at the prospect of company. Her family was relieved to see that my mentor was so well received as they watched Bailey blanket her with kisses and the exuberance of a puppy. Bailey's initial struggles started with arthritis. The sunroom was used at first to limit her need to access the upstairs, but the smell in the room was all too revealing. Although not explicitly stated, the odor and trail of "grease" had proven to be overwhelming and burdensome to the family, and having her in the sunroom was the only solution they could find. The initial reason for the hospice consult was listed as problems related to mobility and arthritic pain, but my mentor would explain that pain management would fall far short in improving Bailey's quality of life and the bond she shared with her family. Bailey's diet was addressed, and secondary bacterial and *Malassezia* infections were treated systemically. An anti-seborrheic shampoo and emollient was used every seven days and an oral fatty acid supplement was added as an adjunct (180 mg EPA/lb). While Bailey's underlying atopy was addressed, an additional set of instructions was left with the family.

The last direction she gave was in the form of a specific prescription written on her pad. Besides the daily care, such as walk and administration of medicine, each family member was ordered to spend 10 minutes a day with Bailey, simply being with her. It took several weeks to improve the condition of Bailey's skin, but only days to improve the family bond. Upon return several weeks later, Bailey still had her room but it was only used at night and the elephant had gladly departed.

Crashing and Failing

From the moment I opened the door, my senses were flooded with the overpowering odor of ammonia. Looking around the house, there was the telltale sign of mental instability with surfaces stacked high in an array of old newspapers and holiday decorations. Mrs Que, a widow who lived alone, had no family nearby. She had called me that morning out of sheer desperation. Rex "was old, very old," he had "some sort of stroke" a few days before and hadn't gotten up. She was too scared to move him out of fear that he may bite her. She needed help now and repeatedly said over tears of anguish that it was time but she didn't want it to be. Rex was lying on the kitchen floor, a skeleton of a mixed-breed Terrier. I could not tell if he was a gray- or black-coated Terrier as what was left of his wiry hair was slicked down and saturated in urine and feces. The muscle atrophy and overall cachexia was astonishing; I could have wrapped my finger around his entire femur. I approached him cautiously, surprised he was able to react. Since his guardian had expressed concern and fear, I decided not to take a chance. I told her I would move slow to check his heart and determine the appropriate medication to make him comfortable. As I suspected, I administered my sedative cocktail with not so much of a flinch from Rex. Within a few minutes, his breathing slowed to a restful state so we could administer the euthanasia solution and end his suffering. As I eased him onto my stretcher, I noticed the floor beneath him was stained and saturated with feces and urine. It was clear that Mrs Que had repeatedly cleaned around him but never had the courage to move him. A flap of skin became dislodged as I moved him onto the stretcher, and a trail of live maggots escaped (Figure 9.3). I did my best to internalize my range of emotions, and I left that day torn between total anger and deep sorrow.

The immediate concern had been addressed, and Rex was no longer suffering, but I felt extremely uneasy, and decided that I would be the one to return the urn and check on Mrs Que. Later that day, I called social services and asked someone to look into helping her. A week later when I brought Rex's urn, her home was only a few degrees removed from squalor. I sat down with her as she rushed to clean off a chair. We sat and spoke and she expressed her fear of judgment, not so much of the house, but the condition of Rex. She thanked me profusely for my kindness and warmth I had shown her that day.

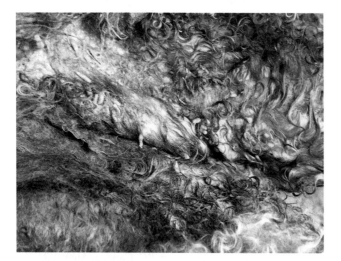

Figure 9.3 Deep pyoderma with maggot infestation in a 14-year-old mixed-breed dog following a prolonged period of immobility (post mortem).

Treating for Quality of Life and the Human–Animal Bond

While veterinary medicine has given us remarkable power to push the limits of mortality, it also comes with the burden of responsibility. Our job is not only to ensure health and survivability, but in essence to acknowledge our limitations and ensure a quality wellbeing. Whatever treatments or patch jobs we may offer, the balance of sacrifices should always tip in favor of improving quality of life and preserving the human–animal bond. We should treat for the treatable, especially if secondary infection is present. Many dermatological exams and samples can be performed and collected bedside, with inexpensive equipment to be examined at the clinic. Treatment options will vary greatly and need to be selected after considering both the patient and guardian factors, thus increasing the rate of compliance. Many of our patients will be on concurrent medications and attention to possible interactions should always be addressed if they cannot be avoided. Antacids may decrease bioavailability and need to be separated, while diphenhydramine may increase sedative effects.

Topical therapies should be selected based on their ease of application. Twice weekly, 10-minute contact baths may not be feasible for large or debilitated patients.

Prevent the preventable and don't assume "across the board" compliance. The presence of fleas, ticks and other parasites are not uncommon, as many guardians will forgo preventatives due to fear of inflicting harm on their pet, who they perceive as too frail to receive parasiticides. Given the higher incidence of allergic dermatitis in our aging pets, it has become increasingly important to stress the necessity of preventative care to limit exposure to the allergens we can actually limit.

Attention to the nails, interdigital, and pad health can improve comfort and mobility and can offer further insight on state of lameness and need for environmental modification. Use of vitamin E cream can help with dry and cracked feet.

There is no one protocol that fits all. Each needs to be tailored to suit the patient and guardian's ability. Creativity and "thinking outside the box" are welcomed but not limited to the use of diapers with holes cut out to accommodate tails, human incontinence pads (often cheaper than pet-specific products), the use of mobile grooming companies that can assist with medicated baths, or the use of crib mattresses that are designed to be waterproof for ease of cleaning while still offering the necessary support.

At the heart of everything is communication and expression of goals and guardian fears or concerns. Those need to be at the forefront with the aim of selecting treatments most likely to maintain or improve patients' comfort and preserve the human–animal bond.

References

Baker, K. P. (1967) "Senile Changes of Dog Skin." *Journal of Small Animal Practice*, **8**(1): 49–54.

Cooley, D. M. and Waters, D. J. (2001) "Cancer in the Elderly Dog." In Clinical Nutrition for the Senior Dog and Cat: Proceedings from a Pre-congress Symposium: World Congress 2001 World Small Animal Veterinary Association, Vancouver, BC, Canada, August 8, 2001. IAMS Company.

Davies, M. (1996) "An Introduction to Geriatric Veterinary Medicine." In *Canine and Feline Geriatrics*, pp. 1–11. Oxford, UK: Blackwell.

Fortney, W. D. (2004) "Geriatrics and Aging." In J. D. Hoskins (ed.), *Geriatric and Gerontology of the Dog and Cat*, 2nd ed., pp. 1–4. Philadelphia, PA: Elsevier Saunders.

Goldston, R. T. (1989) "Preface. Geriatrics and Gerontology." *Veterinary Clinics of North America (Small Animal Practice)*, **19**(1): ix–x.

Moore, P. F., Affolter, V. K., Olivry, T., Schrenzel, M. (1998) "The Use of Immunological Reagents in Defining the Pathogenesis of Canine Skin Diseases Involving the Proliferation of Leukocytes." In K. W. Kwochka, T. Willems, and C. von Tscharner (eds.), *Advances in Veterinary Dermatology*, Vol. 3, pp. 77–94. Oxford, UK: Butterworth-Heinemann.

Mosier, J. E. (1989) "Effects of Aging on Body Systems." *Veterinary Clinics of North America (Small Animal Practice)*, **19**(1): 1–12.

Mosier J. E. (1987) "How Aging Effects the Body Systems in the Dog." In *Geriatric Medicine: Contemporary Clinical and Practice Management Approaches, Proceedings of the Symposium, Kansas City, Missouri, October 4 1987*, pp. 2–5. Lenexa, KA: Veterinary Medicine Pub. Co.

10

Central and Peripheral Nervous System
Laura Devlin Bacon

The Nervous System and Aging

A nervous system that is properly functioning is essential for animals to have the ability to interact and respond to their environment. Proper function requires a complex interaction between the sensory, integrative, and motor components of the nervous system. Disruption of any of these components from aging changes and age-related disease processes can have a significant impact on a pet's normal day-to-day existence.

As a pet ages, the nervous system undergoes natural changes over time. Sensory systems of geriatric pets become less acute, notably hearing, vision, smell, taste, and balance. Cognition declines, spinal reflexes change, and sensory nerves lose myelin, perhaps predisposing to neuropathies.

Within the peripheral nervous system, cell loss occurs, and there is lipofuscin accumulation in ganglia of sympathetic and parasympathetic systems. Segmental demyelination and Wallerian-type degeneration have been described (Davies, 2012). At the level of the neuromuscular junction, age-related degeneration is attributed to many factors, including mitochondrial dysfunction, oxidative stress, inflammation, changes in the innervation of muscle fibers, and mechanical properties of the motor units (Gonzalez-Freire, 2014).

The central nervous system of older mammals (for example, dogs and humans) as compared with younger animals shows anatomical and physiological changes. The brain and the spinal cord gradually atrophy, losing nerve cells and weight. The ventricles enlarge, astrocytes hypertrophy, and senile plaque formation occurs. The number of dendrite branches and interconnections decrease, and nerve impulse amplitude may begin to decrease (Hoskins 2004). Demyelination and neuroaxonal degeneration occur, and there is meningeal fibrosis and/or calcification. Neurotransmitter production can change with age, and neurotransmitter receptors may change in number (Davies, 2012). Functional changes include depletion of catecholamine neurotransmitters (noradrenaline, serotonin, and dopamine), a decline in the cholinergic system, an increase in monoamine oxidase B activity and a reduction of endogenous antioxidants (Dimakopoulos and Mayer, 2002).

Treatment and Care of the Geriatric Veterinary Patient, First Edition. Edited by Mary Gardner and Dani McVety.
© 2017 John Wiley & Sons, Inc. Published 2017 by John Wiley & Sons, Inc.
Companion Website: www.wiley.com/go/gardner/geriatric

In addition to the natural changes of the nervous system that occur through the process of aging, there are a number of neurologic conditions that occur specifically with older age. Age-related disorders of the nervous system are classified based on the location of the nervous system that is affected; that is, central, peripheral or neuromuscular junction. Cranial nerves can be affected both within and outside of the intracranial space as they course to areas of the head. Neurologic disorders can also be classified by the type of disorder that is present, such as degenerative, metabolic, neoplastic, inflammatory or idiopathic.

Neurologic disorders can present with a wide variety of clinical presentation. Many behavioral changes, such as anxiety and depression, and alterations in mental status, as well as pain, stiffness, weakness, gait abnormalities, sensory and motor dysfunction, tremors, and seizures can all be signs associated with neurologic disease. If neurologic deficits are identified, a complete neurologic examination is indicated, which includes testing of reflexes, postural reactions, strength, tone, and sensation, to characterize and localize the disorder (Shull, 2002). However, localizing a neurologic disease process can be especially challenging in the geriatric patient. With respect to postural and spinal reflexes, age-associated muscle atrophy, degenerative joint disease, and generalized weakness can affect reflex assessment and conscious proprioception interpretation. Cognitive decline and age-related mentation changes can affect a patient's response, which may be diminished or exaggerated. If vision or hearing is diminished, the patient may be overly sensitive to other external stimuli. Blind animals may appear to be hypermetric in their gate, and their reflex assessment should be interpreted with caution. When assessing cranial nerves, a diminished response to a menace reflex, olfactory test or auditory stimulus may not indicate a neurologic deficit (Hoskins, 2004).

The neurologic conditions most commonly associated with older dogs and cats are discussed in this chapter. For further classification, the disorders are listed under the corresponding section of the nervous system. While some conditions can lead to problems with more than one section of the nervous system, the disorder is characterized by the system that is most affected (Table 10.1). Laryngeal paralysis is discussed in Chapter 13, and cognitive issues are discussed in Chapter 8.

Disorders of the Central Nervous System

Intracranial Disorders

Cerebral disorders may manifest with a variety of clinical signs, depending on the region that is affected. Patients will present with symptoms such as behavioral changes, altered mental status, circling, head-pressing, focal and generalized seizure activity, and defects in cranial nerves. Brain stem lesions may lead to altered mental status, proprioceptive and gait abnormalities, deficits in cranial nerves III–VII, cardiac and respiratory abnormalities, and central vestibular dysfunction. Cerebellar dysfunctions typically affect the rate, range, direction, and force of motor movements. These symptoms may exhibit themselves as hyper- or hypometria, ataxia, dysmetria, and tremors. Paradoxical head tilt and decerebrate rigidity are two classical signs of cerebellar disease. Lesions of the vestibulocerebellum may cause nystagmus, strabismus, loss of balance, and a head tilt (Hoskins, 2004). Figure 10.1 shows a geriatric cat exhibiting anisocoria.

Table 10.1 Common nervous system disorders of geriatric dogs and cats.

Type	Intracranial	Spinal cord	Peripheral nervous system
Degenerative	Cognitive dysfunction Cerebellar degeneration	Degenerative myelopathy (dogs) Cervical vertebral instability Cauda equina syndrome Spondylosis deformans (clinical)	
Metabolic	Liver disease (hepatic encephalopathy) Renal encephalopathy Hypoglycemia Hyper- and hypothyroidism Electrolyte abnormalities		Diabetic neuropathy Hyper- and hypothyroidism Hypoglycemia Hypoadrenocorticism
Neoplastic	Primary Metastatic Local extension	Primary Secondary Local extension	Primary Secondary Local extension Paraneoplastic
Vascular/ischemic	Hypertension Hyperlipidemia		
Idiopathic	Vestibulitis, central		Laryngeal paralysis Facial paralysis
Inflammatory	Distemper (dog) Feline infectious peritonitis (cat)		Chronic inflammatory demyelinating polyneuropathy

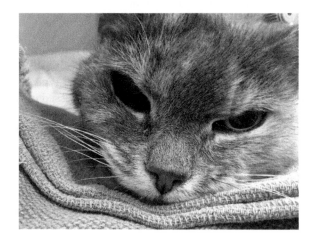

Figure 10.1 Anisocoria in a geriatric cat.

Many of the disease processes that can affect the brain can cause clinical signs that can be very upsetting to owners. Many of these diseases can be treated and palliated, and owners should be cautioned not to rush into making decisions primarily based on the initial clinical appearance.

Because the brain has extremely high metabolic demands, systemic abnormalities that affect the normal energy metabolism of the central nervous system may result in clinical signs of encephalopathy and are termed as metabolic encephalopathies. The cerebral cortex neurons are most susceptible to altered energy metabolism. Clinically, the earliest and most consistent signs are depression of consciousness (confusion, stupor, coma), and generalized seizures. Other neurologic signs will vary with the severity of the metabolic disturbance. Treatment of metabolic encephalopathies is directed at managing the underlying disease and controlling seizures if present.

Hypoglycemic encephalopathy can occur when blood glucose drops below 45–60 mg/dl. Clinical signs of hypoglycemic encephalopathy include altered mental status, compulsive pacing, behavioral change, and seizures. The brain is dependent on circulating blood glucose, as there is limited ability to generate glucose and limited glycogen stores in the brain. The causes of hypoglycemia are many and in the aging patient, the most commonly seen disorders are the overproduction of endogenous insulin or insulin-like substances by pancreatic insulinomas or other neoplasms, sepsis, exogenous insulin overdose in diabetes mellitus patients, and liver failure.

Uremic encephalopathy has been diagnosed in dogs and cats with advanced renal disease. There are numerous proposed mechanisms to explain this condition. Hyperammonemia has been shown to cause symptoms of encephalopathy in four cats with renal azotemia (Adagra and Foster, 2015).

Hypertensive encephalopathy is usually secondary to an underlying disease, although primary hypertension has been recognized. The major causes in cats are chronic renal disease and hyperthyroidism. In dogs, acute and chronic renal failure, glomerulonephritis, hyperadrenocorticism, and pheochromocytomas are often the cause. Treatment is directed toward the primary cause.

Hyperthyroidism (in cats, rarely dogs), hypothyroidism (in dogs, rarely cats), diabetes mellitus, and hyperadrenocorticism may each occasionally lead to clinical signs of encephalopathy. Patients typically exhibit signs of forebrain dysfunction in addition to other clinical signs relating to the underlying endocrine disorder. Hyperthyroid cats are more likely to appear restless and irritable and may exhibit aggressive behavior. A dull or obtunded mental status is commonly appreciated with hypothyroidism and diabetes mellitus. Diagnosis is made by documenting improvement of the clinical signs of encephalopathy when the underlying endocrine disorder is controlled (Cuddon, 1996).

Hepatic encephalopathy is a multifactorial type of neurological disorder that occurs as a result of hepatic insufficiency. It is discussed in Chapter 12.

Neoplasia of the central nervous system can occur in dogs of any age. However, the majority of cases are seen in dogs five years of age and older. Brain tumors are classified as either primary (arising from the brain tissue and its coverings) or secondary (reaching the brain by metastasis or local extension). Meningioma is the most common primary brain tumor diagnosed in dogs and cats. Other common primary tumors of dogs are glioma, astrocytoma, and oligodendroglioma. Lymphosarcoma is the second most common brain tumor in cats, occurring as either a primary neoplasm or as part of a multicentric disease.

Clinical signs of brain tumors depend on the location of the tumor. Diagnosis can be obtained by magnetic resonance imaging (MRI) and computed tomography (CT). Specific tumor type can be determined by biopsy in some cases and by excisional histopathology in others. Treatment depends on the tumor location and type. Surgical excision or debulking, combined with radiation offers the best outcome for most brain tumor patients. Surgical excision is the treatment of choice for meningioma. Radiation therapy can be beneficial in some cases. Lymphomas can have a good response to chemotherapy. Other chemotherapies have limited usefulness in brain tumor therapy because of the inability to penetrate the blood–brain barrier. Supportive therapy includes addressing cerebral edema and use of anticonvulsant therapy. Common drug therapy consists of furosemide dosed at 5 mg/kg intravenously, intramuscularly, subcutaneously, or orally every 6–8 hours, indefinitely; prednisone 2–4 mg/kg orally daily, indefinitely; phenobarbital 2–4 mg/kg orally, intramuscularly, intravenously, every 8–12 hours; zonisamide 5–10 mg/kg orally every 12 hours; or levetiracetam 20 mg/kg orally every 8 hours or 40 mg/kg intravenously. Prognosis depends on the tumor type and location, the treatment elected and the clinical signs. Educate owners to keep a log of any seizure activity (Nelson and Couto. 2014).

Focal ischemic events to the brain are common occurrences. There are multiple potential causes for brain infarcts, including systemic hypertension, cardiac disease, hypercoagulability, increased blood viscosity, infectious disease, and atherosclerosis associated with hypothyroidism, diabetes mellitus, or hyperlipidemia. Causes of thromboembolic disease include hyperadrenocorticism, hypothyroidism, hyperlipidemia, and neoplasia (Dewey, 2009).

Spinal Cord Disorders

Spinal cord tumors, as with brain tumors, can be primary or secondary, and are also further classified as intra- or extramedullary. Metastatic spinal tumors include hemangiosarcoma, adenocarcinoma, and osteosarcoma. Secondary tumors include meningioma, lymphoma, epithelioma, nerve sheath tumors, and multiple myeloma. The majority of all tumors occurred in the T3–L3 spinal cord segments (Pancotto, 2013). Most dogs are middle-aged to older at the onset of symptoms. Clinical signs reflect spinal cord dysfunction such as spinal hyperesthesia, proprioceptive and motor deficits, and compromised deep pain sensation. Figure 10.2 shows abnormal nail wearing in a patient with unilateral conscious proprioception deficits.

Cervical vertebral instability (wobblers) is a collection of abnormalities usually involving the caudal cervical vertebrae of middle-aged to older large-breed dogs. Although several large-breed dogs of any age can be affected, the adult to older Doberman is overrepresented, thereby suggesting a possibly genetic basis. These abnormalities may include stenosis of the cervical vertebral spinal canal, malformation of cervical vertebrae characterized by dorsal angulation of cranial endplates, the proliferation of excessive tissue around articular facets, hypertrophied ligamentum flavum and dorsal annulus fibrosis, degeneration and herniation of the intervertebral disk, and vertebral instability (Dewey, 2009).

MRI, CT, CT/myelography and myelography have all been used to evaluate and confirm a diagnosis of cervical vertebral instability. Survey cervical radiographs may show vertebral changes and may also serve to rule out other differential diagnoses such

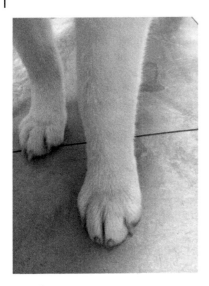

Figure 10.2 Worn nails in a patient with unilateral conscious proprioception deficits.

as diskospondylitis, vertebral fracture, and subluxation. Surgical intervention as early as possible in acute or severe cases leads to the best therapeutic results. Medical treatment is often used before and after surgery and for patients with less severe signs. Conservative management with anti-inflammatory drugs and neck splints may be palliative, but this condition is invariably progressive. Prednisone is often dosed at 1 mg/kg orally every 12–24 hours for three days then tapered to 0.25–0.5 mg/kg orally every 12–24 hours for another week, followed by continued reductions to find the lowest dose that controls clinical signs. Methocarbamol 10–20 mg/kg orally every 8 hours and diazepam 0.5–1.0 mg/kg orally every 8 hours may be used to decrease muscle spasms. Other palliative care for cervical vertebral instability includes the use of a harness instead of a collar, to avoid pulling on the cervical vertebrae and restricting excessive activity.

Degenerative myelopathy is a slowly progressive degeneration of the white matter of the spinal cord. In many dogs, it is caused by a mutation in the superoxide dismutase 1 (SOD1) gene (Awano *et al.*, 2009). Historically, the disease was reported most often in the German Shepherd. Research has centered on the disease in the Pembroke Welsh Corgi, and since the SOD1 mutation was identified, degenerative myelopathy has been confirmed in some other breeds. The disease usually affects older dogs (8–14 years). Pathologically, there is a loss of myelin and axons throughout the spinal cord (Shelton et al., 2009).

Clinical signs typically consist of a slowly progressive, non-painful T3–L3 myelopathy in a middle-aged to the older large-breed dog. Late in the disease process, urinary and fecal incontinence may develop. The disease can progress to involve the thoracic limbs and eventually the brain stem. Unfortunately, no treatment has been shown to reverse the signs.

Supportive therapy for degenerative myelopathy involves physical therapy to maintain muscle mass. Once a dog reaches a non-ambulatory state, nursing care must be instituted to prevent pressure sores and to deal with urinary and fecal incontinence. Long-term prognosis is grave. Larger breed dogs are often euthanized within 18 months of diagnosis, owing to the inability of owners to manage their paraplegia and urinary/fecal incontinence. Smaller breeds may be managed for longer periods of time when owners can provide supportive care that allows an acceptable quality of life.

Spondylosis deformans is a degenerative disorder of the vertebral column in which vertebral osteophytes develop at intervertebral spaces independently of an inflammatory of traumatic processes. The result is bony spurs or complete bony bridges on the ventral, lateral, and dorsolateral borders of the vertebral bodies. The thoracolumbar and lumbosacral junctions are affected more frequently, presumably from increased stress. Older, large-breed dogs are affected most often. This condition is usually a subclinical condition and is often an incidental finding in radiographs obtained for other reasons. Clinical signs typically have an insidious history from spurs of bone impinging on nerve roots or, rarely, compressing the spinal cord. Dogs may present with an acute history if a bone spur suddenly fractures.

Ataxia and paresis from cord compression are possible, and hyperesthesia is the most common clinical sign. Areas of localized discomfort may be identified with deep palpation of the epaxial musculature. At the lumbosacral junction, spondylosis deformans may be part of the wobbler syndrome. Treatment is medical or surgical. Dogs displaying hyperesthesia may be helped by analgesics or glucocorticosteroids. Decompressive surgery can improve signs of spinal cord or nerve root compression (Nelson and Couto, 2014).

Cauda equina syndrome is a collection of clinical signs that arise from compression of the cell bodies or nerve roots of the cauda equina. The compression usually affects the L7, sacral, and caudal nerve roots as they traverse through the lumbosacral area. Lumbosacral diseases most often occur in large-breed dogs such as the German Shepherd and the Labrador Retriever. Pathogenesis involves some degree of lumbosacral instability or stenosis. Clinical signs include pain on palpation dorsal to the lumbosacral area, fecal or urinary incontinence, and lower motor neuron signs in the pelvic limbs. Diagnosis of lumbosacral stenosis and other causes of cauda equine syndrome is based on signalment, history, clinical signs, orthopedic and neurological examinations, spinal radiographs, and specialized spinal imaging. Treatment involves surgical decompression or stabilization of the lumbosacral area. When surgical decompression is not chosen, rest and analgesic agents may be used with varying success.

Disorders of the Peripheral Nervous System

Peripheral nerves can become diseased or damaged anywhere along their pathway, from the cell body in the spinal cord or spinal ganglia, to the small nerve roots that emanate from the spinal cord, or to the lengthy peripheral nerves themselves. If the affected nerve innervates appendicular muscles, then dysfunction of the corresponding muscle occurs. Signs of motor involvement include weakness or paralysis of the muscle, rapid atrophy, and absence of reflex activity of the muscle (typical of lower motor neuron disease). Interruption of the sensory function of the nerve results in decreased sensation.

While there are a number of disease processes that can affect the peripheral nervous system, there are few that are seen primarily in older patients (Table 10.1). Laryngeal paralysis is discussed in Chapter 10.

Diabetes mellitus, hyperthyroidism, and hypothyroidism, hypoglycemia and hypoadrenocorticism have all been associated with peripheral neuropathies in older patients. Clinical signs are those of lower motor neuron dysfunction (muscle weakness, intermittent lameness, cranial nerve dysfunction). Diagnosis is based on clinical improvement when the underlying disease is treated.

Neoplasia affects the peripheral nervous system of geriatric cats and dogs. Nerve sheath tumors commonly involve the peripheral nerves of the thoracic limb in older dogs and less commonly, older cats. Lymphoma can involve nerve roots. Cranial nerves may be involved with hematogenous neoplasia (leukemias) due to direct involvement with the tumor cells. Paraneoplastic neuropathy is occasionally recognized.

Facial nerve paralysis is a condition that affects older animals and may be due to otitis media interna, trauma, hypothyroidism, neoplasia of the middle/inner ear or polyneuropathies. The most common cause of peripheral facial nerve paralysis has been reported to be idiopathic, although all possible causes of facial paralysis should be excluded before this specific diagnosis can be made. Recovery can take three to six weeks, if at all. While there is no specific treatment for facial nerve paralysis, the cornea should be adequately lubricated and monitored for evidence of ulceration (Nelson and Couto, 2009).

General Treatment of Neurologic Disorders

Because neurologic disease in the geriatric canine and feline veterinary patient can affect multiple locations, a multitude of symptoms can be observed. Specific diseases require specific treatments, but general treatment serves to provide pain management, reduce anxiety that may accompany mobility dysfunction, reduce the risk of complications such as decubital ulcers or urinary tract infections, and prevent further injury. Treatments should be directed at maintaining or improving a patient's quality of life and general wellbeing while focusing on maintaining the human–animal bond.

While many dogs and cars with neurologic disease experience pain, it may be challenging to recognize pain in all patients. Some neurologic conditions are not associated with pain, although complications that may arise, such as bed sores or urinary tract infections, can certainly cause discomfort and pain. A pain scoring system should be employed, and pet owners should be taught to observe their pet for symptoms of pain and to seek appropriate treatment if pain is suspected. Multimodal analgesia can better control pain. Additional pharmacological agents can be combined with alternative therapies.

If acute pain is left untreated, it can develop into neuropathic pain. Neuropathic pain is best described as a complex, chronic pain that develops following direct injury to the peripheral or central nervous system. Clinically, neuropathic pain is characterized by the presence of hyperpathia (increasing pain after repetitive stimulation; which includes continued pain after removal of the stimulus and radiating pain to adjacent anatomic areas), allodynia (painful response to a normally innocuous stimulus), and hyperalgesia (a painful response that is interpreted as occurring disproportionate to the initiating stimulus).

Analgesics that may be useful for neurologic pain include non-steroidal anti-inflammatory drugs (NSAIDS), opioids, and N-methyl-D-aspartate receptor antagonists

(NMDA), such as amantadine. NSAIDS are frequently used in the treatment of neurologic pain, although they may not be effective as a sole agent. Tramadol is a weak opioid agonist and norepinephrine and serotonin reuptake antagonist. It may be useful in combination with other analgesics for acute and chronic pain. The initial dose range starts at 2–5 mg/kg orally every 6–12 hours for dogs and 1–2 mg/kg every 12–24 hours for cats, and can be titrated upward as needed. Dysphoria is a common adverse effect in cats. Amantadine (3–6 mg/kg orally every 24 hours) may be beneficial in the treatment of neuropathic pain by dampening or "winding-down" central sensitization.

Acetaminophen and combination products containing acetaminophen and codeine can provide consistent analgesia in dogs with chronic neuropathic pain but must be avoided in cats. Although technically not a NSAID, acetaminophen may function by acting on the COX-3 cyclooxygenase enzyme in central nervous system tissues. Acetaminophen is dosed at 10 mg/kg orally twice daily, and the dose of combination acetaminophen/codeine product should be targeted to achieve 1–2 mg/kg of codeine orally twice daily (Rossmeisl, 2012).

Other classes of drugs may be enlisted to help provide multimodal pain control. Lidocaine dermal patches are frequently used in humans and show promise in dogs and cats. The low systemic concentrations achieved by transdermal lidocaine application suggest that efficacy is achieved via a block of peripheral rather than central nervous system sodium channels.

Tricyclic antidepressants such as amitriptyline, imipramine, fluoxetine, and clomipramine have been used. These drugs function through the variable and in some cases selective inhibition of the reuptake of monoamine neurotransmitters and thus facilitate endogenous descending analgesic mechanisms. Anticonvulsants such as gabapentin (5–10 mg/kg orally every 8–12 hours) and pregabalin may be useful. There is no current established dose for pregabalin. Short use of maropitant may be considered for neuropathic pain as it blocks substance P, a neurotransmitter of pain. Maropitant can be administered at a dose of 1 mg/kg orally every 24 hours for four days, then every other day. More studies are needed to evaluate the benefit of maropitant for neuropathic pain.

Sedation for patients is sometimes necessary to treat anxiety or keep a patient quiet. Anxitane® contains purified L-theanine, a natural amino acid found in green tea that has been clinically proven to reduce the clinical signs associated with fear and anxiety. Zylkene® (alpha casozepine), pheromones (Adaptil and Feliway) and lavender essential oils are natural compounds that may reduce anxiety. Benzodiazepines such as alprazolam are generally safe and can improve wellbeing, and doses at the higher end of the range have sedative effects. Benzodiazepines lacking active metabolites (lorazepam) are recommended for pets with compromised liver function. Gabapentin can also be used for its anxiolytic effects.

Diphenhydramine, phenobarbital, and trazodone can also promote sedation, and melatonin can be given 30 minutes before bedtime to help minimize nighttime waking (Matthews, 2010).

Complementary and alternative medicine for patients with neurologic disease can be used in combination with conventional medicine and may be of particular importance in geriatric patients. The integrative medicine approach can serve to improve the quality of life of the both the patient and the owner, alleviate pain, and provide a more holistic view of the veterinary patient.

Common complementary and alternative medicine modalities in the treatment of neurologic disease are acupuncture, chiropractic, therapeutic ultrasound and laser, and physical therapy, including massage, stretching, and swimming. Traditional Chinese medicine, nutraceuticals, vitamin and mineral supplements, essential fatty acid supplements, and antioxidants should also be considered.

Focus on the Client

Loss of neurologic function in any capacity can be extremely difficult for pets and owners alike. Whereas small declines or deficits may be well tolerated by the pet, pet owners may have difficulties with adjusting to the physical or behavioral changes with their pet. Most conditions that have a significant impact on neurologic function will require owners to provide some degree of nursing care. For example, a pet with facial nerve paralysis will require frequent eye lubrication application and may develop corneal ulcers. Patients with a loss of motor function may need assistance with mobility.

Patients with moderate to severe neurologic deficits will require time-consuming nursing care. It can be physically demanding to manage a large pet that has decreased mobility, or that is paralyzed. The caregivers must commit physically, emotionally, and financially.

When discussing expected progression and outcome of a pet's medical condition with owners, it can be helpful to focus on both the short-term and long-term expectations. It is also helpful to provide as many resources as possible for pet owners. Many online resources are available for owners of pets with a variety of neurologic conditions, including Walkin' Pets (http://www.handicappedpets.com), OrthoPets (http://www.orthopets.com), and DogLeggs (http://www.dogleggs.com).

It can be helpful to also provide owners with information regarding caregiver support and online or community groups of pet owners who are managing similar conditions with their pets.

Humane euthanasia should be considered when owners are unable to manage or maintain their pet's nursing care or when the pet's quality of life declines.

References

Adagra, C., and Foster, D. J. (2015) "Hyperammonaemia in Four Cats with Renal Azotaemia." *Journal of Feline Medicine and Surgery*, **17**: 168–72.

Awano, T., Johnson, G. S., Wade, C. M. (2009) "Genome-Wide Association Analysis Reveals a SOD1 Mutation in Canine Degenerative Myelopathy that Resembles Amyotrophic Lateral Sclerosis." *Proceedings of the National Academy of Science of the United States of America*, **106**: 2794–9.

Cuddon, P. A. (1996) "Metabolic Encephalopathies." *Veterinary Clinics of North America, Small Animal Practice*, **26**: 893–923.

Davies, M. (2012) "Geriatric Clinics in Practice." *Veterinary Focus*, **22**: 15–22.

Dewey, C. W. (2008). "Encephalopthies: Disorders of the Brain." In C. W. Dewey (ed.). *Practical Guide to Canine and Feline Neurology* (2nd ed.), pp. 115–220. Ames, IA: Blackwell Publishing.

Dimakopoulos, A. C., and Mayer, R. J. "Aspects of Neurodegeneration in the Canine Brain." *Journal of Nutrition*, **132**(6 Suppl 2): 1579–82S.

Gonzalez-Freire, M., de Cabo, R., Studenski, S. A., Ferrucci, L. (2014) "The Neuromuscular Junction: Aging at the Crossroad between Nerves and Muscle." *Frontiers in Aging Neuroscience*, **6**: 208.

Hoskins, J. (2004) *Geriatrics and Gerontology of the Dog and Cat* (2nd ed.). St Louis, MO: Saunders.

Matthews, K. A. (2010) "Neuropathic Pain: How to Prevent and Treat." Presented at the International Veterinary Emergency and Critical Care Symposium 2010.

Nelson, R. W., and Couto, C. G. (2014) *Small Animal Internal Medicine* (5th. ed.). St Louis, MO: Elsevier.

Pancotto, T. E., Rossmeisl, J. H., Zimmerman, K., Robertson, J. L., Werre, S. R. (2013) "Intramedullary Spinal Cord Neoplasia in 53 Dogs (1990–2010): Distribution, Clinicopathologic Characteristics, and Clinical Behavior." *Journal of Veterinary Internal Medicine*, **27**: 1500–8.

Rossmeisl, J. H. (2012) "Neuropathic Pain-Modifying Agent." 84th Annual Western Veterinary Conference Notes Online, February 19–23, 2012. Las Vegas, NV.

Shelton, G. D., Snead, E., Kozlowski, M. (2012) "An SOD1 Mutation Associated with Degenerative Myelopathy Occurs in Many Dog Breeds." *Journal of the Neurological Sciences*, **318**: 55–64.

Shull, E.A. (2002) "Neurologic Disorders in Aged Dogs." *Veterinary Medicine*, **97**: 17–19.

11

The Aging Kidney
Shea Cox

Introduction

The scope of geriatric nephrology includes normal age-related renal changes, the clinical consequences of such changes, and the renal diseases that can occur as a result of these changes. Direct evidence and models that study renal aging in healthy animals, however, is lacking; we have an understanding of kidney function and how disease can affect it, but a very limited understanding of what happens to the canine and feline kidney as it ages. Because of this, information regarding specific age-related changes is often inferred from human studies. Despite these limitations, it is suggested that age-related decline in renal function may occur similarly in dogs and cats as it does in humans (Syme, 2010). To understand the renal-related disease processes that can occur in a geriatric pet, one must first understand the general physiology behind the aging kidney, and information must be procured from both human and veterinary resources.

Aging at the Glomerular Level

Glomeruli are the functional units in the kidney that filter urine from the blood, and as the kidney ages, glomerulosclerosis can occur. In human studies, age-related glomerulosclerosis occurs when the glomeruli are replaced by fibrous tissue, which in turn causes a decrease in glomerular filtration rate (GFR) and the effective renal plasma flow.

Glomerular hypertension can develop as a result of these progressive changes. There is an increase in single-nephron GFR required to maintain total GFR. This occurs because of reduced glomerular arteriolar resistance following vasodilation of the afferent arteriole. As renal mass decreases, surviving nephrons cannot autoregulate, and systemic arterial pressure is transmitted to the glomerulus resulting in glomerular hypertension and hyperfiltration, the net effect being increased GFR. Over time, glomerular hypertrophy develops and results in loss of filtration barrier integrity (via podocyte damage), proteinuria, glomerulosclerosis and ultimately, reduced GFR (Korman, 2014).

In one animal study, the GFR was found to not vary with age in dogs, except possibly in the very small breeds. Similarly, GFR was not correlated with age in a study performed in cats (Syme, 2010). In another study in the adult dog, aging seemed to have a limited effect as shown in both longitudinal and cross-sectional studies. In the cat, plasma clearance of creatinine, but not iohexol, was about 25% lower in 9–12-year-old cats compared with 7–12-month-old cats. In another study involving 51 cats, no correlation between plasma clearance of iohexol or creatinine and age was evidenced (Lefebvre, 2010). Although a decline in renal function with aging seems limited in healthy dogs and cats, the potential clinical relevance of a GFR decrease in the aged animal needs further study.

In small animal medicine, GFR is usually estimated on the basis of assessment of plasma/serum creatinine concentrations. However, this approach may be flawed in aged patients since creatinine production is directly related to muscle mass. It has been shown that both dogs and cats have a reduction in lean body mass with advancing age, and because of this, creatinine concentrations may decrease, resulting in the underdiagnosis of chronic kidney disease in geriatric patients (Syme, 2010).

Aging at the Renovascular Level

Human studies reveal that arterioles in the renal vasculature show subendothelial deposition of hyaline and collagen fibers that produce intimal thickening. In the small arteries, the intima is thickened due to proliferation of the elastic tissue, showing atrophy. Another characteristic of the aging kidney is the formation of aglomerular circulation (the formation of a direct channel between afferent and efferent arterioles) and dysfunction of the autonomic vascular reflex (Musso *et al.*, 2007). Studies show that there are several consequences of renal vascular changes, which can include:

- renovascular atherosclerosis, which can lead to renovascular hypertension, ischemic nephropathy, and chronic kidney disease (Cameron, 1995)
- intrarenal atheroembolism, which can occur when plaque material breaks free from the diseased renal artery and enters the renal circulation; the kidney rarely recovers from this acute insult (Cameron, 1995)
- renal dysautonomia, which can lead to kidney damage during hypotensive and/or hypertensive states (Musso, 2002).

Aging at the Tubular–Interstitial level

Renal tubules undergo fatty degeneration and irregular thickening of their basal membrane. In response, diverticula arise from the distal and convoluted tubules, and in the human geriatric patient it has been suggested that these may serve as reservoirs for recurrent urinary tract infections. In addition, the aged kidney in humans also shows increasing zones of tubular atrophy and fibrosis (Silva, 2005).

In animals, tubulointerstitial fibrosis is the most common lesion occurring early in the course of chronic kidney disease. Sustained glomerular injury causes glomerular hypertension, increased single-nephron GFR, glomerular hypertrophy and proteinuria.

Proteinuria is accompanied by cytokine production (for example, transforming growth factor-β1), initiating renal fibrogenesis. Activated fibroblasts then produce matrix components such as collagen, which disrupt surviving tubules. Chronic hypoxia also occurs, contributing to continuing inflammation (Korman, 2014). The physiological and clinical consequences of these changes in the aging renal tubules can be summarized in three groups: tubular dysfunction, medullary hypotonicity, and tubular frailty.

Tubular Dysfunction

In healthy geriatric patients, tubular handling of many substances becomes modified.

Sodium

Although the proximal nephron behaves similarly in both the young and old, reabsorption of sodium is reduced in the ascending loop of Henle with age in human studies. This phenomenon has two important consequences: first, the amount of sodium loss is increased; and second, the capacity of the medullar interstitium to concentrate is also diminished (medullary hypotonicity). Thus, geriatric patients exhibit both an increased sodium excretion and an inability to maximally concentrate the urine (water saving). The basal plasma concentrations of renin and aldosterone and the response to their stimuli are also diminished in old age, which is another mechanism for enhanced sodium loss. It should be noted, however, that despite exaggerated natriuresis, total body sodium is generally not significantly decreased with age (Alvarez Gregori *et al.*, 2009; Fish *et al.*, 1994).

Potassium

It has been shown that in healthy aged people, total body potassium content is lower than it is in the young, and the correlation with age is linear. This phenomenon is explained in part by reduced muscle mass, which is the main potassium stores in the body. Additionally, renal excretion of potassium is significantly lower in the geriatric population, and despite having a lower total body content of potassium, there remains a predisposition for geriatric patients to develop hyperkalemia. This trend can be explained by reduced serum aldosterone and reduced tubular response to this hormone. Studies have also shown that there is an increase in the activity of the hydrogen potassium ATPase pump (potassium reabsorption) in the intercalated cells of the aged collecting ducts in rats (Andreucci *et al.*, 1996), which may further explain this finding.

Urea, Creatinine and Uric Acid

In the geriatric population, fractional excretion of urea is increased and this phenomenon is thought to be due to a reduced distal urea reabsorption secondary to diminished urea channels. With regards to the handling of creatinine, it has been shown in human studies that the net creatinine tubular reabsorption is similar in both the young and old populations. The level of serum uric acid and its urinary fractional excretion are also similar in the young and the old (Musso *et al.*, 2009).

Calcium, Phosphate, and Magnesium

Serum calcium, phosphorus, and magnesium levels and their urinary fractional excretion are similar in the healthy young and old. However, even though the renal handling of calcium, phosphate and magnesium are not altered in the elderly, a lower intestinal absorption can easily lead to hypocalcaemia, hypophosphatemia, and hypomagnesaemia (Musso *et al.*, 2009).

Erythropoietin

Erythropoietin is produced mainly by the peritubular interstitial cells near the proximal convoluted tubules, and production does not appear to be affected by age. Plasma levels are found to be normal in the *healthy* geriatric population and the normal aging process does not explain the presence of anemia (Musso *et al.*, 2004).

Medulla Hypotonicity (Water Handling)

Total body water diminishes with age. In people, water comprises 65% of total body weight in the young population, whereas it comprises only 54% in the elderly population. Since the reduction in senile water content takes place in the intracellular compartment, hypovolemia always represents a pathological state in the geriatric population.

Senescence reduces the capacity of the kidney to concentrate the urine. This phenomenon can be explained by aglomerular circulation, the defect in sodium reabsorption in the ascending limb of the loop of Henle and the reduced distal urea reabsorption. Another mechanism for the impairment of the urine concentration ability is the decrease in responsiveness of tubular epithelium of the collecting tubules to antidiuretic hormone. Finally, concentration of angiotensin is lower in the geriatric population (Sands, 2008).

Tubular Frailty

Tubular cells are frail in the aged kidney, and because of this, progression to acute tubular necrosis and acute kidney injury can easily occur, with recovery from insult slow. If the kidney does not recover after approximately three months, it remains as chronic kidney disease (Musso, 2002).

Diseases of the Aged Kidney

A summary of the common diseases that geriatric patients may experience is outlined below.

Glomerulonephritis

Glomerular disease is an important cause of chronic renal failure in human patients and has been increasingly recognized in veterinary medicine in recent years (Figure 11.1). Most animals with glomerular disease are middle-aged or older at presentation. Animals with glomerular disease may present in one of six possible ways (DiBartola, 2012):

1) Signs may be related to the presence of chronic renal failure if more than 75% of the nephron population has become non-functional (most common).
2) Signs may be related to an underlying infectious, inflammatory or neoplastic disease.

Figure 11.1 Sunny, with glomerulonephritis.

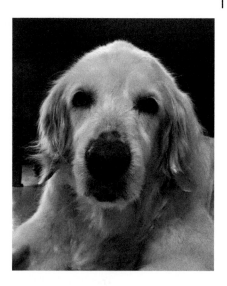

3) Proteinuria may be an incidental finding detected during diagnostic evaluation of another medical problem.
4) Signs may be related to classical nephrotic syndrome (e.g., ascites, subcutaneous edema).
5) Signs may be related to thromboembolism (such as sudden onset of dyspnea with pulmonary thromboembolism, sudden onset of paraparesis with iliac or femoral artery embolism).
6) Sudden blindness may occur due to retinal detachment resulting from systemic hypertension.

Glomerulonephritis is an important cause of chronic renal failure in dogs (common) and cats (less common), and is characterized by morphologic and functional abnormalities in the glomeruli. Glomerulonephritis is usually caused by the presence of immune complexes in the glomerulus. These complexes initiate damage characterized by glomerular cell proliferation, thickening of capillary walls, hyalinization, and glomerulosclerosis. There are many different disease processes associated with immune complex formation and subsequent development of glomerulonephritis. In most cases, however, the antigen source or underlying disease process is not identified and the glomerular disease is referred to as idiopathic (DiBartola, 2012). See Table 11.1 for a summary of age-related diseases that are associated with glomerulonephritis.

Non-immunologic glomerular insult can also occur. This is generally the result of hemodynamically mediated injury from hyperperfusion (systemic hypertension or glomerular hyperfiltration due to various causes) or hypoperfusion. Secondary disease involving the renal tubules/interstitium can also occur as the disease progresses (Yaphe, 2004).

The mean age for the development of glomerulonephritis in dogs is seven years, while the mean age in cats is four years. Most glomerular diseases will eventually progress and involve the renal interstitium, resulting in the development of chronic renal failure (Yaphe, 2004). Glomerulonephritis has a variable course and a poor prognosis

Table 11.1 Age-related diseases associated with glomerulonephritis (Langston et al., 2008).

Type	Dog	Cat
Infectious	Bacterial endocarditis	Feline leukemia virus
	Pyometra	Feline infectious peritonitis
	Chronic bacterial infections	Feline immunodeficiency virus
	Septicemia	
Inflammatory	Pancreatitis	Pancreatitis
	Polyarthritis	Immune-mediated diseases
	Prostatitis	Chronic skin diseases
Neoplasia	Hemangiosarcoma	Leukemia
	Hepatocellular carcinoma	Lymphoma
	Leukemia	
	Mastocytosis	
	Lymphoma	
	Transitional cell carcinoma	
	Bronchogenic adenocarcinoma	
Other	Idiopathic	Idiopathic
	Hyperadrenocorticism	Familial diseases
	Long-term steroid therapy?	Vascular insults
	Vascular insults	Non-immunologic hyperfiltration?
	Non-immunologic hyperfiltration?	Diabetes mellitus
	Diabetes mellitus	

should not be given unless there is evidence of progression to chronic renal failure. Various outcomes may occur in dogs and cats with glomerulonephritis: spontaneous remission, stable course with ongoing proteinuria for several months to years, or progression to chronic renal failure over months to years (DiBartola, 2012).

Urinary Tract Infection/Pyelonephritis

Urinary tract infections and pyelonephritis can be common in the geriatric population. The incidence of bacteriuria has been shown to increase with advancing age because of changes in anatomy (such as vaginal and urethral atrophy), changes to mucosal defense barriers, changes to composition of urine, and changes in frequency or amount of voiding (Nicolle, 2008). The incidence of pyelonephritis is unknown in companion animals, but is thought to be a common cause of acute renal failure and the deterioration of more stable chronic renal disease (Goldstein, 2015).

It is not uncommon for geriatric patients to experience comorbidities that further predispose them to infection. These can include urinary and/or fecal incontinence, decreased frequency of urination or an inability to completely empty the bladder during voiding (for example, secondary to underlying mobility issues), increased urinary glucose (for example, diabetes mellitus), cancer, decreased immunity and low urine osmolality secondary to chronic kidney disease. With regards to urinary tract infections in patients with underlying chronic kidney disease, the increase in occurrence is likely caused by ascending infections that become more easily established due to dilute urine providing a more favorable medium in which contaminant bacteria can more easily survive and multiply.

Geriatric patients should be closely monitored for the development of urinary tract infections. Bacterial infections can increase the risk for the development of ascending pyelonephritis, which can cause further and significant deterioration in renal function (Cannon, 2014). Untreated infections can also lead to lower urinary tract dysfunction, prostatitis, urolithiasis, sepsis, pyelonephritis, and scarring.

Acute Kidney Injury

Acute kidney injury, previously known as acute renal failure, is a sudden and severe decrease in renal function. The use of the word "injury" over "failure" helps to imply the potential of reversibility and recovery, which is not indicated by the term "failure".

Acute kidney injury may be caused by a variety of insults, resulting in marked reduction in glomerular filtration rate, tubular function and urine production. Overall, this results in failure of waste product excretion and fluid, electrolyte and acid-base balance (Korman, 2014). The most common causes in the geriatric population include:

- pre-renal causes: dehydration (main-cause), hypotension, hypovolemic shock, hemorrhage
- renal causes: acute tubular necrosis due to the persistence of pre-renal causes, nephrotoxins (such as aminoglycosides, non-steroidal anti-inflammatory drugs), damage due to primary or secondary glomerular disease, acute interstitial nephritis, infectious diseases, ischemic causes/thrombosis
- post-renal (obstructive) causes: including calculi, tumor, stricture, prostatic hypertrophy.

Development of acute kidney injury occurs through a series of steps that include initiation, extension, maintenance, and recovery. The initiation phase occurs with exposure to the toxin or the ischemic event. Extension occurs during the response to injury and the subsequent renal damage that exacerbates the response to the initial insult. The maintenance phase consists of established tubular lesions and nephron dysfunction. The recovery phase occurs with nephron repair and return to function, with compensatory hypertrophy of the remaining functional nephrons. In general, renal recovery occurs over 6–8 weeks following establishment of renal failure (Kerl, 2015).

The cause is often multifactorial, and its incidence can be higher in the geriatric population due to the presence of comorbidities (such as diabetes mellitus), use of polypharmacy, or because of the renal aging process itself. However, age *per se* is not an important determinant of survival in patients with acute kidney injury. Because acute injury may progress to a chronic condition, an acute injury from any cause can lead to chronic kidney disease.

Recognizing the possibility of renal injury and administering appropriate therapy during the initiation phase help prevents the establishment of renal failure and/or lessens the severity of injury. Many causes of injury are reversible if diagnosis is made early and if treatment is initiated in a timely manner.

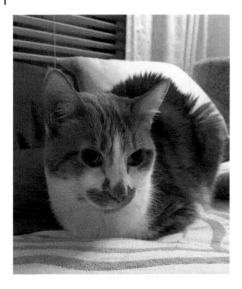

Figure 11.2 Renal failure in a cat, Mr Barney.

Chronic Kidney Disease

Chronic kidney disease is an important clinical problem in both dogs and cats, and is encountered most frequently in geriatric patients (Figure 11.2). It is a syndrome that is characterized by progressive and generally irreversible deterioration of renal function, owing to the reduction of the nephron mass. It is reported that kidney disease is approximately three times as common in the cat as it is in the dog, and is most often seen in elderly patients. In one study, the average age of cats with chronic kidney disease without reported clinical signs was 8.3 ± 1.5 years, and with clinical signs, 14.4 ± 0.7 years; in feline patients with end-stage renal disease, the average age was 12.5 ± 0.9 years. In a study of 38 dogs with chronic kidney disease, the average age for disease development was 8.0 ± 4.2 years (Syme, 2010).

Known causes of chronic kidney disease are many, and the most common age-related etiologies are summarized in Table 11.2.

Kidney diseases can be broadly divided into two main histological types: glomerular disease and tubulointerstitial disease. Glomerular disease is more frequently encountered in younger animals (although it is still prevalent in older populations), while tubulointerstitial disease seems to increase in prevalence in older patients (Syme, 2010). It should be noted that the glomerular, tubulointerstitial, and vascular lesions found in animals with generalized chronic kidney disease are often similar, regardless of the initiating cause, and renal histology generally only reveals marked interstitial fibrosis. Interstitial fibrosis is often referred to as chronic interstitial nephritis or tubulointerstitial fibrosis, and these terms describe the morphologic appearance of kidneys with end-stage chronic disease of any cause (Brown, 2016).

Renal Neoplasia

The incidence of neoplasia can increase as a pet ages. With regards to the kidney, 90% of renal tumors are malignant, and metastatic tumors are far more common than primary tumors (likely due to significant perfusion of kidneys). The mean age of dogs with primary malignant renal neoplasms is seven to nine years, and there is an increased

Table 11.2 Common age-related causes of chronic kidney disease.

Compartment	Cause
Microvascular	Systemic and glomerular hypertension
	Glomerulonephritis
Macrovascular	Systemic hypertension
	Chronic hypoperfusion
Interstitial	Pyelonephritis
	Progressive interstitial fibrosis
	Neoplasia
	Obstructive uropathy
Tubular	Tubular reabsorptive defects
	Chronic low-grade nephrotoxicity
	Obstructive uropathy

incidence in males. Dogs with renal neoplasia often do not present with signs referable to the urinary tract, but rather present with vague signs of systemic illness such anorexia, weight loss, fever, or vomiting. Lameness may occur in some cases, due to hypertrophic osteopathy, and less often, signs referable to the urinary tract (such as hematuria). The most common primary malignant renal neoplasm in the dog is renal cell carcinoma, which generally occurs unilaterally, and accounts for 69% of primary renal neoplasms. This tumor is highly malignant and often metastasizes to the lungs, lymph nodes, liver, brain or bone.

In cats, renal lymphoma is the most common renal neoplasia, and it is reported in 16% of felines with chronic kidney disease. Unlike the presentation in dogs, 60% of cats with renal lymphoma present with signs referable to the urinary tract, including azotemia and bilateral renomegaly (Korman, 2014). About 50% of affected cats are positive for feline leukemia virus, and there can be central nervous system involvement in about 40% of this population (Polzin, 2010).

Monitoring the Health of the Kidney

Early detection and appropriate intervention is key in maintaining the health of the kidney in the geriatric pet; thus, serial evaluation of a patient's chemistry profile, complete blood cell count, urinalysis, and blood pressure are recommended for assessing and monitoring the health of the kidney. Abdominal ultrasound is of additional benefit, allowing assessment of the architecture of the kidney and its associated structures.

Therapies

Therapies are directed at slowing the primary disease process affecting the kidneys and at controlling factors influencing progression, including dehydration, systemic hypertension, proteinuria, infection, activation of the renin-angiotension-aldosterone system, hyperparathyroidism, hypoxia, anemia and oxidative stress. Specific therapies that ameliorate the clinical signs of disease should also be implemented. These include the management of nausea, vomiting, inappetance, dehydration, and discomfort.

Special Considerations in the Aging Kidney

Medication

Many pharmacokinetic parameters are affected by the natural aging process of the kidney. These include the amount of drug that reaches the systemic circulation (and therefore the amount at the site of action, or bioavailability), the distribution size of the drug (volume of distribution), its renal excretion (GFR), and the length of time needed to reach steady-state serum concentration or to eliminate the drug. Owing to these pharmacokinetic changes, the geriatric population is predisposed to drug toxicity, and treatment should take into account these factors (Bennet, 2008). Drug dosages need to be altered appropriately in animals with hypoalbuminemia or decreased GFR, such as with glomerulonephritis, as these changes can influence both drug binding and clearance.

Diet

Dietary protein restriction helps to delay the onset of uremia in the aging kidney, and has been shown to extend survival in dogs and cats with chronic kidney disease stages 2–4. In addition to reduced protein, other important components of a renal diet should include a reduced phosphorus, sodium and net acid content while supplementing with omega-3 fatty acids and antioxidants. Free access to fresh water at all times is imperative.

Although initially counterintuitive, patients with glomerulonephritis should be fed a moderately protein-restricted diet. Studies in people with protein losing nephropathies have shown that feeding a high protein diet is associated with increased mortality. Patients fed a low protein diet and lived longer and suffered lower morbidity. The reason for this paradox is unclear but is likely due to the increased loss of protein into the tubule (Acierno, 2014).

How an Aging Kidney Affects Life for the Pet

The chronic changes that occur within the normal aging kidney in the healthy pet are not considered painful, nor do they generally interfere with overall quality of life. However, if complicating factors develop, such as urinary tract infections or renal failure, a different clinical picture can emerge and directly affect quality of life. Infection of the urinary tract can cause discomfort and therefore directly affect patient quality of life. In addition to antibiotic therapy, appropriate pain management needs to be considered in order to maintain optimal patient comfort.

If glomerular or chronic kidney disease develops, the full clinical picture of uremia will eventually emerge, and will ultimately affect the quality of life for the pet. Early signs of compromise include loss of appetite or anorexia, with the appearance of nausea or vomiting. As disease progresses, other systems will become more dramatically affected. With regards to the musculoskeletal system, cachexia and weakness can develop. Within the cardiorespiratory system, hypertension, heart failure, pulmonary edema, coronary disease, and arrhythmia may be seen. Neurologically, the patient may develop polyneuropathy, seizures and the potential for uremic coma in the advanced stage of the disease. Secondary hyperparathyroidism is a potential endocrinological abnormality. Impaired cellular immunity, clotting alterations and anemia can also be present. Each of these comorbidities can contribute to a decreased quality of life, depending upon the severity of signs experienced and the stage of disease.

How an Aging Kidney Affects Life for the Owner

Management of a chronic disease, with its inherent waxing and waning periods of clinical improvement and decline, can be an emotionally, physically, and financially challenging course for families to navigate (Figure 11.3). The development of chronic kidney disease in an aging pet can be an exacting disease to regulate, and meeting the demands of care may ultimately affect owner quality of life far more intensely than the pet's quality of life. Because of this, the considerations in Table 11.3 should be explored when developing a plan of care.

Figure 11.3 Quality of life.

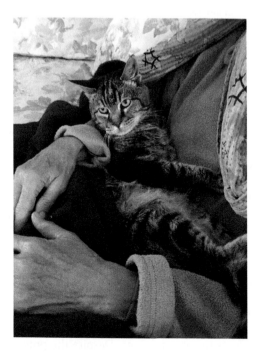

Table 11.3 Considerations around the development of chronic kidney disease in an aging pet.

Considerations	Questions for the client
Delivery of care	How easy is your pet to medicate?
	Would medication delivery cause any distress to you or your pet?
	Would you be comfortable with delivering (potentially) daily subcutaneous fluid therapy? Would administration cause any distress to you or your pet?
	Do you feel that diagnostics are stressful for your pet? Does this cause you distress?
	If your pet will not be amendable to a prescription renal diet, would home cooking be a realistic alternative for you to consider?
Owner lifestyle and work schedule	Is your current lifestyle and/or work schedule amendable to delivering the level of care needed? (Such considerations include free access outdoors for increased frequency of urination due to polyuria/polydipsia.)
	What are your current thoughts and feelings about experiencing the emotional roller coaster with the potential for ups/down throughout progression of disease?
	What do you want for your pet? What don't you want?
	What do you want yourself and your family? What don't you want?
	Do you have help in care? Do you need help in care?
	Do you have any limitations or challenges with regards to providing care? (physical/emotional/time)?
Anticipated costs of care when managing a potentially long-term disease	Considerations around the cost of medications and prescription diets.
	Considerations regarding the cost and frequency of diagnostics.
	Considerations around the potential need for hospitalization if a severe acute on chronic crisis develops.
	Considerations with regard to managing and monitoring secondary complications of disease, such as the development of hypertension.

End of Life Considerations

If a pet develops chronic kidney disease, it will continue to progress and will eventually be terminal, and the decision for euthanasia versus allowing for a hospice-supported natural death will ultimately need to be made. In addition to worsening metabolic derangements, outward physical changes will begin to occur and progress. Box 11.1 gives signs and symptoms that may indicate that a pet is nearing the end stage of renal disease, and may help guide families when making end of life decisions.

Conclusion

Age-related renal changes affect many geriatric patients. Further research is needed in the field of veterinary nephrology in order to increase our limited understanding of its effects in cats and dogs. Despite the potential for development of disease associated

---

Box 11.1 Signs and Symptoms which may Indicate that a Pet is Nearing the End Stage of Renal Disease

- Change in behavior, such as a progressive loss of daily happiness, or an increase in withdrawing or hiding behaviors.
- A continued dull expression or "lack of brightness" in the eyes.
- Progressive and continued lack of appetite and/or water consumption.
- Nausea and/or vomiting that cannot be adequately managed despite therapies.
- Progression of dehydration, despite therapies, which can be reflected by dull, sunken eyes; reduced urination; poor skin turgor.
- Generalized weakness that progresses to a change in gait or inability to walk.
- Change in breath or body odor from a uremic state.
- Development of oral ulcers, which is due to increasing gastrin due to reduced renal clearance.
- Development of pruritus; uremic pruritus is described in human medicine, and it is a symptom that develops in patients with end-stage renal disease as a result of the excessive uremia. It is thought to be a combination of factors, including dry skin, abnormal metabolism of calcium and phosphorus/raised parathyroid hormone, accumulating of toxins, sprouting of new nerves, systemic inflammation and additional comorbidities.
- Progressive hypothermia; in cases of renal failure, hypothermia is usually directly related to anemia; the reduction in red blood cells reduces the amount of oxygen being delivered to the tissues and organs, and as a result, glucose cannot be oxidized to produce; dehydration and decreased circulation also contributes to hypothermia.
- Reduced blink response; patients are often found to begin to "sleep with their eyes open" when they are nearing death.
- Mental confusion or difficulty rousing, owing to a continued build up of toxins in the blood.
- Restlessness.
- Twitching that may progress to seizure activity, owing to electrolyte abnormalities or potentially hypertension.

---

with these changes, a good quality of life can often be maintained for both pet and family with appropriate management and care.

References

Acierno, M. (2014) "Proetin Losing Nephropathy – The Latest Treatment Recommendations." Presented at Atlantic Coast Veterinary Conference, 2014. Baton Rouge, LA.

Alvarez Gregori, J., Musso, C., Macías Nuñez, J. F. (2009) "Renal Ageing." In J. Sastre, R. Pamolona, J. Ramón (eds), *Medical Biogerontology*, pp. 111–23. Madrid: Ergon.

Andreucci, V., Russo, D., Cianciaruso, B., Andreucci, M. (1996) "Some Sodium, Potassium and Water Changes in the Elderly and their Treatment." *Nephrology Dialysis Transplantation*, **11**(Suppl 9): 9–17.

Bennet, W. (2008) "Geriatric Renal Pharmacology: Practical Considerations." In E. Friedman, D. Oreopoulos, J. Sands (eds), *Geriatric Nephrology: An Epidemiologic and Clinical Challenge*, pp. 205–13. Postgraduate Education Course of the American Society of Nephrology.

Brown, S. A. (2016) "Renal Dysfunction in Small Animals." Merck Veterinary Manual, Available at http://www.merckvetmanual.com/urinary-system/noninfectious-diseases-of-the-urinary-system-in-small-animals/renal-dysfunction-in-small-animals.

Cameron, J. S. (1995) "Renal Disease in the Elderly: Particular Problems." In G. D'Amico, and G. Colasanti (eds), *Issues in Nephrosciences*, pp. 111–17. Milan: Wichting.

Cannon, M. (2014) "Chronic Kidney Disease – Why All the Fuss About Proteinuria?" Presented at International Society of Feline Medicine Asia Pacific Conference, 2014.

DiBartola, S. (2012) "Glomerular Disease." In Conference Proceedings, Atlantic Coast Veterinary Conference, February 19–23 2012, Las Vegas, NV.

Polzin, D. J. (2010) "Chronic Kidney disease." In Ettinger, S., and Feldman, E. *Textbook of Veterinary Internal Medicine: Disease f the Dog and Cat, Volume* **2**, pp. 1990–2020. St Louis, MO: Elsevier Saunders.

Fish, L. C., Murphy, D. J., Elahi, D., Minaker, K. L. (1994) "Renal Sodium Excretion in Normal Aging: Decreased Excretion Rates Lead to Delayed Sodium Excretion in Normal Aging." *Geriatric Nephrology and Urology*, **4**: 145–51.

Goldstein, R. (2015) "Canine and Feline Urinary Tract Infections and Pyelonephritis." Preseanted at Pacific Veterinary Conference, June 18–21, 2015, Long Beach, NY.

Kerl M. (2015) Recognizing and Managing Acute Kidney Injury. Presented at ACVIM Forum 2015, June 3–6, Indiana Convention Center.

Korman, R. (2014) "Chronic Kidney Disease – Aetiology, Diagnosis and Staging." Presented at International Society of Feline Medicine Asia Pacific Congress, 2014.

Lefebvre, H. (2010) "Glomerular Filtration Rate in Dogs and Cats: Where are we Now?" ACVIM 2010. Toulous, France.

Musso, C. G. (2002) "Geriatric Nephrology and the 'Nephrogeriatric Giants'." *International Urology and Nephrology*, **34**: 255–6.

Musso, C. G., Musso, C. A., Joseph, H., De Miguel, R., Rendo, P., Gonzalez, E., *et al.* (2004) "Plasma Erythropoietin Levels in the Oldest Old." *International Urology and Nephrology*, **36**: 259–62.

Musso CG, Macıas Núñez JF. "Feedback Between Geriatric Syndromes: General System Theory in Geriatrics." *International Urology and Nephrology*, 2006;**38**: 785–6; 34:255-6.

Musso, C. G., Macías Núñez, J. F., Oreopoulos, D. G. (2007) "Physiological Similarities and Differences Between Renal Aging and Chronic Renal Disease." *Journal of Nephrology*, **20**: 586–7.

Musso, C. G., Michelángelo, H., Vilas, M., Reynaldi, J., Martinez, B., Algranati, L., Macías Núñez, J. F. (2009) "Creatinine Reabsorption by the Aged Kidney." *International Urology and Nephrology*, **41**: 727–31.

Nicolle, L. (2008) "Urinary Infection in the Elderly. When Does it Matter?" In E. Friedman, D. Oreopoulos, J. Sands (eds), *Geriatric Nephrology: An Epidemiologic and Clinical Challenge*, pp. 249–60. Postgraduate Education Course of the American Society of Nephrology.

Sands, J. (2008) "Changes in Urine Concentrating Ability in the Aging Kidney." In E. Friedman, D. Oreopoulos, J. Sands (eds), *Geriatric Nephrology: An Epidemiologic and Clinical Challenge*, pp. 85–94. Postgraduate Education Course of the American Society of Nephrology.

Silva, F. G. (2005) "The Ageing Kidney: A Review – Part I." *International Urology and Nephrology*, **37**: 185–205.

Syme, H. (2010) "The Aging Kidney." In *British Small Animal Veterinary Association Congress*. Quedgley, UK: BSAVA.

Yaphe, W. (2004) Small Animal Medicine Course. Lecture 8 and 9: Glomerulonephritis and Amyloidosis. vin.com.

12

The Hepatic System

Laura Devlin Bacon

The liver is the largest internal organ and performs many essential functions related to digestion, metabolism, immunity and the storage of nutrients within the body. Specifically, the liver is responsible for the manufacture of proteins, bile and cholesterol; metabolism of fats and carbohydrates; storage of substances such as fats and iron; breakdown of toxins, drugs and other metabolites; integrity of the immune system; and for contributing to the maintenance of a steady glucose concentration. The gall bladder is closely associated with the liver, and functions to store bile produced by the liver, and as needed, secrete it into the intestine to aid in the digestion of food. The blood supply of the liver is unique among all organs of the body, owing to the hepatic portal vein system. The liver also has an incredible ability to regenerate dead or damaged tissues and has an enormous reserve capacity, with liver failure occurring only when two-thirds of the function is lost.

Like other organ systems, there are age-dependent changes of the liver. Liver size and weight decrease with age. Both liver blood flow and microsomal enzyme activity are decreased, and there is a decline in regeneration rate and detoxification (Schmucker, 2005). There are also many aging changes present at a cellular level. Cytological changes in the liver in older dogs include significantly greater hepatocyte cell sizes, a decreased nuclear: cytoplasm ratio, increased frequency of neutrophils and increased number of nuclei per cell. The larger cell size and an increase in the number of nuclei could be associated with nodular hyperplasia, which is known to increase with age. Cytoplasmic volume increases as nuclear size remains constant. Additionally, the higher frequency of neutrophils is a change seen in both young and older dogs, as compared with middle-aged dogs, and may reflect a response to nonspecific reactive hepatitis (Stockhaus *et al.*, 2002). Older dogs and cats are at greater risk for the development of liver disease. This is most likely owing to the decline in weight, blood flow, regeneration rate and detoxification of the liver. These same changes have been related to an increased risk of liver abnormalities in elderly people (Schmucker, 2005).

Patients with liver disease can present with a variety of clinical signs, none of which is pathognomonic for liver disease. Patients often have non-specific signs of lethargy, decreased appetite, anorexia, weight loss, polyuria and polydipsia, and intermittent vomiting and diarrhea. More specific signs of liver disease are icterus, ascites with a low

Treatment and Care of the Geriatric Veterinary Patient, First Edition. Edited by Mary Gardner and Dani McVety.
© 2017 John Wiley & Sons, Inc. Published 2017 by John Wiley & Sons, Inc.
Companion Website: www.wiley.com/go/gardner/geriatric

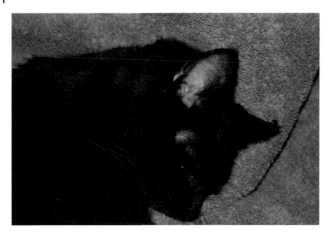

Figure 12.1 Patient whose only sign of liver disease was icterus on the ear pinnae.

protein level, encephalopathy, and coagulopathies. Patients may present with a chronic history while others have an acute history. Most patients will show signs of clinical disease when more that 80% of the liver has been affected. However, some animals with liver disease will not show any clinical signs (Figure 12.1).

Diagnosis of hepatic disease can pose difficulties for the clinician. The presence of liver disease can be detected with physical examination and laboratory screening tests. Subsequent testing may include a liver function test, radiographic or ultrasonographic imaging studies, hepatic fine-needle aspiration, and liver biopsy. A definitive diagnosis of a specific disease requires histopathology in most cases (Nelson and Couto, 2014). However, cytological evaluation of hepatic cells obtained by fine-needle aspiration is being used with increasing frequency in small animal medicine. Advantages over largebore percutaneous needle biopsies include minimal invasiveness, ease of technique, the need for minimal sedation, and faster result time. A 2013 retrospective study showed the cytological evaluation of focal liver disease had a high degree of accuracy for diagnosing neoplasia. Cytology was less reliable than histopathology for excluding the potential for neoplasia, detecting inflammatory disease, and confirming a diagnosis of vacuolar change, hyperplasia, and necrosis (Bahr *et al.*, 2013).

There are many possible causes of liver disease in an older pet, including viral and bacterial infections immune disease, toxins, changes in blood flow due to heart disease. A general description of common liver diseases of geriatric dogs and cats is provided below. Additional supportive therapies for liver disease are further described at the end of this chapter.

Hepatic Diseases of the Dog

Chronic hepatitis is the most common liver disease in dogs (Lawrence and Steiner, 2015). In most cases of canine chronic hepatitis, the cause is unknown. Histopathologically, chronic hepatitis is characterized by hepatocellular necrosis, a variable mononuclear or mixed inflammatory cell infiltrate, regeneration, and fibrosis. While certain breeds, such as the Doberman, West Highland White Terrier, Labrador Retriever, and American and English Cocker Spaniel, are predisposed to chronic hepatitis, any breed can be affected. Most cases are idiopathic. Known causes of canine chronic hepatitis are drug related (carprofen, phenobarbital, trimethoprim/sulfadiazine), infectious (canine adenovirus type 1, herpesvirus, leptospirosis), genetic (alpha-1-proteinase inhibitor deficiency) and various toxins, autoimmune and copper hepatotoxicosis. Acute and chronic hepatitis typically affects middle-aged to older dogs, with an on average earlier onset in copper-associated forms (Poldervaart *et al.*, 2009).

General treatment principles for canine chronic hepatitis include immunosuppressive therapy to control the inflammatory process, antioxidant therapy to prevent oxidative stress, and antifibrotic therapy to inhibit fibrosis.

Symptomatic therapy is aimed at mitigating symptoms and slowing the progression of fibrosis. Treatment mainstays are antiemetic and antacid therapy, inhibition of renin-angiotensin system, and appropriate dietary therapy. Appropriate antimicrobial agents and chelation therapies are employed for cases of infectious hepatitis and copper hepatotoxicosis (Lawrence and Steiner, 2014).

Copper accumulation can be a primary or secondary disorder. Copper accumulation of hepatocytes occurs due to damage of a protective mechanism that functions to release copper from the cell. The condition is self-perpetuating with further hepatocyte damage, leading to increased copper accumulation. Secondary copper hepatotoxicity occurs secondary to inflammation in the liver. Primary copper hepatotoxicity is seen more commonly in Bedlington Terriers, West Highland White Terriers, Skye Terriers, and Doberman Pinschers, although any breed can have the primary disorder.

Copper hepatotoxicity is diagnosed by quantification of copper levels of liver tissue, with normal copper tissue levels less than 400 µg/g of dry weight. Patients with copper levels above 750 µg/g dry weight should be treated with copper reduction therapy. Therapy includes a low copper diet such as Hill's® Prescription Diet® l/d®. Copper can be chelated with D-penicillamine, trientine, and tetramine. Elemental zinc can be given orally to induce synthesis of intestinal mucosal metallothionein, which has a high affinity for copper and binds dietary copper and limits its absorption (Nelson and Couto, 2014).

Portal hypertension is an important consequence of chronic hepatitis and fibrosis and can occasionally be seen in dogs with acute liver disease. Portal hypertension is a sustained increase in blood pressure in the portal system. It is caused by the increased resistance to blood flow through the sinusoids of the liver or obstructions in the portal vein or cauda vena cava. The increased pressure results in intestinal wall edema and ulceration, ascites, and acquired portosystemic shunt formation. Addressing the primary condition, preventing and treating gastrointestinal ulceration, and avoiding ulcerogenic drugs are the mainstay of treatment for portal hypertension (Nelson and Couto, 2014).

Cirrhosis is the loss of the normal liver structure, with fibrous tissue replacing the normal functional liver cells. Cirrhosis occurs at the end stage of chronic liver disease and typically occurs in older animals. The long-term prognosis in these cases is grave, as the disease is caused by the loss of functional liver tissue, and regeneration is unlikely. Supportive care with low protein diet, B vitamins, and, if necessary, anabolic steroids can help to maintain a decent quality of life for several months.

Chronic Infiltrative Disease

Alterations in hepatic structure and function may occur when hepatocytes are infiltrated with lipid, glycogen, amyloid, or other substances. Hepatic lipidosis is a common histopathologic finding in dogs with diabetes mellitus, although it seldom becomes a clinical problem associated with liver dysfunction. Steroid hepatopathy is often caused by exogenous glucocorticoids and naturally occurring hyperadrenocorticism in older dogs. Severe steroid hepatopathy can cause impairment of liver function, but most dogs do not develop signs referable to hepatic dysfunction. Amyloidosis is another infiltrative disease that is less commonly seen.

Hepatocutaneous Syndrome

Hepatocutaneous syndrome (also known as superficial necrolytic dermatitis) is a skin condition reported in association with certain liver diseases. While the pathophysiology and underlying causes in dogs remain unclear, patients have low circulating amino acids levels. The disease is usually reported in older dogs of small breeds, with males being overrepresented (Outerbridge *et al.*, 2002). Skin lesions may wax and wane for several months. Lesions consist of interdigital erythema, crusting, erosions, and hyperkeratosis of the footpads, nose, periorbital, perianal and genital areas. Signs of liver disease may be present, and diabetes mellitus may develop later in the disease process. Treatment includes the elimination of any hepatotoxic drugs, supplementation with amino acids and proteins, antibiotics for secondary skin infection, and zinc and fatty acid supplementation. Hepatocutaneous syndrome carries a very poor prognosis.

Hepatic Encephalopathy

Hepatic encephalopathy is a complex neurologic syndrome resulting in cerebral dysfunction from severe liver disease (Figure 12.2). It typically occurs when over 70% of liver function is lost. While it is most commonly seen in younger patients with

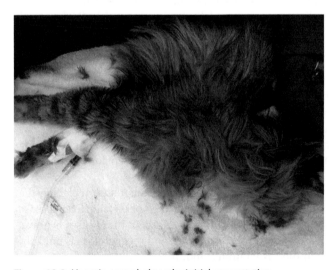

Figure 12.2 Hepatic encephalopathy initial presentation.

portosystemic shunts, in the geriatric patient hepatic encephalopathy is most often associated with hepatic neoplasia. Other causes include liver failure secondary to chronic active hepatitis and metastatic neoplasia.

In addition to cerebral dysfunction symptoms, neurologic abnormalities noted with hepatic encephalopathy may include pacing, circling, drooling, apparent blindness, and head pressing, followed by stupor, seizure activity or coma. Diagnosis is based upon documenting hepatic dysfunction in a patient with neurologic deficits and the response to treatment (Hoskins, 2005). Medical management is directed toward minimizing the signs of hepatic encephalopathy and includes reduction of dietary proteins, avoidance of medications that can worsen the signs, and the use of enemas, lactulose and antimicrobials, such as metronidazole and amoxicillin, to reduce toxin formation.

Hepatic Neoplasia

Primary hepatic tumors are most common in dogs that are ten years of age or older. Hepatocellular carcinoma is the most prevalent primary hepatic tumor. Metastatic neoplasia is also common and can particularly arise from primary neoplasms in the spleen, pancreas and gastrointestinal tract. Systemic malignancies such as lymphoma can also affect the liver. Surgical resection is the treatment of choice for single tumors involving one liver lobe. The prognosis for diffuse hepatocellular carcinomas and other malignant tumors is poor because there is no effective therapy. The response of metastatic liver tumors depends on the type and location of the primary tumor and can vary from very good to excellent with the multicentric form of hepatic lymphoma to poor in dogs with metastatic carcinomas (Nelson and Couto, 2014).

Gall Bladder Mucocele

A gall bladder mucocele is a distension of the gallbladder by an inappropriate accumulation of mucus. This condition can lead to gall bladder rupture and bile peritonitis. The average age for its formation is 11 years. Gall bladder mucoceles have been associated with endocrinopathies, and one study has shown that the odds of mucocele development in dogs with hyperadrenocorticism are 29 times that of dogs without hyperadrenocorticism. Mucoceles have also been associated with hypothyroidism, pancreatitis, hyperlipidemia, and a high-fat diet (Mesich, 2009). Figure 12.3 shows the ultrasound appearance of a gall bladder mucocele discovered during an abdominal ultrasound of a geriatric dog suspected to have hyperadrenocorticism.

Vascular Disease

Heart failure can result in circulatory changes in the liver as blood collects and vessels become congested. Any cause of right ventricular dysfunction can be associated with severe hepatic congestion. The primary pathophysiology involved in hepatic dysfunction is either passive congestion from increased filling pressures or low cardiac output resulting in impaired perfusion. Passive hepatic congestion owing to increased central venous pressure may cause elevations of liver enzymes and serum bilirubin. Severe decreases in perfusion may be associated with acute hepatocellular necrosis, with marked elevations in serum aminotransferases (Alvarez and Mukherjee, 2011).

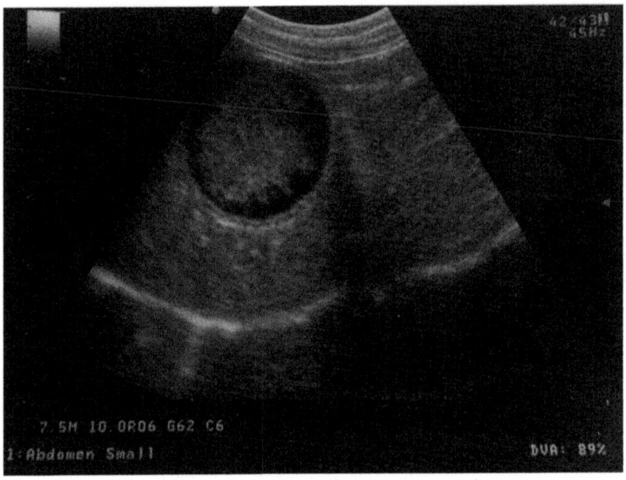

Figure 12.3 Gall bladder mucocele formation in a geriatric patient with suspected hyperadrenocorticism. Gall bladder mucoceles may display echogenic membranes or striations often described as a stellate or striated pattern, similar to that of a sliced kiwi fruit ("kiwi sign").

Hepatic Diseases of the Cat

Inflammatory Liver Disease

Inflammatory liver disease is the second most commonly diagnosed form of liver disease in cats. Whereas neutrophilic (acute) cholangitis/cholangiohepatitis is most commonly diagnosed in the young-to-middle-aged feline patient, lymphocytic (chronic) cholangitis/cholangiohepatitis is more commonly diagnosed in geriatric feline patients. The etiology of the chronic cholangiohepatitis is unknown, and the role of bacteria in this condition is unclear. A combination of antimicrobial and corticosteroid therapy is often used, either concurrently or with the corticosteroids dosed two weeks after starting the antibiotic therapy. A dosage of 1–2 mg/kg every 24 hours of prednisolone given orally is used initially and slowly tapered to as low as possible for long-term maintenance. Ursodial 10–15 mg/kg every 24 hours orally may also be used (Nelson and Couto, 2014).

Hepatic Lipidosis

Hepatic lipidosis may be primary or secondary to another disease. It usually affects obese cats and is associated with a high mortality unless the patient is intensively fed. The pathogenesis of primary lipidosis is poorly understood but seems to involve a combination of lipid mobilization to the liver, deficiency of dietary proteins and other nutrients, and disturbances in appetite. Secondary lipidosis may occur in association with any disease causing anorexia but has been most commonly recognized in cats with pancreatitis, diabetes mellitus other hepatic disorders, inflammatory bowel disease and neoplasia. Most affected cats are middle-aged but secondary hepatic lipidosis is seen more frequently in older cats.

Diagnosis is made through histopathology of a wedge biopsy of the liver, although hepatic lipidosis is typically recognizable on the cytological evaluation of fine-needle aspiration samples. Treatment is directed at restoring nutritional status and managing the underlying cause of the systemic illness. The single most important factor in reducing mortality is early and intensive feeding of a high protein diet. Enteral nutritional support using nasoesophageal, esophagostomy, or gastrostomy tube feeding is recommended (Nelson and Couto, 2014).

Copper Accumulation

While there is a paucity of availability information about copper storage disease in the cat as compared with the dog, research suggests that copper accumulates in livers of cats as primary and secondary processes. Long-term management of cats with primary copper hepatopathy was possible. Findings from a 2013 study indicated that hepatic copper accumulation also may develop secondary to various liver disorders in cats and may contribute to liver injury (Hurwitz *et al.*, 2014).

Hepatic Neoplasia

Metastatic neoplasia of the liver in cats is more common than primary neoplasia. Malignant lymphoma is the most frequent type of hematopoietic neoplasia diagnosed. Hepatocellular adenomas are the most common primary benign tumors of cats. They are a consideration when lobar liver enlargement is found in an older cat on palpation, radiographs, or ultrasonographic examination. The most common primary malignant tumors are bile duct carcinomas (see Figure 12.4). Both adenomas and carcinomas of the liver may form cystic structures in cats, which can grow very large, eventually causing clinical signs such as vomiting and anorexia. Hepatic neoplasms localized to one or

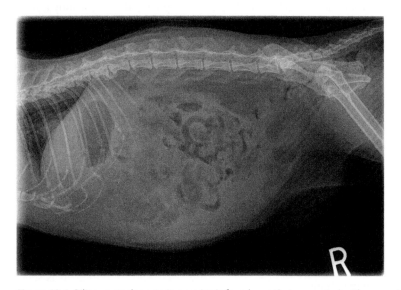

Figure 12.4 Biliary cystadenoma in a geriatric female cat that presented with anorexia and icterus.

two lobes of the liver may be amenable to surgical resection. Cats with low-grade well-differentiated lymphocytic lymphoma have a good prognosis for long-term survival with oral prednisone and chlorambucil (Armstrong 2007).

Reactive Hepatopathies

Reactive hepatopathies are changes in the liver that occur secondary to a primary non-hepatic disorder, such as inflammatory bowel disease, hyperthyroidism and cardiac disease. Usually, there is also a degree of secondary lipidosis in the reactive hepatopathies.

Treatment

Management of liver disease requires treatment of the underlying liver disease, as well as management of the clinical signs and complications of liver disease (such as ascites, gastroduodenal ulceration, and hepatic encephalopathy; Box 12.1). Liver disease can have a profound effect on a patient's quality of life. Coagulopathies are common in cats whereas portal hypertension with ascites, acquired portosystemic shunts and risk of gastrointestinal ulceration is frequently observed in dogs with chronic liver disease. Hepatic encephalopathy and protein-calorie malnutrition are common in both species. Effective management of these problems is essential to maintain comfort and general wellbeing of patients with liver disease and failure. Depending on the disease process and the stage of the disease, a good quality of life can be maintained for some time with supportive and symptomatic therapy.

Dietary therapy is important for the management of liver disease and failure. As a general recommendation, the dietary protein should represent 17–22% of digestible calories. Protein restriction should only be initiated in the patient that has clinical evidence of protein intolerance (such as in hepatic encephalopathy). Carbohydrates should provide most of the energy requirements, and fat levels should not be excessive.

Box 12.1 Common Problems and Complications of Liver Disease and Failure

- Vomiting
- Diarrhea
- Anorexia
- Polydipsia and polyuria
- Hepatomegaly
- Icterus
- Ascites
- Hepatic encephalopathy
- Gastrointestinal ulceration
- Protein-calorie malnutrition
- Coagulopathies
- Portal hypertension
- Acquired portosystemic shunts

The diet must be palatable and it may be necessary to warm the diet or "top dress" with a small amount of protein or carbohydrate that the pet will eat. Diets low in copper are recommended for the dogs that have copper-associated liver disease. A commercially available prescription diet (such as Hill's l/d) may be ideal for some patients, or a diet can be formulated by a veterinary nutritionist. Patients with ascites may need to be managed with a low sodium diet, and those with reduced albumin levels may require higher amounts of dietary protein. There is evidence that fiber is beneficial for patients with liver disease. Psyllium, as a source of soluble fiber given at a dose of 1–3 teaspoons/day, can be used as a dietary supplement (Twedt, 2015).

There is increasing interest in the use of nutraceuticals in the treatment of liver disease. High concentrations of bile acids, accumulation of heavy metals, and inflammation cause free radical generation in the liver. Antioxidants have been shown to improve chronic hepatocyte damage that causes oxidative damage. Vitamin E (alpha-tocopherol) has proven to be effective in humans with chronic hepatitis, and it is suspected to be beneficial in cats and dogs as well. The dose most commonly recommended is 10–20 IU/kg orally or 400–600 IU/day orally. Milk thistle (silymarin) and S-adenosyl-L-methionine (SAMe) have also been shown to protect hepatocytes from damage due to toxins and corticosteroid-induced hepatopathy. Silymarin has antioxidant, anti-inflammatory, anti-fibrotic and hepatoprotective effects. SAMe provides the hepatocyte with glutamine, which is necessary for metabolic reactions within the hepatocyte to maintain the function of the liver. The current recommended oral dose for silymarin is 20–50 mg/kg/day and for SAMe is 17–20 mg/kg in dogs and 200 mg/day in cats (Webb and Twedt, 2008).

Acetylcysteine may function as an important methyl donor and to augment intracellular concentrations of glutathione. It functions directly as a free radical scavenger and is most commonly used to treat severe oxidant injury, especially by acetaminophen toxicosis. The recommended dosing is 140 mg/kg intravenously initially, then 70 mg/kg intravenously or orally for three to six treatments, given at eight to twelve-hourly intervals.

Antifibrotics may be useful to prevent collagen deposition during inflammation and stimulate collagenase activity to prevent cirrhosis. Colchicine is often used for this purpose, although its effectiveness in dogs has not been studied. The dose rate is 0.025–0.03 mg/kg once daily. Zinc has an antifibrotic action and can be dosed at a rate of 1–10 mg/kg elemental zinc every 24 hours in dogs and 7 mg/kg every 24 hours in cats. Ursodeoxycholic acid (ursodiol) is recommended for dogs and cats with all types of inflammatory liver disease. It has anti-inflammatory, immunomodulatory, and antifibrotic properties, and can increase the fluidity of biliary secretions. Ursodeoxycholic acid has safely been administered to dogs and cats at a dose of 10–15 mg/kg orally every 24 hours. Adverse effects are uncommon and usually limited to mild diarrhea. A dose of 0.03 mg/kg/day has been suggested. It has been found that the angiotensin II inhibitor losartan (Zestril™, 0.25–0.5 mg/kg/day) has effects in reducing or preventing fibrosis in humans by effecting function of stellate (fibrosis producing) cells.

Because the diseased liver has reduced function to clear bacteria from the intestines, antibiotics can be useful to prevent septicemia and to decrease the risk of bacterial colonization that may take place in a diseased liver. Amoxicillin, cephalosporin, or metronidazole are suggested. Metronidazole may have some immunosuppressive properties as well as antibacterial mechanisms. For liver disease, a reduced dose of 7.5–10 mg/kg orally twice daily is recommended of hepatic metabolism of the drug.

Gastroprotectants are recommended for the treatment of gastrointestinal ulceration. Sucralfate is the mainstay of treatment of gastrointestinal ulceration and is effective for healing of erosions and ulceration by binding to the tissue and forming a barrier against gastric acid penetration. The usual dose is 1/30 kg in dogs, and 250 mg/cat orally three times daily. Additionally, H2 blockers (ranitidine, famotidine) may be used, although there is some evidence that gastric pH is normal to increased in liver disease, so they may be unnecessary. Cimetidine should be avoided. Omeprazole is a very potent inhibitor of gastric secretion and is given at a dose of 0.7 mg/kg (0.2–1.0 mg/kg) orally once daily.

Diuretics and therapeutic paracentesis can be useful in cases with ascites. Spironolactone is generally the most effective diuretic to use in liver disease due to the activation of the renin-angiotensin-aldosterone system. The usual dose is 1–2 mg/kg PO BID, and it takes at least 2–3 days to work. Furosemide can be added if needed although it is essential to monitor for hypokalemia. Therapeutic paracentesis should generally be avoided and performed only if ascites is life threatening, causing respiratory compromise or causing obvious discomfort (Nelson and Couto 2014).

Vitamin K1 supplementation is recommended for all cholestatic (hyperbilirubinemic) patients with liver disease. Parenteral administration of a 0.5–1 mg/kg dose subcutaneously is given for three to five days and then weekly if the primary cholestatic disorder is not corrected. Fresh frozen plasma and recombinant factor V11a can be administered to patients with active bleeding (Twedt, 2015).

Integrative medicine can be beneficial to the patient with liver disease. There are several Chinese herbal formulas that may be effective in managing small animal liver disease (Marsden, 2013). Acupuncture has a normoregulatory effect on gastrointestinal motility and is an excellent adjunct to the treatment of any vomiting or diarrhea. It is very useful in stimulating the appetite and decreasing the nausea associated with various hepatopathies (Schoen, 2001).

Focus on the Client

There are many different types of liver disease, all with different expected outcomes and prognoses. Some pet owners may elect not to pursue invasive or extensive diagnostics. The lack of a diagnosis can make it difficult to provide accurate treatment or to provide an owner with the expected disease course and prognosis.

Difficulties for owners caring for patients with liver disease and failure can be many. Treatment of liver disease can be costly for owners. Prescription diets or home cooking, together with any medication and supplements, can cost several hundreds of dollars a month for larger-breed dogs. Medicating with polypharmacy can be very time consuming, particularly when various medications must be divided and given throughout the day. Nursing care for pets and maintaining a clean environment can also be time consuming when pets have vomiting, diarrhea, and polyuria. Anorexia can be discouraging for owners and symptoms such as vomiting, diarrhea, and polyuria can be stressful for pets and owners. Frustration can develop from the waxing-waning nature of many types of liver disease.

For pets with a poor to grave long-term prognosis, owners should be counseled on ways to maintain quality of life and how to recognize complications from liver failure. Hospice and humane euthanasia are options for patients with severe ascites, hepatic encephalopathy, intractable vomiting and diarrhea, anemia from coagulopathies and gastrointestinal blood loss. Pain management can be difficult in patients with advanced liver disease because of the necessity to avoid ulcerogenic and hepatotoxic drugs, and because of changes in the ability of the liver to metabolize and process drugs. Concurrent osteoarthritis and other painful conditions that cannot be properly managed due to liver disease can significantly impact a patient's comfort.

Humane euthanasia should be considered for pets when owners are financially or otherwise restricted from providing care that would maintain quality of life.

References

Alvarez, A. M., and Mukherjee, D. (2011) "Liver Abnormalities in Cardiac Diseases and Heart Failure." *International Journal of Angiology*, **20**: 135–42.

Armstrong, P. J. (2007) "Neoplasms of the Feline Liver and Pancreas." Presented at the 79th Western Veterinary Conference, Las Vegas, Nevada, 2007.

Bahr, K. L., Sharkey, L. C., Murakami, T. (2013) "Accuracy of US-Guided FNA of Focal Liver Lesions in Dogs: 140 Cases (2005–2008)." *Journal of the American Animal Hospital Association*, **49**: 190–6.

Hoskins, J. D. (2005) "Liver Disease in the Geriatric Patient." *Veterinary Clinics of North America Small Animal Practice*, **35**: 617–34.

Hurwitz, B. M., Center, S. A., Randolph, J. F., McDonough, S. P. (2014) "Presumed Primary and Secondary Hepatic Copper Accumulation in Cats." *Journal of the American Veterinary Medical Association*, **244**: 68–77.

Lawrence, Y., and Steiner, J. (2015) "Canine Chronic Hepatitis." *Today's Veterinary Practice*, **5**: 32–39.

Marsden, S. (2013) "An Integrative Approach to Hepatic Disease." In *Proceedings of the Australian Veterinary Association Annual Conference 2013 Proceedings Online*, May 26–31. Cairns, Queensland, Australia.

Mesich, M., Mayhew, P. D., Holt, D. E., Brown, D. C. (2009) "Gall Bladder Mucoceles and their Association with Endocrinopathies in Dogs: a Retrospective Case–Control Study." *Journal Of Small Animal Practice*, **50**: 630–5.

Nelson, R. W., and Couto, C. G. (2014) *Small Animal Internal Medicine* (5th ed.) St Louis, MO: Elsevier, Saunders.

Outerbridge, C. A., Marks, S. L., Rogers, Q. R. (2002) "Plasma Amino Acid Concentrations in 36 Dogs with Histologically Confirmed Superficial Necrolytic Dermatitis." *Veterinary Dermatology*, **13**: 177–86.

Poldervaart, J. H., Favier, R. P., Penning, L. C., Van Den Ingh, T. S. G. a. M., Rothuizen, J. (2009) "Primary Hepatitis in Dogs: A Retrospective Review (2002–2006)." *Journal of Veterinary Internal Medicine*, **23**: 72–80.

Schmucker, D. (2005) "Age-Related Changes in Liver Structure and Function: Implications for Disease?" *Experimental Gerontology*, **40**: 650–9.

Schoen, A. (2001) *Veterinary Acupuncture, Ancient Art to Modern Medicine* (2nd ed.). St Louis, MO: Mosby.

Stockhaus, C., Teske, E., Van Deh Ingh, T., Rothuizen, J. (2002) "The Influence of Age on the Cytology of the Liver in Healthy Dogs." *Veterinary Pathology*, **39**: 154–8.

Twedt, D. C. (2015) "Treatment Considerations for Liver Disease." Presented at the 2015 Ontario Veterinary Medical Association and Trade Show Proceedings, Ontario, Canada.

Webb, C. and Twedt, D. (2008) "Oxidative Stress and Liver Disease." *Veterinary Clinics of North America Small Animal Practice*, **38**: 125–35.

13

The Respiratory System
Cheryl A. Braswell

This chapter addresses the purpose of the respiratory system, the changes that occur with "healthy aging," the disease states commonly encountered as the pet ages, including general therapeutic recommendations for those conditions, followed by explanations as to *why* these disease conditions occur in the geriatric canine and feline population. Rescue therapy for hospice patients suffering from dyspnea is also be discussed.

In the healthy young mammal, the respiratory system provides essential oxygen to the alveoli of the lungs, which diffuses across membranes and is subsequently delivered to the cells of the body via the blood (primarily hemoglobin). Oxygen is required for efficient mitochondrial adenosine triphosphate production by the cells of the body, which is the bedrock of cellular function. The respiratory system is also the means by which the end product of cellular metabolism, carbon dioxide, is expelled into the external environment. The flow of air and the oxygen–carbon dioxide exchange, is accomplished by controlled rhythmic contractions and relaxation of the respiratory muscles (diaphragm, intercostal, and accessory muscles) as well as the tone of bronchial smooth muscles (Lalley, 2013). In the young healthy individual, when the diaphragm contracts downward and the intercostal muscles expand the chest wall outward, the intrapleural pressure decreases, causing air to flow into the lungs. Alveolar surfactant reduces elastic recoil so that the alveoli are open during inspiration. During expiration of quiet breathing, which is mainly passive, the chest wall muscles return to their resting position and elastic recoil of the lungs permit expiratory airflow (Lalley, 2013).

Healthy Aging of the Respiratory System

A significant amount of research has been conducted regarding changes in the respiratory system of people as they age. Although not all of this research is translational to our species of interest, common logic dictates that many of these concerns will apply. Changes in the spine, muscles, and ribs over time can impact normal function. Decrease in intervertebral spaces can decrease the space between ribs and impact the contraction of intercostal muscles making them less efficient. Intrinsic changes of the muscles

Treatment and Care of the Geriatric Veterinary Patient, First Edition. Edited by Mary Gardner and Dani McVety.
© 2017 John Wiley & Sons, Inc. Published 2017 by John Wiley & Sons, Inc.
Companion Website: www.wiley.com/go/gardner/geriatric

themselves occur with age decreasing their strength of contraction and reducing inspiratory/expiratory muscle strength. A decline in muscle strength can impact the ability to respond to increased ventilatory demands when the patient is ill, leading to an increased risk of ventilatory failure (Lowery, 2013). Calcification of the ribcage cartilage and vertebral articulations contributes to reduced chest wall compliance, which also impacts the patient's ability to respond to increased ventilatory demands (Lowery, 2013).

As one ages, there is a decrease in the ability to clear mucus from the lungs. This is attributed to reduced cough strength and an altered ability to clear particles from the airways (Lowery, 2013). The reduced cough strength is related to changes in muscles discussed earlier. The decreased ability to clear particles is related to a change in the mucociliary apparatus. The nasal mucociliary cells work to clear large particles before they enter smaller airways. The lower airway mucociliary cells remove fine particles from the airway over time. The association between age and decreased mucociliary clearance may be related to the "beat frequency" of the cilia. Notably, cigarette smoke, to which many of our patients are exposed via their owners, has a huge negative impact on beat frequency (Lowery, 2013).

With age, respiratory resistance in the airways increases and lung elasticity declines. When this is considered in the context of decreased chest wall compliance and decreased respiratory muscle strength, it is not surprising that respiratory reserves in older individuals are reduced and significantly worsen in the face of illness or insult (Lowery, 2013). In humans, the average reduction in lung function until the age of 70 years is about 20% (Petersen, 2014). The decline in lung function is more dramatic in patients with respiratory disease and those exposed to environmental factors such as cigarette smoke. It has been documented that efficiency in gas exchange decreases with age, even in healthy non-smoking human patients, due to shrinkage and loss of lung tissue plus loss of elasticity (Petersen, 2014). These changes occur despite the maintenance of overall fitness and general wellbeing.

It is well recognized in geriatric small animals that despite normal oxygen diffusion in the lung, mechanical changes associated with aging result in disruption of the precise matching of ventilation and perfusion required for optimal oxygenation (Mosley, 2005). These changes mirror those documented in humans: decreased thoracic compliance, atrophy of intercostal muscles and diaphragm and decreased alveolar elasticity (Mosley, 2005). The ventilatory response to hypoxia and hypercarbia is markedly blunted. There is also evidence that protective laryngeal and pharyngeal reflexes are reduced (Mosley, 2005).

In the aged patient, pulmonary immune responses are exaggerated. In an animal model study of lung injury (Alvis and Huges, 2015), the pulmonary inflammatory response in older animals was found to be delayed but ultimately worse than in younger animals. This leads to a more severe lung injury in the geriatric population when faced with an inflammatory respiratory disease.

The Suffering of Dyspnea

One must consider the term "dyspnea" and its implications. In veterinary medicine, dyspnea has come to mean labored or difficult breathing (Mellema, 2008). However, in human medicine, the definition is focused on the unpleasant sensory experience, recognizing that dyspnea is, indeed, a form of suffering. "While pain represents a response to a threat to tissue integrity, dyspnea represents a response to the threat of adequate ventilation" (Mellema, 2008). There is ample documentation in human literature that verbal hospice patients equate the suffering associated with the feeling of breathlessness to the suffering of uncontrolled pain. As advanced care providers, we are compelled to alleviate the suffering of dyspnea in our patients, regardless of its etiology.

The Larynx

Laryngeal disease varies in the degree of severity of upper airway obstruction. Both dogs and cats may be affected with laryngeal paralysis, laryngeal collapse and laryngeal masses. The larynx of the cat differs from that of the dog in that the arytenoid cartilage lacks cuneiform and corniculate process. The sides of the cat epiglottis connect directly to the cricoid lamina by laryngeal mucosa. The intrinsic muscles of the larynx are responsible for all laryngeal function, which includes regulation of air flow, protection of the lower airway from aspiration during swallowing, and control of phonation (Macphail, 2014). The cricoarytenoideus dorsalis muscle is responsible for enlarging the glottis during inspiration. The caudal laryngeal nerve is the terminal segment of the recurrent laryngeal nerve and is responsible for the innervation of all intrinsic laryngeal muscles except the cricothyroid muscle (innervated by the cranial laryngeal nerve; Macphail, 2014).

Laryngeal paralysis is not uncommon in older large- and giant-breed dogs. Most often, this is an acquired disease later in life (over nine years) and proposed etiologies include accidental trauma, iatrogenic trauma, cervical masses, and neuromuscular disease. In most dogs, it is classified as idiopathic, although it has been shown that many of these dogs develop generalized neuropathy within one year of the diagnosis of laryngeal paralysis. Dogs with idiopathic laryngeal paralysis may, in fact, have a progressive generalize polyneuropathy (Macphail, 2014).

Geriatric onset laryngeal paralysis polyneuropathy has been suggested as a more appropriate term for this condition. In this condition, the arytenoid cartilages and the vocal folds do not lateralize on inspiration, thus creating an upper airway obstruction. These patients will have noisy inspiratory breathing (stridor) and exercise intolerance, with the earliest signs being a voice change and mild coughing or gagging. Progression of the disease is variable with individuals sometimes having signs for several months to years before developing significant respiratory distress. Heavy exercise, heat and humidity will exacerbate the condition. As the patient breathes with increased rate and effort, the arytenoid mucosa can become inflamed and edematous making the airway obstruction worse. Laryngeal paralysis patients are at significant risk for aspiration pneumonia. It is noteworthy that some patients with this condition will also have progressive esophageal dysfunction, which is most likely associated with the progressive polyneuropathy.

Definitive diagnosis requires direct laryngeal examination and the visualization of the lack of movement in the arytenoid cartilages. During this examination, it is very important to pay attention to the depth of the sedation as false positive results are common due to the influence of anesthetics and sedatives (Macphail, 2014). Many advocate the use of doxapram hydrochloride (1 mg/kg intravenously) to exaggerate the movement of the larynx on inspiration and to confirm the diagnosis. It is also recommended that the patient have a thyroid panel and supplementation be instituted if appropriate (although it rarely improves the clinical signs).

Medical management goals for unilateral laryngeal paralysis is improvement in quality of life through environmental changes, decreased exercise activity, owner education, weight loss, and consideration of anti-inflammatory drugs. An occasional sedative may be of benefit.

Severely affected dogs (bilateral) may be candidates for a surgical procedure. Many different surgical techniques have been described. Aspiration pneumonia is the most common complication in surgically treated patients occurring in 10–20%. However, it has been reported that owner satisfaction postoperatively is high. Most owners believe that their pet's quality of life has been significantly improved after surgery (Macphail, 2014).

Laryngeal disease in cats is not a common finding, but when it does occur it is predominantly left sided. The signs are very similar to those seen in dogs, such as inspiratory dyspnea, change in meow, gagging, and stridor (Thunberg and Lantz, 2010). The cause of this condition in cats is often undetermined, but it has been reported to be associated with trauma, neoplasia, and iatrogenic trauma following thyroidectomy. Cats may be medically managed, as with canines, or if severe, may require surgery (Thunberg and Lantz, 2010).

Laryngeal collapse is classically associated with brachycephalic airway obstruction syndrome. This condition exists with varying severity, depending on the individual's unique degree of compromise. Some patients have relatively minimal affect, while others have significant symptoms that can intensify with age. Stenotic nares, elongated palate, everted laryngeal saccules and a hypoplastic trachea are the hallmarks of this constellation of genetic abnormalities. Owing to their anatomic differences, brachycephalic patients have increased resistance to airflow and an increased intraluminal pressure gradient compared with other dogs (Macphail, 2014). Decreasing the diameter of the airways by 50% results in a 16-fold increase in resistance (Poiseuille's law). The increased negative pressure generated to overcome the airway resistance in these dogs is the major factor in the progression of the disease.

Stage 1 is the eversion of the laryngeal saccules into the glottis, narrowing the airway. Increased effort to breathe causes turbulent air flow, which in turn results in tissue edema and inflammation of the saccules, further narrowing the airway. In Stage 2, the arytenoid cartilages lose their rigidity and collapse into the lumen. In Stage 3, the corniculate process of each arytenoid fatigues and then collapses toward the midline, causing complete laryngeal collapse. Early stages of laryngeal collapse are amenable to surgical treatment. With late disease, permanent tracheostomy is the recommendation, although many owners find this unacceptable (Macphail, 2014).

It is important to note that brachycephalic airway patients also have gastrointestinal disease that parallels their degree of airway compromise. A relationship has been identified between digestive (for example, esophageal deviation, cardiac atony, gastroesophageal and duodenogastric reflux, hiatal hernia, gastric stasis, mucosal hyperplasia, esophagitis, duodenitis) and respiratory (upper airway noises, snoring) signs in brachycephalic dogs. This is most likely secondary to chronic negative intrathoracic pressure from upper airway obstruction. Interestingly, gastrointestinal signs resolved in 91–100% of cases following surgical correction of the airway (Hoareau *et al.*, 2011; Meola, 2013).

Unfortunately, gastrointestinal disease can lead to regurgitation and/or vomiting. Because these patients do not "protect" their airway well, they are prone to aspiration. Once a brachycephalic patient develops aspiration pneumonia, it can be extremely challenging for them to recover (Hoareau *et al.*, 2011). Emergency management of a brachycephalic patient with acute respiratory distress should focus on oxygenation, ventilation, and temperature management. Mild sedation is often helpful.

Laryngeal neoplasia is uncommon in either dogs or cats. Prognosis is guarded because most cases are advanced at the time of diagnosis. Benign laryngeal masses secondary to inflammatory disease have been documented in dogs and cats but is extremely rare.

The Airways

Airway collapse is a common cause for coughing in dogs, and can involve the cervical trachea, intrathoracic trachea, and/or bronchial walls. Bronchial walls can be the main bronchi or other smaller airways supported by cartilage (Maggiore, 2014). The cause of this condition is unknown. It may be primary (congenital) or acquired (inflammatory). The classic "collapsing trachea" is usually seen in older miniature and toy breeds of dog that exhibit paroxysmal (waxing/waning) respiratory signs often described as a dry, harsh or "honking" cough. These signs usually worsen with excitement, drinking or eating, or by pulling on a neck lead.

Tracheal collapse is caused by a softening of the tracheal cartilage and is characterized by a dorsoventral flattening of the tracheal rings with prolapse of the tracheal membrane into the lumen. (Maggiore, 2014). The softening of the tracheal rings is secondary to a reduction of glycosaminoglycans and chondroitin sulfate. Changes to the tracheal matrix and an inability to retain water lead to a decreased ability to maintain functional rigidity (Maggiore, 2014). The prolapse of the tracheal membrane leads to narrowing of the lumen whenever extraluminal pressure exceeds intraluminal pressure, causing airway collapse.

Cervical collapse occurs on inspiration, and intrathoracic collapse occurs on expiration, owing to the changes in pressure of the respiratory cycle. Dynamic collapse of the airway perpetuates additional inflammation, tracheal edema, alterations or failure in the mucociliary apparatus, increased mucous secretion and mucous trapping in the airway (Maggiore, 2014). Cats and large-breed dogs are rarely diagnosed with tracheal collapse.

While tracheal collapse occurs almost exclusively in small dogs, bronchomalacia (bronchial collapse) can affect any breed of dog. This condition causes narrowing and loss of luminal dimensions in intrathoracic airways and a reduction in the ability to clear secretions. This results in a chronic cough, wheezing and intermittent or chronic respiratory difficulty. Bronchmalacia has been reported in 45–83% of dogs with tracheal collapse (Maggiore, 2014). Both bronchomalacia and intrathoracic tracheal collapse results in increased expiratory effort. Close observation can sometimes reveal cranial lung herniation through the thoracic inlet during expiration in some dogs with intrathoracic airway collapse.

A thorough examination of patients with collapsing airway disease is mandatory as comorbidities often exist such as laryngeal paralysis which has been reported in up to 60% of tracheal collapse patients (Maggiore, 2014). Mitral regurgitation was found significantly more often in patients with airway collapse than without. Hepatomegaly is also common (Maggiore, 2014). The gold standard for diagnosis of airway collapse is a thorough visual laryngeal exam and bronchoscopy. Medical management involves weight loss, environmental control (temperature), treatment of inflammation and/or infection, cough suppressants and bronchodilators.

When medical management fails, surgical interventions should be considered. If cervical collapse is present, extraluminal tracheal rings is the therapy of choice. Postoperative laryngeal paralysis is commonly anticipated with this procedure. Intrathoracic tracheal collapse is managed with the placement of an intraluminal stent and can be life saving. Extensive medical management is often required with tracheal stenting, and complications can include bacterial infections, stent fracture or migration, and obstructive granulation tissue.

A patient with a collapsing airway that is in respiratory distress is a medical emergency and should be stabilized with a cool environment, oxygen supplementation, antitussive medication, and careful sedation.

Bronchitis

Canine chronic bronchitis is an inflammatory condition that results in coughing and can lead to exercise intolerance and respiratory distress (Rozanski, 2014). It is considered to be a syndrome in the dog, and not a definitive diagnosis. It is also considered to be a condition of the older small-breed dog with bronchiectasis being the sequel to poorly controlled disease. Most canine chronic bronchitis patients are systemically well, with a persistent "productive" cough as their only complaint. A respiratory arrhythmia is often present in these patients and thought to be due to increased vagal tone. It is important to remember that canines with chronic tracheobronchial disease may also have pulmonary hypertension, which can also lead to syncope (Rozanski, 2014).

In chronic bronchitis, narrowing of the airway develops from a combination of airway thickening and excessive mucus production, which results in increased airway resistance. This is pronounced on expiration. There may also be expiratory airway collapse leading to hyperinflation. Hyperinflation increases the work of breathing and perpetuates lung dysfunction (Rozanski, 2014).

Bronchoscopy is the preferred diagnostic modality. Cytology from a bronchoalveolar lavage typically reveals a neutrophilic infiltrate with excessive mucus. This chronic disease results in bronchial wall thickening and malacia, which contributes to worsening airflow obstruction and progressive inflammation. The inflammatory response perpetuates coughing and contributes to progressive decline in lung function. Chronic pulmonary disease results in pulmonary hypertension.

Treatment goals for dogs with chronic bronchitis include reducing inflammation, limiting cough, and improving exercise tolerance. Treatment also hopefully prevents or slows disease progression and the associated airway remodeling. Any environmental pollutants should be eliminated (such as cigarette smoke or other airborne irritants). Obesity should be treated as it markedly worsens cough, lung function and limits activity. A harness should be used in place of a collar. Glucocorticoids are the mainstay of treatment because they reduce inflammation which reduces the cough. Inhaled glucocorticoids have been used widely in people and are used with growing frequency in dogs with chronic bronchitis. There is limited evidence for efficacy with the use of broncho-dilators. Antibiotics are only warranted in dogs with an acute exacerbation of chronic bronchitis and a reasonable suspicion of infection. Cough suppressants are helpful for improving the quality of life for the patient and their family (Rozanski, 2014).

Asthma

Although there is a plethora of triggers for human asthma, there is little evidence that stimuli other than allergens are important risk factors for asthma in cats (Reinero, 2011). Cats spontaneously develop a syndrome similar to human asthma. The species similarities between people and cats have led to the development of feline models of allergic asthma for preclinical studies applicable to both felines and humans (Reinero, 2011).

When a cat is exposed to an inhaled allergen, it is processed by the immune system so that cytokines are produced, which then orchestrate the allergic inflammatory response system and lead to immunoglobulin E (IgE) production. Upon reexposure to the allergen, bound IgE is cross-linked, leading to degranulation and further exacerbation of the inflammatory cascade. The patient develops hallmark features of asthma: eosinophilic airway inflammation, airway hyperresponsiveness/airflow obstruction and airway remodeling (Reinero, 2011). Although asthma is thought to be a feline disease, certain dogs (racing sled dogs in particular) exhibit an exercise-triggered airway inflammation and airway hyperreactivity, which models cold exercise-induced asthma in people.

It is now believed that asthma and chronic bronchitis are the most common feline lower airway disorders and should be considered as two distinct entities (Reinero, 2011). Chronic bronchitis is caused by a previous insult, such as infection or inhaled irritants. It is described as a neutrophilic inflammation of the lower airways accompanied by edema and hypertrophy of the respiratory mucosa and excessive mucus production. Feline asthma is a T-cell induced hypersensitivity reaction characterized by eosinophilic airway inflammation and bronchoconstriction (Schulz, 2014). Specific differentiation of these two diseases requires advanced diagnostics such as a bronchoalveolar lavage.

In people, pulmonary function tests are tremendously helpful. A measured positive response to a bronchodilatory medication is an important means by which to distinguish asthma from other forms of lower airway disease. In certain areas of the country, heartworm-associated respiratory disease complex or airway parasites (*Aelurostongyla abstrusus*) can mimic the same clinical signs of asthma and can also cause eosinophilic airway inflammation.

Asthmatic felines usually respond to one, or a combination of, the following: oral glucocorticoid, inhaled fluticasone or flunisolide, and bronchodilators (methylxanthines, short- and long-acting beta-2 agonist and anticholinergics). Daily consumption of omega 3 polyunsaturated fatty acids with the antioxidant luteolin has been advocated to blunt production of bioactive eicosanoids. One study showed this supplementation to reduce airway hyperresponsiveness but it is not effective enough to use as a stand-alone therapy. Lidocaine has received interest in human medicine as a potential treatment for severe asthma, and it has been investigated in an experimental feline asthma model (Trzil and Reinero, 2014). In the feline study, nebulized lidocaine (2 mg/kg every 8 hours) was administered to healthy and experimentally asthmatic cats for two weeks. Lidocaine decreased airway hyperresponsiveness without decreasing airway eosinophilia. Importantly, no adverse effects were noted in cats. (Trzil and Reinero, 2014)

It is noteworthy that all current treatments for feline asthma act fairly late in the allergic inflammatory cascade and are, indeed, only palliative. The only potentially curative therapy for any type of allergy is allergen-specific immunotherapy (Reinero, 2011). The difficulty with this therapy is appropriately identifying the allergens for a given individual. Only closely matched allergens have the potential to induce an immunologic cure by induction of tolerance, which could potentially allow discontinuation of therapy with permanent benefit (Trzil and Reinero, 2014). Further studies are desperately needed.

The Pulmonary Parenchyma

Pneumonia

Bacterial pneumonias are most often associated with either aspiration of acidic gastric contents (aspiration pneumonitis), secondary to viral infection or subsequent to inhalation of a foreign body. The diagnosis of bacterial pneumonia is more common in dogs than cats (Dear, 2014). Healthy animals (and people) have factors that reduce the potential for aspiration. During swallowing, the epiglottis retracts and the arytenoid cartilages adduct to occlude the trachea and protect the airway. Anything that affects the normal swallowing reflexes predisposes aspiration, and anything that inhibits a normal cough reflex when aspiration occurs will contribute to more diffuse pulmonary infiltrates and acute lung injury. Conditions predisposing aspiration are esophageal disease, chronic vomiting, laryngeal dysfunction, brachycephalic airway syndrome, neurologic disorders (including seizures) and general anesthesia (Dear, 2014).

The initial injury to the lungs upon aspiration of gastric contents is one of irritation and inflammation (aspiration pneumonitis) owing to the acidity of the aspirate. This injury to the respiratory tract sets the stage for colonization by the bacteria (gut flora) in the gastric contents. Using antacids have been advocated for those patients at risk of aspiration and remains controversial as more alkaline stomach pH increases the resident bacterial colony count (Dear, 2014).

Infectious canine and feline pneumonias often begin with viral infection of the upper respiratory tract (Dear, 2014). These conditions are often acute and self-limiting; however, in some patients, the inflammation associated with viral disease affects the patient's immune defenses and allows bacterial pathogens to establish lower respiratory infection (pneumonia). Such is the case with canine infectious respiratory disease, previously termed "kennel cough," in which canine respiratory coronavirus, herpesvirus, pneumovirus and parainfluenza virus have been implicated.

These viral infections set the stage for bacteria such as streptococcus, mycoplasma and bordetella pneumonia (Dear, 2014). In cats, viral respiratory infections can also lead to bacterial pneumonias in a subset of patients. Bacteria commonly identified in feline patients are *Pasteurella, Escherichia coli, Staphylococcus, Streptococcus, Pseudomonas, Bordetella* and *Mycoplasma* spp. (Dear, 2014).

Any systemic virus, such as feline leukemia or feline immunodeficiency virus, can potentiate the severity of the respiratory infection. Immune suppression caused by various medications such as chemotherapy and immunosuppressives can enhance the potential for, and severity of, infection. Overcrowding and/or stressful environments have been associated with increased risk.

Clinical signs and physical exam findings can be vague and varied depending on the etiology, severity and chronicity of the disease. Often, dogs and cats with mild disease will have no abnormalities on physical examination. An early clue is a change in respiratory pattern with increased rate and a modest increase in effort. Auscultation often only reveals harsh or "increased" breath sounds. Less than 50% of the patients will exhibit a fever (Dear, 2014). There may or may not be a soft cough. Feline owners often interpret their cats cough as gagging or vomiting. Radiography is the primary diagnostic modality but it is important to remember that radiographs lag behind clinical disease. Therefore, repeat radiographs are not beneficial early in the disease course but may be useful to document resolution before discontinuing antibiotics.

In stable patients with mild clinical signs, antibiotic monotherapy is indicated. Patients with moderate clinical signs may need dual therapy, and those with severe clinical signs may need escalation of their medication to antibiotics not routinely used, such as carbenicillins. The need for mucolytics, nebulization and coupage or supplemental oxygen should be considered for some. Cough suppressants are not recommended.

Interstitial Pulmonary Disease

Interstitial lung diseases are a heterogeneous group of conditions that affect the pulmonary interstitium. They are noninfectious and nonmalignant (Heikkilä-Laurila and Rajamäki, 2014). This group includes eosinophilic pneumonia, lymphocytic interstitial pneumonitis, bronchiolitis obliterans, and pulmonary fibrosis, among others. Extensive review of all of these conditions is beyond the scope of this chapter. Pulmonary fibrosis is discussed as a representative disease process that occurs mostly in dogs, of which the West Highland White Terrier is particularly predisposed. Pulmonary fibrosis has been documented in cats as well as humans. Immune-mediated diseases, infections, chronic inflammation, environmental chemicals, and other primary insults to the lungs, as well as inherited defects, may lead to secondary pulmonary fibrosis in humans. The feline model of pulmonary fibrosis most closely resembles the human disease when compared with other spontaneous or induced animal models.

Idiopathic pulmonary fibrosis is a chronic progressive interstitial lung disease of unknown etiology. (Heikkilä-Laurila and Rajamäki, 2014). The nature of the disease process manifests as slowly progressive clinical signs and can be confused with aging. Pathogenesis of the disease and role of genetics is poorly understood.

Pulmonary fibrosis causes thickening of the pulmonary interstitium leading to impairment in gas exchange. In humans, it is thought to arise from a chronic, repetitive insult to the distal lung parenchyma, leading to injury and apoptosis of alveolar epithelial cells (Heikkilä-Laurila and Rajamäki, 2014). Following injury, there is an abnormal healing process with fibroblast and myofibroblast accumulation and deposition of excess extracellular matrix, leading to the final archetectural changes (Heikkilä-Laurila and Rajamäki, 2014). The disease usually affects middle-aged to older smaller-breed dogs, being especially prevalent in the West Highland White Terrier. The median survival of Westies with idiopathic pulmonary fibrosis has been reported to be 16 months from onset of clinical signs and 7 months from diagnosis (Lilja-Maula *et al.*, 1999).

Initially these patients seem quite well except for their exercise intolerance and chronic cough (not all affected dogs cough). Progression in clinical signs include syncope, gagging, panting and tachypnea. This condition is inevitably progressive with advance stages experiencing respiratory distress, cyanosis, and respiratory failure (Heikkilä-Laurila and Rajamäki, 2014). Of note, pulmonary neoplasia (carcinoma) coincident with pulmonary fibrosis, has been documented in dogs, cats, and people.

On physical examination, these patients are usually bright and alert with bilateral inspiratory "Velcro" crackles. A low-grade, right-sided, systolic murmur may be present if there is pulmonary hypertension causing tricuspid regurgitation. Hypoxemia is often present becoming more severe as the disease progresses. Despite low oxygen levels, most dogs remain bright, adapting to their chronic slowly progressive disease. Changes on radiographs are not specific or sensitive for this condition.

There is no effective treatment for pulmonary fibrosis. Goals of care are to reduce the clinical signs and to try and mitigate possible complications (Heikkilä-Laurila and Rajamäki, 2014). Various medications that may be tried for our species of interest are corticosteroids, bronchodilators, and antitussives. In humans, a new drug, pirfenidone, has been approved in Europe and Asia. This medication is anti-fibrotic, antioxidant and anti-inflammatory. A Japanese study indicates it slowed the decline in lung function of patients with pulmonary fibrosis (Heikkilä-Laurila and Rajamäki, 2014). Sometimes, an acute worsening in respiratory function may due to pneumonia, and it is very important to address contributory problems; however, at times, no cause can be determined for acute exacerbations. In humans, acute exacerbations of pulmonary fibrosis have a mortality up to 50%. In patients with pulmonary hypertension, efforts target reducing the pulmonary arterial pressure. Sildenafil and tadalafil are phosphodiesterase-5 inhibitors and have been shown to be of benefit.

Pulmonary Vasculature and Pulmonary Hypertension

Although there are many conditions that result in pulmonary hypertension, in this chapter consideration is limited to those that involve the respiratory system specifically. Heartworm disease is usually considered a primary obstructive vascular disease but is also documented to cause pulmonary inflammation (Kellihan and Stepien, 2010) Chronic pulmonary parenchymal disease, such as chronic bronchitis, or pulmonary fibrosis, can lead to destruction of pulmonary capillary beds and elevated pulmonary vascular pressures (Kellihan and Stepien, 2010). In people, regional or global hypoxia can lead to reactive pulmonary hypertension (Kellihan and Stepien, 2010). Regional or global hypoxia in dogs can be caused by chronic bronchitis, bronchiectasis, laryngeal paralysis, and collapsing trachea. Pulmonary inflammation, destruction of pulmonary capillary beds, reactive vasoconstriction with structural alterations in the pulmonary vascular arteries from hypoxia and restrictive pulmonary conditions can all ultimately lead to pulmonary hypertension.

This condition is most often reported in middle-aged to older small-breed dogs (Kellihan and Stepien, 2010). Presenting clinical signs are varied from cough to dyspnea to lethargy, but there is a high incidence of exercise intolerance and syncope in these patients.

Physical examination findings reflect pulmonary pathology. Auscultation reveals harsh breath sounds to fine crackles. Tricuspid murmurs, mitral murmurs, and gallop rhythms have all been reported. Diagnostic modalities include thoracic radiographs, electrocardiography, and echocardiography. In advance stages, signs of right-heart failure are present with evidence of right-heart enlargement and ascites. In human patients, the recognition of right-heart failure in the context of pulmonary hypertension is associated with a life expectancy of less than six months (Kellihan and Stepien, 2010).

Therapeutic goals are increased exercise tolerance, decreased pulmonary arterial pressure, decreased right ventricular workload, and increased quality of life. Treatments aimed at the underlying disease are a priority. If the condition is considered to be idiopathic or treatment of the underlying disease is insufficient, pulmonary vasodilators are indicated. Selective phosphodiesterase-5 inhibitors (such as sildenafil or tadalafil) have shown positive results (Kellihan and Stepien, 2010; Kellihan *et al.*, 2015).

The Pleural Space

Pleural Effusions

The pleural space is a potential cavity formed by the visceral and parietal pleura which normally contains a small amount of fluid to minimize friction and provide mechanical coupling between chest wall and lungs for normal respirations (Dempsey and Ewing, 2011). Increased fluid in the pleural space occurs when there is increased capillary hydrostatic pressure, widening of the oncotic pressure gradient, increased endothelial permeability, or loss of lymphatic drainage. (Dempsey and Ewing, 2011). This increased fluid is referred to as pleural effusion and, by convention, is divided into transudates, modified transudates, and exudates. Differentiation is accomplished by analysis of the fluid with respect to cell count and protein levels. Transudates and modified transudates are a consequence of an increase in capillary hydrostatic pressure or a decrease in capillary colloid osmotic pressure (that is, altered fluid dynamics; Dempsey and Ewing, 2011; Epstein, 2014). They are characterized by low cell counts and either low (transudate) or high (modified transudate) protein concentration (Dempsey and Ewing, 2011).

Exudates usually result from an inflammatory condition and associated mediators, or obstruction of lymphatic drainage (Epstein, 2014). They are usually the result of the presence of a foreign material be it infectious, neoplastic, exogenous material, or rupture of a vessel as in hemorrhagic or chylous effusion (Dempsey and Ewing, 2011). It is duly noted that felines can have chylous effusion from primary cardiac disease.

Thoracocentesis is both diagnostic and therapeutic. This procedure is well within the purview of the attending veterinarian, whether a general practitioner or hospice provider. The conditions that can result in a pleural effusion are numerous, varied and beyond the scope of this chapter. Those that may be encountered in the geriatric population may include cardiac disease, protein-losing nephropathy or enteropathy, liver disease, and neoplasia, to name a few. Determination of the type of effusion will guide the investigation of the etiology, and ultimately, the therapy to address the underlying cause.

Spontaneous Pneumothorax

Secondary pneumothorax is a common sequel to blunt force trauma. Therefore, when pneumothorax occurs, trauma is often assumed. Documentation in the scientific literature of spontaneous pneumothorax exists in dogs as well as cats (Liu and Silverstein, 2014). The condition of pneumothorax is usually divided into primary or secondary. Although primary pneumothorax (without underlying etiology) exists in people, this has not been documented in our species of interest. The spontaneous pneumothoraxes of veterinary medicine are secondary; that is, associated with a primary underlying disease. The respiratory conditions that lead to pneumothorax in cats are varied and usually chronic. Documented causes of secondary spontaneous pneumothorax (SSP) include asthma, heartworm infection, neoplasia, thromboembolism, pneumonia secondary to bacterial and parasitic infections, among others. In cats, asthma alone has accounted for up to 26% of cases (Liu and Silverstein, 2014). The prevalence of asthma as a cause of SSP in cats has led to one author categorizing the patients as asthma-associated SSP vs. non-asthma-associated SSP. The generalized nature of the underlying disease in cats rarely lends itself to surgical correction. Medical management provides a good quality of life for a short time in most cases. Long-term survival is not expected, owing to the progressive nature of the underlying pathology.

SSP in dogs is most commonly caused by bullous emphysema. Surgical management offers lower reoccurrence rates and better prognosis than medical management in these cases. Other causes of SSP in the canine population are pulmonary abscesses, bacterial pneumonia, migrating foreign bodies, parasites (including heartworm), chronic obstructive pulmonary diseases, and thromboembolism (Liu and Silverstein, 2014). Dogs with generalized pulmonary disease have an unfavorable long-term prognosis.

Medical management of these cases can be conservative at times, or may require intensive care. Some may do well with a simple thoracocentesis; others will require thoracostomy tubes. There have been some patients whose pneumothorax was so mild that thoracocentesis was not required.

Additional diagnostics to determine the underlying disease are recommended. Continuing therapy is based on the definitive diagnosis. With generalized pulmonary parenchymal disease, short-term prognosis may be good, but ultimately the progressive nature of the underlying disease usually does not allow long-term survival.

The Thoracic Wall

Although the thoracic wall and the diaphragm are vital to the function of the respiratory apparatus, conditions that affect these structures can be overlooked in the geriatric patient. Non-traumatic rib fractures and acquired hiatal hernia can cause significant morbidity. Other documented chest wall/diaphragm abnormalities include neoplasia and neuromuscular disease. The purpose of this section is to highlight the potential of non-traumatic rib fractures as a cause of respiratory difficulty in the geriatric patient.

The diagnosis of multiple rib fractures in the absence of known trauma should alert the clinician to consider underlying disease (Hardie *et al.*, 1999). Conditions that may predispose the elderly to non-traumatic rib fractures include prolonged severe respiratory effort and excessive coughing, with predisposing comorbidities such as metabolic disease or neoplastic disease (Hardie *et al.*, 1999; Adams *et al.*, 2010) Secondary renal hyperparathyroidism and renal osteodystrophy are well-known effects of chronic kidney disease (Adams *et al.*, 2010). Plasma cell tumors can invade bone, resulting in lytic lesions, diffuse osteoporosis and pathologic fracture (Adams *et al.*, 2010). Historically, patients with non-traumatic rib fracture are older, have multiple rib fractures that are more caudal (9th to 13th rib) and they occur in the middle third of the rib. Traumatic fractures tend to occur in younger animals and in the proximal one-third of the rib with variable location in the rib cage.

Clinical signs of rib fractures, especially in cats, may be subtle, and may be overlooked as part of their respiratory disease. Although no definitive therapy is usually necessary for these fractures, they are considered painful and quality of life is affected if the animal's pain is not appropriately addressed (Adams *et al.*, 2010).

The Why

What has been described as healthy aging is only homeostatic outside the context of disease or injury. Having decreased chest wall compliance, decreased intercostal muscle strength, less effective coughing, impaired mucociliary apparatus, and less than optimal oxygen and ventilation only becomes a significant problem for the geriatric patient in the face of illness, injury or increased demand. In their day-to-day existence, these patients are able to compensate for age-related changes, but when faced with challenges, it becomes difficult for them to recover. What then predisposes this population to illness in which the healthy aging process influences the course of disease and the prognosis? The answer may lie at the cellular and subcellular level.

Aged lungs become highly susceptible to endogenous and exogenous insults or stress, which facilitates progression of disease. One theory is that aging results in an increase in free radicals that cause oxidative stress thereby promoting various disease processes (Nho, 2015). Oxidative stress is an imbalance between the production of reactive oxygen species and the body's natural antioxidant defenses. Increased oxidative stress leads to premature induction of cellular aging and senescence (Nho, 2015). The ability to withstand oxidative stress has been correlated with enhanced longevity in several species. Because aging increases chronic hypoxia, excessive amounts of free radicals are formed. There is a close relationship between chronic hypoxia and pulmonary fibrosis (Nho, 2015).

Micro-ribonucleic acids (miRNAs) represent an important epigenetic mechanism for the regulation of various messenger RNA function. They are endogenous, small noncoding 21–25-nucleotide, single-stranded RNAs that play a crucial role in almost every aspect of biology (Nho, 2015). It is well established that miRNAs are linked to aging and they have been implicated in various types of human diseases. miRNAs are closely associated with brain aging, declining brain function and neurodegenerative disease in people. Findings of various studies indicate that certain miRNAs are associated with aging in the lung, and the alterations of these can lead to aging-associated lung disease. miRNA dysregulation was originally thought to be only associated with cancer development but has been implicated in cardiovascular, pulmonary disease, and inflammatory disease (Nho, 2015). The balance of miRNAs and anti-miRNA can alter pathways controlling metabolism, endocrine signaling, nutrient sensing and stress resistance (Nho, 2015).

Sirtuins 1–7 (SIRTs 1–7) are mammalian homologs of yeast. The SIRT family plays a crucial role in various biological processes including cell apoptosis, muscle and adipose cell differentiations, chromatin condensation and metabolism. (Nho, 2015). Persistent DNA damage from oxidative/carbonyl stress is linked to the onset of chronic obstructive pulmonary disease (COPD) in humans, suggesting that the deregulation of SIRT 1 is linked to the progression of lung disease (Nho, 2015). Studies have linked the sirtuin family members, especially SIRT 3, to mitochondrial integrity, mitochondrial DNA damage repair and aging. (Kim *et al.*, 2015). There are current conceptual models of how SIRTs modulate reactive oxygen species driven mitochondrial metabolism that may be important for tumor suppression function. (Kim *et al.*, 2015). Current research into the pathobiology underlying alveolar epithelial cell mitochondrial DNA damage and apoptosis suggesta novel therapeutic targets for the management of age-related disease, including pulmonary fibrosis and lung cancer (Kim *et al.*, 2015).

Age-related declines in immune function (immunosenescence) likely play a significant role in the manifestation of age-related pulmonary diseases such as infection, asthma, and chronic airway disease. Features of mammalian aging include genomic instability, epigenetic changes, modified cell communications, and dysregulated immune function (Murray and Chotirmali, 2015). The immune systems of older individuals declines with advancing age, increasing their susceptibility to infection and cancer. The aging pet suffers more severe community-acquired infections and tend to have poorer outcomes. They also have decreased response to vaccination. Such physiologic decline in immune function is termed "immunosenescence". More correctly defined, immunosenescence is the impairment of both cellular and adaptive immunity as a result of age related changes. (Murray and Chotirmali, 2015). Aging is also associated with a chronic low-grade inflammatory state that is inhibited in "healthy aging" individuals by cytokines such as interleukin-10 (Murray and Chotirmali, 2015). This chronic low-grade inflammatory state shapes the clinical phenotype observed in many respiratory diseases, including asthma, chronic airway disease, and pulmonary fibrosis.

Acute Management of the Patient Suffering from Dyspnea

General recommendations for management of respiratory conditions in our geriatric canine and feline patients has been presented in the preceding sections. Our focus now turns to the suffering dyspneic patient, particularly those patients in the palliative care and hospice population. These recommendations are valid regardless of the etiology of the patient's condition. These rescue therapies will not address the underlying cause of the patient's difficulties but will, at least for a time, alleviate their distress. By alleviating the pet's distress, the family or caregiver is comforted.

One intervention that is easily administered in the home consists of placing a fan in front of the dyspneic pet and blowing cool air in their face. Facial cooling, in a well-ventilated room, has been reported to be beneficial by human patients (Williams, 2006). Although the mechanism is still speculative, it is suspected that the temperature of the air (cool) ameliorates the feeling dyspnea via stimulation of thermoreceptors in the airways. Anxiety is always part of the feeling of breathlessness. A calm, comfortable environment for the pet will help during this difficult time. Anxiolytics can be beneficial in some patients.

There have been studies in human hospice and palliative care that document benefit from acupuncture and acupressure for patients with chronic respiratory disease, particularly chronic obstructive COPD (Williams, 2006). These patients reported clinically significant benefits when their standard of care was supplemented with complementary and alternative therapies. A systematic review of complementary and alternative therapies near end of life, in patients with COPD, found these interventions to be beneficial (Williams, 2006).

In the human hospice movement, it is common knowledge that the first drugs of choice for the dyspneic patient are opioids. There is a plethora of studies documenting that the appropriate administration of opioids will alleviate dyspnea and *will not* hasten death. Granted the adage to "start low and go slow" is a well-accepted axiom, opioids (pure mu agonists) should not be withheld from the dyspneic hospice patient. A typical hydromorphone dose in an otherwise healthy trauma patient is considered to be 0.1–0.2 mg/kg intravenously or intramuscularly. In the geriatric dyspneic hospice patient, this author typically starts with a dose of 0.01–0.02 mg/kg intravenously or intramuscularly. The dose of opioid is repeated every 15 minutes until relief is noted. Although hydromorphone is used as an example, any opioid (fentanyl, oxycodone, morphine) may be used. If the partial mu agonist, kappa antagonist, buprenorphine, is considered, please be reminded that the onset of action is quite delayed (up to 40 minutes if given intramuscularly). Many advocate the use of butorphanol in the patient with respiratory distress. One may consider using the agonist/antagonist butorphanol, but if it is administered and found lacking, the effect of subsequent dosing with a pure mu agonist will be significantly decreased. This applies to buprenorphine as well.

Another novel therapy is the nebulization of magnesium sulfate ($MgSO_4$) and furosemide (Figure 13.1). $MgSO_4$ is a smooth-muscle relaxant and therefore a bronchodilator. Nebulized $MgSO_4$ has no contraindications to its use and there are no significant complications. $MgSO_4$, diluted with sterile water, is nebulized for approximate 10–12 minutes, then typically followed with a nebulized dose of furosemide at 5 mg/kg. Only 20% of nebulized furosemide is systemically absorbed, so a diuretic effect is not appreciated.

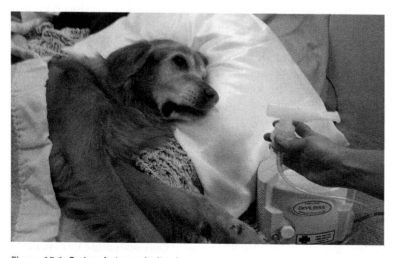

Figure 13.1 Patient being nebulized.

Box 13.1 Nebulization of Magnesium Sulfate (MgSO₄)

- Mix 1 mL of 50% $MgSO_4$ with 6 mL sterile water.
- Use half of the mixture (3.5 mL) for one nebulization treatment.
- Save the remaining 3.5 mL for the next treatment.
- Nebulization time will be approximately 10–12 minutes
- Mix 5 mg/kg of furosemide with either sterile water or 0.9% sodium chloride (NaCl) to make a total volume of approximately 3.5 mL.
- Nebulization time will be 10–12 minutes.

It is important that you do not attempt to mix the $MgSO_4$ with the furosemide as crystallization will occur.

    This treatment may be repeated as needed.

It has been this author's experience that the patient becomes much more comfortable, and is able to rest and sleep, even before the nebulization process is complete (Box 13.1).

In the airways and pulmonary parenchyma, there exists receptors named "slow-adapting receptors" and "rapid-adapting receptors". During the course of normal breathing, the slow-adapting receptors increase their firing and the rapid-adapting receptors decrease firing, sending a neural signal to the brain that a normal comfortable breath was achieved. With dyspneic patients who are not getting a normal "breath," these receptors fire aberrantly, sending a neural signal that results in the feeling of breathlessness and air hunger.

Simply put, nebulization with furosemide causes the receptors to fire normally, regardless of the condition or severity of illness. The author has administered this rescue therapy to multiple animals with diverse disease including metastatic lung cancer, terminal bronchiectasis, consolidating pneumonia, brachycephalic airway obstruction syndrome stage 3, among many others. It has not failed to alleviate the patient's clinical signs but, admittedly, the duration of effect has varied. The longest a patient has been able to rest comfortably after a treatment has been 6 hours.

In the hospice patient with a significant respiratory condition, their comfort is predicated on being able to breathe without feeing air hunger or breathlessness. In human medicine, once therapies no longer alleviate the patient's dyspnea, proportionate palliative sedation is employed until natural death occurs. Because proportionate palliative sedation is not routine in veterinary medicine, although plausible from this author's perspective, humane euthanasia is the kindest choice. No one should die suffering because they cannot get a breath of air.

> Treat often, cure sometimes, comfort always.
>
> *Hippocrates*

References

Adams, C., Streeter, E. M., King, R., Rozanski, E. (2010) "Cause and Clinical Characteristics of Rib Fractures in Cats: 33 Cases (2000–2009)." *Journal of Emergency and Critical Care*, **20**(4): 436–40.

Alvis, B., and Huges, C. (2015). "Physiologic Considerations in Geriatric Patients." *Anesthesiology Clinics*, **33**: 447–56.

Dear, J. D. (2014) "Bacterial Pneumonia in Dogs and Cats." *Veterinary Clinics of North America Small Animal Practice*, **44**: 143–59.

Dempsey S. M., and Ewing, P. J. (2011) "A Review of Pathophysiology, Classification and Analysis of Canine and Feline Cavitary Effusions." *Journal of the Animal Hospital Association*, **47**: 1–11.

Epstein, S. E. (2014) "Exudative Pleural Disease in Small Animals." *Veterinary Clinics of North America Small Animal Practice*, **44**: 161–80.

Hardie, E., Ramirez, O. III, Clary, E. M., Kornegay, J. N., Correa, M. T., Feimster, R. A., Robertson, E. R. (1998) "Abnormalities of the Thoracic Bellows: Stress Fracture of the Ribs and Hiatal Hernia." *Journal of Veterinary Internal Medicine*, **12**: 279–87.

Heikkilä-Laurila, H. P., and Rajamäki, M. M. (2014) "Idiopathic Pulmonary Fibrosis in West Highland White Terriers." *Veterinary Clinics of North America Small Animal Practice*, **44**(1): 129–42.

Hoareau, G., Mellema, M. S., Silverstein, D. C. (2011) "Indication, Management, and Outcome of Brachycephalic Dogs Requiring Mechanical Ventilation." *Journal of Veterinary Emergency and Critical Care*, **21**(3): 226–35.

Kellihan, H. B., and Stepien, R. L. (2010) "Pulmonary Hypertension in Dogs: Diagnosis and Therapy." *Veterinary Clinics of North America Small Animal Practice*, **40**: 623–41.

Kellihan H. B., Waller, K. R., Pinkos, A., Steinberg, H., Bates, M. L. (2015) "Acute Resolution of Pulmonary Alveolar Infiltrates in 10 Dogs with Pulmonary Hypertension Treated With Sildenafil Citrate: 2005–2014." *Journal of Veterinary Cardiology*, **17**: 182–91.

Kim, S. K. Cheresh, P., Jablonski, R. P., Williams, D. B., Kamp, D. W. (2015) "The Role of Mitochondrial DNA in Mediating Alveolar Epithelial Cell Apoptosis and Pulmonary Fibrosis." *International Journal of Molecular Sciences*, **16**(9): 21486–519.

Lalley, P. M. (2013) "The Aging Respiratory System - Pulmonary Structure, Function and Neural Control." *Respiratory Physiology and Neurobiology*, **187**(3): 199–210.

Lilja-Maula. L. I., Laurila, H. P., Syrjä, P., Lappalainen, A. K., Krafft, E., Clercx, C., Rajamäki, M. M. (2014) "Long-Term Outcome and Use of 6-Minute Walk Test in West Highland White Terriers with Idiopathic Pulmonary Fibrosis." *Journal of Veterinary Internal Medicine*, **28**: 279–385.

Liu, D. T., and Silverstein, D.C. (2014) Feline Secondary Spontaenous Pneumothorax: A Retrospective Study of 16 Cases (2000–2012). *Journal of Veterinary Emergency and Critical Care*, **24**(3): 316–25.

Lowery, E. M., Brubaker, A. L., Kuhlmann, E., Kovacs, E. J. (2013) "The Aging Lung." *Clinical Interventions in Aging*, **8**: 1489–96.

Macphail, C. (2014) "Laryngeal Disease in Dogs and Cats." *Veterinary Clinics of North America Small Animal Practice*, **44**: 19–31.

Maggiore, A. D. (2014) "Tracheal and Airway Collapse in Dogs." *Veterinary Clinics of North America Small Animal Practice*, **44**: 117–27

Mellema M. (2008) "The Neurophysiology of Dyspnea." *Journal of Veterinary Emergency and Critical Care*, **18**: 561–71.

Meola, S. D. (2013) "Brachycephalic Airway Syndrome." *Topics in Companion Animal Medicine*, **28**(3): 91–6.

Moseley, C. (2005) "Anesthetic Management of the Geriatric Patient." *Proceedings of the North American Veterinary Conference, January 8–12, 2005, Orlando, Fl,* Vol. 19, pp. 63–66. Gainsville, FL: Eastern States Veterinary Association.

Murray, M. A., and Chotirmali, S. H. (2015) "The Impact of Immunosenescence on Pulmonary Disease." *Mediators of Inflammation,* **2015**; 692546. doi: 10.1155/2015/692546.

Nho, R. S. (2015) "Alterations of Aging-Dependent MircoRNAs in Idiopathic Pulmonary Fibrosis." *Drug Development Research,* **76**: 343–53.

Petersen, S., von Leupoldt, A., Van den Bergh, O. (2014) "Geriatric Dyspnea: Doing worse, Feeling Better." *Aging Research Reviews,* **15**: 94–99.

Reinero, C. R. (2011) "Advances in the Understanding of Pathogenesis, and Diagnostic and Therapeutics for Feline Allergic Asthma." *Veterinary Journal,* **190**: 28–33.

Rozanski, E. (2014) "Canine Chronic Bronchitis." *Veterinary Clinics of North America Small Animal Practice,* **44**: 107–16

Schultz, B. S., Richter, P., Weber, K., Mueller, R. S., Wess, G., Zenker, I., Hartmann, K. (2014) "Detection of Feline Mycoplasma Species in Cats with Feline Asthma and Chronic Bronchitis." *Journal of Feline Medicine and Surgery.* **16**(12): 943–49.

Trzil, J. E., and Reinero, C. R. (2014) "Update on Feline Asthma." *Veterinary Clinics of North America Small Animal Practice,* **44**: 91–105.

Thunberg, B., and Lantz, G. (2010) "Evaluation of Unilateral Arytenoid Lateralization for the Treatment of Laryngeal Paralysis in 14 Cats." *Journal of the American Animimal Hospitals Association,* **46**: 418–24.

Williams, C. M. (2006) "Dyspnea." *Cancer Journal,* **12**(5): 365–73.

14

Mobility Issues
Tammy Perkins Johnson

The physical components most directly involved with mobility issues in the geriatric patient include the skeletal, muscular, and nervous systems. The skeleton forms the rigid internal framework of the body. Muscles and nerves together, in conjunction with the skeleton, are responsible for motion and also referred to as the musculoskeletal system. Difficulties in maintaining normal or previous levels of movement are often the first indicators of aging.

Musculoskeletal Changes

Sarcopenia

As a patient ages or is less active, loss of muscle mass and function in the absence of disease can occur. This loss of lean body mass is very common in geriatric and arthritic patients. Sarcopenia refers to the progressive decrease in muscle mass and strength that occurs with aging. Sarcopenia reflects loss of myofibers due to apoptosis, as well as decreases in myofiber size. Overall muscle circumference is often maintained during early sarcopenia, as lost myofibers are replaced with adipose and fibrous tissue (Freeman, 2012).

In humans, sarcopenia has been indicated as a reliable marker of frailty and poor prognosis among older individuals. The European Consensus recommends using the criteria of both low muscle function (strength or performance) and low muscle mass for the diagnosis of sarcopenia (Cruz-Jentoft *et al.*, 2010). Resistance exercises are effective in increasing muscle mass and strength. Endurance exercises are superior for maintaining and improving maximum aerobic power. Recommendations for frail older patients include a balanced program of both endurance and strength exercises, performed at least three days a week (Landi *et al.*, 2014). Instituting a three-day-a-week balanced endurance and strengthening program for our small animal patients is beneficial both physically and mentally.

Muscle fibers are generally classified as type I (slow twitch) or type II (fast twitch). Type I fibers have a slow contraction time, resist fatigue and use oxidative pathways. Type II fibers have a quick reaction time, fatigue more easily and rely on glycolytic pathways (Shmalberg, 2014).

Treatment and Care of the Geriatric Veterinary Patient, First Edition. Edited by Mary Gardner and Dani McVety.
© 2017 John Wiley & Sons, Inc. Published 2017 by John Wiley & Sons, Inc.
Companion Website: www.wiley.com/go/gardner/geriatric

Loss of muscle fiber number is the principle cause of sarcopenia, although fiber atrophy, particularly among type II fibers, is also involved. Multiple mechanisms have been implicated in the development of sarcopenia. A significant contributor is the anabolic resistance of older skeletal muscles to protein nutrition that can be ameliorated with dietary supplementation and resistance exercises (Farnfield *et al.*, 2012). Other areas of intense research are related to oxidative damage and the loss of innervation. Denervation is a characteristic of aging muscle cells with changes occurring at many levels, in the peripheral and central nervous system and the skeletal muscle tissue. Changes include diminished function and loss of motor neurons in the central nervous system, demyelination of the axons, and withdrawal of the nerve terminals from the neuromuscular junction (Chai *et al.*, 2011). A decrease in the production of anabolic hormones such as testosterone, growth hormone and insulin-like growth factor-1 impairs the capacity of skeletal muscle to incorporate amino acids and myosin heavy chain proteins. An increase in the release of catabolic agents, specifically interleukin-6, amplifies the rate of muscle wasting among the elderly (Morley *et al.*, 2001; Deschenes, 2004).

A patient can be overweight but still have muscle loss. Figures 14.1 and 14.2 illustrate a body condition and muscle condition scoring system from the World Small Animal Veterinary Association nutritional toolkit, that can aid in the assessment of geriatric patients. This muscle condition scoring system should be used as only one of the tools to aid in assessment. It does not necessarily correlate with other measures of body composition and does not consider "overcoat syndrome."

Clinically, body and muscle condition scores are not directly related, because of the "overcoat syndrome". This occurs when an animal has less muscle and more fat, making a muscle condition score of 1 or 2 appear relatively normal. Overcoat syndrome is suspected when the history and physical examination do not concur. Palpation is required for diagnosis. Although some areas of the body may feel relatively normal, marked wasting is felt over bony prominences of the head, scapulae, epaxial muscles over the thoracic and lumbar vertebrae, and pelvic bones.

Sarcopenia results in decreased muscle strength and early fatigue, causing reduced physical activity and starting a vicious cycle. The cycle can be slowed down by concentric exercises (exercises causing a muscle contraction that shortens the muscle) like walking on the underwater treadmill, wearing weights on the legs, use of therapy bands, and other methods. Often, the only early indicator of sarcopenia may be a decrease in performance. As the muscle fibers atrophy there is loss of elasticity and reduced oxygen transport to the muscles. Care should be taken to differentiate this syndrome from cachexia, neoplasia, and osteoarthritis, as these are processes that also occur in the musculoskeletal system. Cachexia is also loss of lean body mass but is associated with a chronic illness. Osteoarthritis is a chronic degenerative joint disease that is common in aging animals, but which can also occur in young animals.

Myofascial Pain Syndrome

Pain and mobility issues caused by the skeletal system and the nervous system are often easily recognized. However, recognition of muscle and myofascial pain is less commonly recognized. Myofascial pain syndrome is a chronic disorder in which pressure on sensitive points in the muscles (trigger points) cause pain in apparently unrelated parts of the body (referred pain). Myofascial pain syndrome typically occurs after a muscle

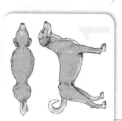
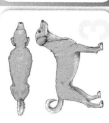
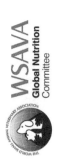
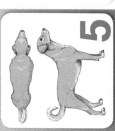
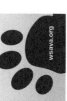
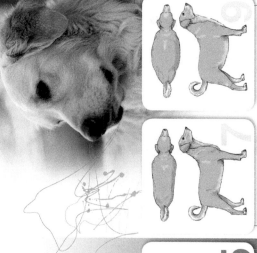

Figure 14.1 WSAVA body condition score (© 2013, WSAVA).

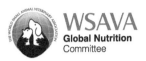

Muscle Condition Score

Muscle condition score is assessed by visualization and palpation of the spine, scapulae, skull, and wings of the ilia. Muscle loss is typically first noted in the epaxial muscles on each side of the spine; muscle loss at other sites can be more variable. Muscle condition score is graded as normal, mild loss, moderate loss, or severe loss. Note that animals can have significant muscle loss if they are overweight (body condition score > 5). Conversely, animals can have a low body condition score (< 4) but have minimal muscle loss. Therefore, assessing both body condition score and muscle condition score on every animal at every visit is important. Palpation is especially important when muscle loss is mild and in animals that are overweight. An example of each score is shown below.

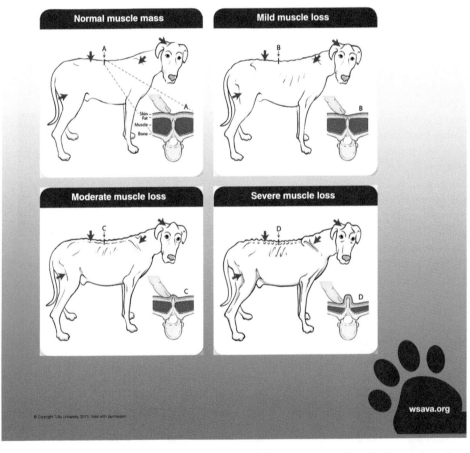

wsava.org

© Copyright Tufts University, 2013. Used with permission

Figure 14.2 WSAVA muscle condition score (© 2013, Tufts University; reproduced with permission).

has been contracted repetitively (Mayo Clinic, 2014). Myalgia is defined as pain in a muscle group or muscle that can come from myofascial pain, overuse, inflammation, trauma, poor nutrition, or metabolic and endocrine disorders. Myofascial trigger points (MTPs) are hyperirritable spots located within a band of skeletal muscle. An MTP can be identified by using a flat hand to palpate perpendicular to the muscle fiber direction (or a pincer palpation for muscles with large bellies), to find a taut band. A "knot" contraction within the taut muscle band is the MTP. Application of slight pressure to this point will often cause the dog to demonstration a pain response (Wall, 2014).

In geriatric medicine, there is an opportunity to help regain some muscle function and strength, and to definitely decrease a potential source of pain if myofascial pain syndrome can be diagnosed and treated (Simons *et al.*, 1999). Myofascial pain syndrome is most often the result of a constant low-grade contraction of the affected muscle. Constant contraction ultimately results in depletion of the adenosine triphosphate (energy) required to release the muscle. Pressure on local blood vessels causes a localized ischemia that prevents oxygenated blood from reaching the area where it is most needed. This can become a lingering pattern, resulting in trigger points that can last for months. Consider osteoarthritis affecting the hind limb of a dog causing decreased weight bearing and slight contraction of the muscles (iliopsoas, sartorius, or rectus femoris) when the dog is standing. The arthritic joint is protected but the constant contraction causes trigger points to form, often several within a single muscle (Petty, 2012).

Trigger points are either active or latent, and when these palpable nodules are stimulated mechanically, local pain and referred pain can be induced, together with visible local twitch response. An active MTP is one that refers pain either locally to a large area and another remote location, the local and referred pain can be spontaneous or reproduced by mechanical stimulation that elicits a patient-recognized pain (Ge *et al.*, 2011).

A latent MTP is defined as a focus of hyperirritability in a taut muscle band that is clinically associated with local twitch response and tenderness and referred pain upon manual examination. Treating latent MTPs in patients with musculoskeletal pain may not only decrease pain sensitivity and improve motor functions, but may also prevent latent MTPs from transforming into active MTPs, and hence, may prevent the development of myofascial pain syndrome (Ge and Arendt-Nielsen, 2011).

There is an increased intramuscular electromyography activity at MTPs in an antagonist muscle during an agonist muscle contraction, suggesting an association of a reduced efficiency of reciprocal inhibition with MTPs. This result has important clinical implications in that latent MTPs may be an important initiator to motor dysfunctions in musculoskeletal pain syndromes. (Ibarra *et al.*, 2011). These likely lead to poor motor control and possibly increase the likelihood of injuries.

In humans, it is suggested that the development of muscle fatigue at latent MTPs is approximately four times faster than at non-MTPs. Elimination of latent MTPs and inactivation of active MTPs may effectively reduce muscle fatigue and prevent overload spreading within a single muscle in musculoskeletal pain conditions (Ge *et al.*, 2012). This suggests that if latent trigger points can be identified and treated in geriatric patients, it may be possible to decrease how quickly their muscles fatigue.

Latent MTPs are also associated with a reduced efficiency of reciprocal inhibition. Reciprocal inhibition is interference of spinal cord motor neurons innervating muscles whose contraction would oppose an initiated movement; for example, when flexing the elbow to lift a weight, the elbow extensors are relaxed. The term was introduced in the 1890s by Charles Sherrington (British neurophysiologist and Nobel prize winner) and later came to be known as Sherrington's law (Jennett, 2008). Thus, trigger points play a major role in the control of voluntary movements and have been studied in animals and human models at rest, during contraction, and after electrical stimulation in different groups of muscles (Crone, 1993; Hamm and Alexander 2010).

Treatment of MTPs can be with a therapeutic laser, therapeutic ultrasound, digital compression, and dry needling. Digital compression is the most practical; laser and ultrasound are effective but require equipment that may not always be readily available. Dry needling is considered to be the most effective and least expensive treatment of MTPs in dogs (Petty, 2012). An acupuncture needle is used to make contact with the trigger point. When contact is made, an involuntary twitch occurs that involves a spinal reflex loop. This occurs even if the animal is anesthetized, and instantly releases the contraction. Trigger points can remain latent for weeks, months or years but have the potential to become active again.

Osteoarthritis

Osteoarthritis is by far one of the most common causes of chronic pain in canine and feline patients. A single definition of osteoarthritis remains elusive. At a 1995 workshop, the American Academy of Orthopedic Surgeons proposed the following consensus definition:

> Osteoarthritic diseases are a result of both mechanical and biologic events that destabilize the normal coupling of degradation and synthesis of articular cartilage chondrocytes, extracellular matrix, and subchondral bone. Although they may be initiated by multiple factors, including genetic, developmental, metabolic, and traumatic factors, osteoarthritic diseases involve all of the tissues of the diarthrodial joint. Ultimately, osteoarthritic diseases are manifested through morphologic, biochemical, molecular, and biomechanical changes in both cells and matrix that lead to softening, fibrillation, ulceration, articular cartilage loss, sclerosis and subchondral bone eburnation, and osteophyte production. When clinically evident, osteoarthritic diseases are characterized by joint pain, tenderness, movement limitation, crepitus, occasional effusion, and variable degrees of inflammation without systemic effects.
>
> (Brandt, 2010)

Osteoarthritis, in essence, is thinning and damage of articular cartilage, subchondral bone sclerosis, marginal bone, and cartilage growth as osteophytes, and periarticular muscle wasting. Cartilage is a unique tissue with viscoelastic and compressive qualities, owing to its extracellular matrix, which is composed of predominately type-II collagen and proteoglycans. Under normal conditions, the extracellular matrix is subjected to dynamic remodeling processes in which low-level synthetic and degradative enzymatic activities are balanced. In cartilage affected by osteoarthritis, the matrix degrading enzymes are overexpressed, shifting the balance toward net degradation, resulting in loss of collagen and proteoglycans from the matrix (Krüger *et al.*, 2012).

Chondrogenic differentiation of human subchondral progenitor cells is affected by synovial fluid from donors with osteoarthritis or rheumatoid arthritis. Owing to this loss, chondrocytes proliferate and produce supplemental amounts of proteoglycans and collagen. However, as the disease proceeds, the progressive cartilage degradation overwhelms the reparative processes. Initially, fibrillation, cracking, and erosion appear in the superficial layers of the cartilage, eventually resulting in larger clinically observable erosions. Several differences between osteoarthritic cartilage and aging cartilage exist, suggesting that osteoarthritis is more of a disease rather than just a natural process of aging. Denatured collagen is found both in natural aging cartilage and osteoarthritis cartilage, but it is more predominant in osteoarthritis. Osteoarthritis is a disease of the joints, although the pain is mostly felt at the periarticular structures, not at the joint surface. Pain is caused by the inflamed synovium and the tension placed on a joint capsule that has become fibrotic. This is a disease of the entire joint, caused by synovitis, joint fibrosis, and atrophy.

Patients with arthritis can have decreased mobility, a decreased range of motion, muscle atrophy, reduced activity, and increased stiffness and pain, which can, in turn, lead to more decreased mobility, more muscle loss, worsened pain, and diminished flexibility.

Feline Osteoarthritis

Cats are notoriously difficult subjects when it comes to pain assessment. Consequently, feline pain recognition and intervention have historically been deficient (Muir *et al.*, 2004). Feline osteoarthritis is particularly challenging for owners and veterinarians to identify, purportedly because signs such as overt lameness are rare (Hardie *et al.*, 2002; Lascelles, 2010). In one of the first studies designed to determine the prevalence of degenerative joint disease in cats, radiographs of 100 cats more than 12 years old (taken as part of a diagnostic work-up for multiple reasons) were retrospectively reviewed; 90% of them showed radiographic evidence of degenerative joint disease (Hardie *et al.*, 2002). Overweight cats have an increased risk of non-injury-related lameness, which may include osteoarthritis (Scarlett and Donoghue, 1998; Bennett and Morton, 2009). Studies show differences in demeanor, activity, mobility, self-grooming, and elimination habits between cats with and without osteoarthritis, and in cats with osteoarthritis before and after treatment. These findings confirm the presence of osteoarthritic pain in cats, and the resultant disability affecting their quality of life, and also that signs can be detected by cat owners (Clarke and Bennett, 2006; Bennett and Morton, 2009).

Canine Osteoarthritis

Osteoarthritis is a common problem affecting up to 60% of dogs (Millis *et al.*, 2014). Passive stretching has been shown to increase range of motion in affected dogs. Owners of Labrador Retrievers with osteoarthritis and restricted joint motion were given instructions for a home stretching program. Owners performed ten passive stretches with a hold of ten seconds twice daily. After 21 days, goniometric measurements showed that the passive stretching had significantly increased the range of motion of the joints by 7% to 23% (Crook *et al.*, 2007).

Although it is still under some debate, there is a theory that sarcopenia and osteoarthritis go hand in hand and maintain a vicious cycle. The injection of botulinum type-A toxin in knee extensor muscles of rabbits induced muscle weakening by partial inhibition of acetylcholine at the neuromuscular junction. After four weeks, initial signs of articular cartilage degradation could be observed, with obvious changes observed in the patellofemoral region, indicating that muscle weakness could be a risk factor for joint degeneration leading to osteoarthritis (Youssef *et al.*, 2009). In the initially healthy joint surrounded by muscle, when the muscle becomes weak, altered muscle mass and quality, altered protein synthesis and myonuclear apoptosis possibly precipitate osteoarthritis. The joint develops cartilage degradation; chondrocyte apoptosis, inflammation, subchondral bone remodeling, bone marrow lesions, and osteophyte activity lead to further muscle weakening.

Treatment Goals

In both feline and canine patients, the goals of treating the arthritis are to decrease pain, preserve range of motion, and to maintain function and quality of life. In the past, the limited treatment options available to veterinarians would have included surgery, lifestyle changes, and anti-inflammatories to negate the lameness and pain from osteoarthritis. Now, as physical rehabilitation is emerging in the veterinary field, there are many more options to combat both sarcopenia and osteoarthritis. The medical treatment of sarcopenia and arthritis is multifaceted and includes physical modalities, controlled therapeutic exercises, changes in the home environment, and disease-modifying osteoarthritic agents.

Physical Treatment Modalities

Cryotherapy

Cryotherapy is a method in physical therapy that refers to the application of cold. Local application of cold reduces blood flow through vasoconstriction, thus reducing the response to acute inflammation or injury. The response includes edema, hemorrhage, histamine release, local metabolism muscle spindle activity, nerve conduction velocity, pain and spasticity. It is a superficial treatment but can have effects of up to 3 cm of tissue depth. The depth of cold penetration depends on the amount of adipose tissue and the blood flow at the site. Therefore, cryotherapy may be more effective in the extremities where joints, tendons, and ligaments are more superficial, and there is less adipose tissue present (Palmer and Knight, 1996).

In veterinary medicine, cryotherapy is primarily used locally. It temporarily increases connective tissue stiffness and decreases tensile strength; it also increases muscle viscosity temporarily, which decreases rapid movement performance. Effects of cooling therapy include:

- vasoconstriction, which leads to decreased cell metabolism, diminished blood flow, and avoidance of secondary cellular hypoxic injury
- increased cold receptor activity, followed by decreased nerve conduction velocity of primary afferent fibers, which together act as a counter irritant providing pain gating to decrease pain and increase pain tolerance

- decreased gamma motor neuron activity resulting in decreased muscle spindle activity and subsequent decreased muscle spasm.

Cryotherapy should be applied within the first 48 hours following an acute musculo-skeletal injury, or anytime there is heat or swelling in a muscle or joint. The cold pack can be left on for 10–20 minutes and with application repeated every 2 hours; if left in place longer there is a possibility for skin tissue damage. The effects occur when the tissue temperature reaches 59–66 degrees F. Cold packs can be crushed ice packs (preferred), gel packs, artificial ice packs, or crushable chemical packs (not preferred because they usually do not get the area cold enough). Homemade options are to place liquid dishsoap in a ziplock bag, or a mix of 50% isopropyl alcohol and 50% water in ziplock bag and put in the freezer; it stays cold for a while and bends around the joint nicely. It is recommended that a towel be placed between the skin surface and the ice pack when using gel packs. Commercially available cold compression systems are made by Game Ready™ and Cryo Cuff®. A cold pack can also be made using a crushed ice pack and elastic bandage (Vetrap®). Vapocoolant sprays are not recommended.

Cryotherapy is safe to apply over inflamed tissue, diseased skin areas, irradiated tissues, areas of known malignancy, epiphyses, and implants. It is safe to use on the lower back or abdomen of pregnant animals, and on the chest, heart, and head. Cold packs should not be used in areas of impaired circulation, over chronic wounds, or over regenerating nerves. They should be used with caution in areas of impaired sensation, on damaged skin, and near or over the eyes. Intensity and size of application should be reduced in patients with cardiac failure and those with hypertension.

Thermotherapy

Thermotherapy refers to the therapeutic use of heat. Heating agents can be superficial (less than 2 cm tissue depth) or deep (greater than 2 cm tissue depth). Effects of heat therapy include:

- vasodilation, which in turn increases cell metabolism and blood flow, aids in soft tissue healing and facilitates removal of chemical irritants from nociceptors
- activation of thermoreceptor activity, which promotes a counter-irritant effect, through the pain gate mechanism decreasing pain and promoting relaxation
- decreased tissue viscosity, leading to warming of intra-articular tissues, thereby reducing joint stiffness.

Local application of heat decreases blood pressure, muscle spasm, and pain. It increases body temperature, respiratory rate, and possibly heart rate, if applied for long enough. The application of heat also increases capillary pressure, leukocyte migration into the heated area, local circulation, local metabolism, muscle relaxation, and tissue elasticity (Hayes, 1993).

Application of thermotherapy is best after the acute inflammation stage. Superficial heat directly penetrates to about 1 cm tissue depth. Optimal effects occur when the tissues reach 105–113 degrees F. The skin and subcutaneous tissue can reach this range after about 5 minutes of superficial heat while it takes 15–30 minutes for deeper tissues to reach the same temperatures. Heat sources are classified as:

- radiant transfer of energy in the form of rays, waves or particles (for example, an infrared lamp)

- conductive transfer of heat between two objects of different temperatures after coming into contact with each other (as in use of a hot pack)
- convection transfer of heat to or from an object by passage of fluid or air past its surface (a dryer or whirlpool for instance)
- conversion — when a form of energy other than heat (mechanical, electricity, chemical) is converted to heat within the body; conversion is the only way of increasing the temperature of deep tissues to therapeutic levels.

Some indications for use of heat would be for pain relief, to increase circulation, decrease muscle spasm, facilitate tissue healing, to help release tissue scars, and to prepare stiff muscles or joints for exercise. In geriatric patients, often a hot pack is applied for ten minutes before passive range of motion of the joints. Thermotherapy is safe to use over active epiphyses, over superficial or regenerating nerves, and over implants. It is safe near chronic wounds, near the head, chest, and heart, and for patients with hypertension.

Thermotherapy should not be used on an area so large that it would increase the body temperature in pregnant patients or cardiac patients. It should not be used over areas of impaired sensation, actively bleeding tissues, the testes, recently irradiated tissues, or on areas of edema or inflamed tissues. It should be used cautiously in areas over the eyes, and in pregnant animals and cases of cardiac failure.

Chiropractic

Chiropractic is commonly and successfully used for the geriatric patient. Regular chiropractic adjustments are recommended for musculoskeletal issues, stilted gait, neurologic disorders, or animals with amputations. Chiropractic treatments can also improve overall mentation, attitude and sometimes resolve other chronic ailments. Chiropractic adjustment is a procedure that uses controlled force, leverage, direction, amplitude, and velocity, directed at specific joints or areas. These adjustments are used to influence joint and neurophysiological conditions.

Laser therapy

Low-level laser therapy (LLLT) refers to the use of cold lasers. Laser is an acronym for light amplification by stimulated emission of radiation. Lasers emit radiation in the form of a flow of photons. There are four different classes of laser:

- Class I (<0.5 mW) lasers can emit visible or nonvisible light; they provide no heat or effect on tissue. These are the lasers common in everyday life, such as used in supermarket scanners and remote controls.
- Class II lasers (<1 mW) include items such as laser pointers and some therapy lasers. All emit visible light, are safe on the skin for extended periods, and are safe for the eyes for short periods.
- Class IIIa (<5 mW) lasers emit visible light and include some therapy lasers; class IIIb (>5 mW) lasers emit nonvisible light, and include some survey lasers and therapy lasers. Class IIIb lasers are hazardous to the eyes but not the skin. These lasers can be helium neon, infrared, galium arsenide, or galium aluminum arsenide.
- Class IV lasers (carbon dioxide, argon, neodymium-doped yttrium aluminum garnet) increase tissue temperature. The high-powered class IV lasers are used to cut through tissues; these are the surgical lasers. Low-powered class IV lasers are used to stimulate tissue repair through a process of photobiomodulation.

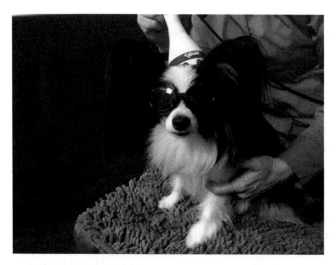

Figure 14.3 Therapeutic laser.

The first law of photobiology states that, for low-power visible light to have any effect on a living biological system, the photons must be absorbed by electronic absorption bands belonging to some molecular chromophore or photoacceptor (Sutherland, 2002). The method of action of photobiomodulation is still questioned among many scientists. There are likely many mechanisms of action depending on the target cell and the type of cell being modulated. The most published and recognized is the cytochrome c system, which is a photoreceptor found in the inner cell membrane of the mitochondria

Low-powered class IV therapeutic lasers deliver specific red and near-infrared wavelengths of laser light to induce a photochemical reaction and therapeutic effect (Figure 14.3). The laser light interacts with tissue at the cellular level increasing metabolic activity within the cell, causing a cascade of reactions that increase cellular function and enhance tissue repair. Physiological effects include increased circulation, reduced inflammation, pain reduction, and enhanced tissue healing. Laser therapy should not be used over areas of malignancy or the thyroid gland, and care must be taken to protect the eyes from exposure.

Therapeutic ultrasound

Ultrasound refers to high-frequency acoustic waves. When used clinically, these sound waves are produced by the transducer head of the instrument. Ultrasound provides heat to deeper tissues and in a more localized area than can be attained with a hot pack. The most common therapeutic ultrasound frequencies are 1 and 3 MHz, used in either continuous or pulsed mode. Continuous waves heat the tissues to 104–112 degrees F, which lasts for only five to eight minutes after the cessation of treatment. The effects of continuous ultrasound are similar to those described for superficial heat, as well as increasing soft tissue (collagen) extensibility, pain tolerance, macrophage activity, nerve conduction velocity, tissue repair, restoring motion lost from a scar and relieving muscle spasm.

Pulsed ultrasound is used to reduce swelling and for tissue and bone repair; 1 MHz frequency penetrates to 2–5 cm; it is a longer wavelength, so has poorer absorption due to attenuation. Higher intensity is needed to affect the deeper tissue. The shorter wavelength of 3 MHz penetrates to 0.5–2 cm and has better absorption at lower intensities for more superficial target areas (Fyfe and Bullock, 1985).

Therapeutic ultrasound is used to treat muscle spasms, wound healing, tendonitis, bursitis, capsulitis, trigger points, adhesions, calcifications, and fracture healing. Therapeutic ultrasound is safe over metal implants as long as there is no compromised skin overlying the implant. It is contraindicated in pregnant animals and on testes. It should not be used over malignancy, the eyes, epiphyses in young animals, irradiated tissue, or on a laminectomy site or any tissue with decreased circulation.

Electrical Stimulation

Electrical stimulation modalities include transcutaneous electrical neuromuscular stimulation (TENS) and neuromuscular electrical stimulation (NMES; Figure 14.4). TENS is the application of an electrical current to provide pain relief by depolarizing sensory nerves. Evidence supports the opiate system for pain modulation when set at specific settings. When human patients whose pain was being relieved by TENS treatment were given naloxone, an inhibitor of endogenous and endogenous opiates, the pain returned rapidly (Mannheimer and Lampe, 1984; Wall, 1994). Low-frequency TENS activates opioid, gamma-aminobutyric acid, serotonin, and muscarinic receptors to reduce dorsal horn neuron activity and nociception and stimulates a release of endogenous opiates. High-frequency TENS stimulates larger-diameter peripheral nerve fibers that help block nociceptive activity in smaller afferent fibers. Higher frequency also increased endorphin release into the bloodstream and cerebrospinal fluid, and enkephalins into the cerebrospinal fluid. It decreased the release of the excitatory neurotransmitters glutamate and substance P in the spinal cord dorsal horn in patients with inflammation (Maeda *et al.*, 2007).

Contraindications for veterinary use of TENS include any animal with a pacemaker. TENS should not be applied near cervical ganglia, the eyes, ears, or the heart. It must be avoided in the lumbar area of pregnant animals, around any growths or tumors, areas of desensitization, and in animals with seizure disorders (Johnson and Levine, 2004).

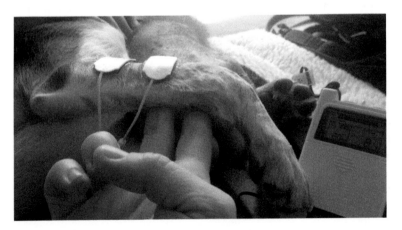

Figure 14.4 Neuromuscular electrical stimulation.

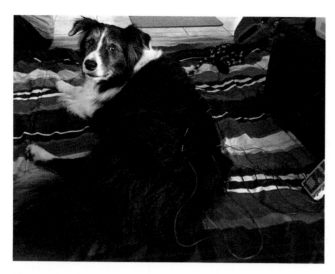

Figure 14.5 Electro-acupuncture.

When TENS is used on the veterinary patient, the hair over the area to which the electrodes will be placed should be clipped and wiped with alcohol. If the animal has short hair, it may not be necessary to clip it, but a proper coupling medium should be used. The electrodes should be positioned around the painful area, or over a nerve or nerve root. Acupuncture points can be incorporated (Figure 14.5; Vance *et al.*, 2014).

NMES is used for strengthening and to minimize muscle atrophy in patients when it is not possible or contraindicated for them to bear weight. It is commonly used in patients recovering from cranial cruciate ligament surgery or femoral head osteotomy. Other indications are disuse atrophy, pain, neurological atrophy, joint effusion, improper muscle firing sequences, and tendon or fracture healing (Canapp, 2007).

The frequency used for NMES can be 2–60 Hz; 20 Hz has been shown to prevent atrophy of slow-twitch muscle fibers; 30 Hz has been shown to prevent fast-twitch muscle fiber atrophy and 2–10 Hz is best for disuse atrophy.

Hyperbaric Oxygen Therapy

The goal of hyperbaric oxygen therapy is to increase oxygenation in diseased or injured tissue to support function and healing. This goal is accomplished through increased oxygenation of the blood via the pulmonary system. Some increased local tissue oxygenation can also occur through open wounds devoid of epidermal tissue. Typically, a hyperbaric oxygen chamber is used to deliver 100% oxygen under pressure. Such chambers are now available for the small animal practice. Currently there are only a handful of veterinary hospitals in the United States that offer hyperbaric oxygen therapy for small animals (Veterinary Specialty Care, n.d.).

Conditions in the geriatric veterinary patient that could potentially benefit from hyperbaric oxygen therapy include trauma, wound healing, fibrocartilaginous embolism, and intervertebral disc disease. Hyperbaric therapy is contraindicated in untreated pneumothorax, tension pneumothorax, seizure disorders, chronic emphysema with CO_2 retention, high fevers, history of spontaneous pneumothorax, thoracic surgery, otosclerosis, viral infections of the respiratory tract, and optic neuritis. It is also contraindicated if the patient is being treated with mafenide acetate cream for burn patients, or concurrent treatment with cis-platinum, disulfiram or doxorubicin.

Physical Rehabilitation

The goals of veterinary physical rehabilitation are to maintain, restore, and promote optimal function and quality of life as they relate to movement. A major emphasis is to minimize clinical signs and functional limitations that may be brought about by diseases, injuries or disorders. Whether the diagnosis is sarcopenia or osteoarthritis, both can benefit from many of the same therapeutic exercises. Therapeutic aspects of physical rehabilitation may include modification of the home environment, therapy to improve flexibility, exercises to improve range of motion and muscle strength, techniques to improve balance and massage therapy.

Home Environment

At home, most owners will first notice the pet's inability to walk, stand, or lie down easily. It is difficult for the owner to determine whether the pet is in pain, and many owners will perceive weakness as pain. The majority of owners have the primary concern of ensuring their pet is not in pain.

There are some things can be changed in the home environment that will make a difference. One is the surface that the pet has to walk on. Wood floors and slick tile or marble are the most challenging for a mobility impaired pet; it is very difficult for the pet to get up or feel comfortable walking when they tend to slip or slide. Placing carpet runners or yoga mats in strategic areas can help. Sometimes, even with carpet runners, the pets will choose to be on the slick surface, probably to get cool, so setting a small fan next to their bed or favorite spot on the carpeted surface will help them stay cool and motivate them to navigate areas with better footing. If the house has stairs, they should be carpeted or have stair tread mats or in some cases be bypassed with a pet ramp or wheelchair ramp.

Hair should be trimmed from between the paw pads to aid in traction. Products applied directly to the paws such as Biogroom Show Foot™ anti-slip spray, or Dr Buzby's™ toegrips (www.toegrips.com) will provide more traction, so the pet feels more confident in walking (Figure 14.6).

When the owner is home, setting a timer and encouraging the pet to get up every two hours is very beneficial, even if the pet just gets up, turns around and lies back down. If the pet has difficulty getting up from the floor or walking, use of a towel under the abdomen or a harness can be helpful. The Help'em up™ harness, which has a handle between the shoulder blades and a handle over the pelvis, can be of great assistance(Figure 14.7).

If pets are unable to move around or find it difficult, they can become frustrated and depressed. Efforts to enrich their environment can help. Enrichment techniques usually fall into four categories (with some overlap) – sensory, novelty, social, and alternate types of exercise. Sensory enrichments can address sight, smell, hear, taste, and touch. Giving the pet an area where they can see out of a window, and hiding treats around the house for them to find, are examples. Using a wagon or stroller to take the pet on walks

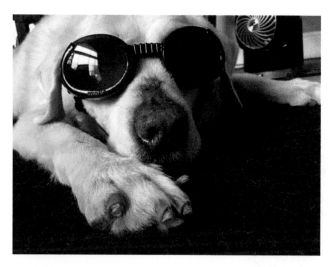

Figure 14.6 Dr. Buzby's ToeGrips.

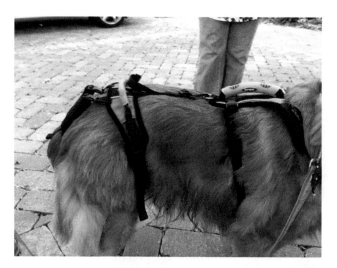

Figure 14.7 HelpEmUp Harness.

is also beneficial (Figure 14.8). Creating novelty in the animal's environment is another form of enrichment. This could include periodically changing out the toys and beds in the area where the pet spends most of its time. Toys specifically designed for mental stimulation (Figure 14.9) can be especially helpful (such as those designed for dogs by Nina Ottosson, www.nina-ottosson.com).

If the pet likes dogs, cats or people make sure they get to socialize and maintain exposure to their "friends". This can be accomplished by taking the pet for a ride in a wagon or stroller to visit a neighbor, or by arranging to have pets and people come visit the animal at home.

Light physical exercise, such as teaching a new trick like a nose touch or giving a paw, may not be strenuous but it is good mental exercise. Several of the products made by

Figure 14.8 Stroller.

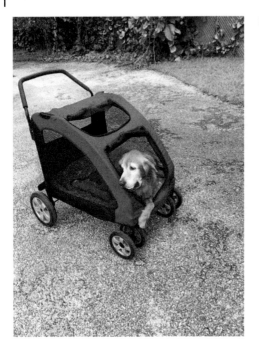

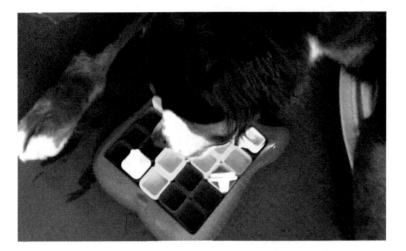

Figure 14.9 Brain game.

FitPAWS® (K9Fitbone™, balance disks; www.fitpawsusa.com) can be used at home to teach new tricks, as well as to perform exercises as recommended to maintain strength and flexibility (Figure 14.10). Indoor treadmills especially designed for dogs can also be used to provide controlled physical exercise. Treadmills in different sizes are available from DogTread (www.dogtread.com).

Figure 14.10 Cat on the balance disk.

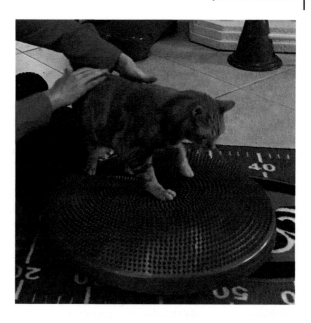

Flexibility and Range of Motion

There is a difference between range-of-motion and flexibility. Range of movement refers to joint movement; flexibility refers to muscle and tendon elasticity. Often, flexibility issues appear in two-joint muscles rather than one-joint muscles. Once the affected muscle has been determined, therapeutic exercise that focuses upon stretching that muscle can be initiated. In the ambulatory patient, some form of warm-up is recommended before initiating any stretching work. In the non-ambulatory patient, electrical stimulation, or therapeutic ultrasound may be used for the warm-up.

Stretches can be done actively or passively (Table 14.1). An active stretch is one that is initiated by the patient. One of the most common forms of active stretching techniques – "biscuit stretches" – involves the use of treats to encourage the patient to reach into positions that will stretch the affected muscle. Examples include supporting the dog while holding a treat near one hip. The dog will stretch the contralateral epaxial muscles in an effort to reach the treat. Active stretches can also be accomplished through active exercise, such as walking through weave poles or around cones set in a tight pattern.

The therapist performs passive stretches. The patient must be relaxed and willing to accept this stretching work. This work is generally well accepted by the patient once they gain confidence in the therapist. An example of a passive stretch is the therapist extending the hip joint, stretching the quadriceps muscle.

Arthritic joints can commonly lose range of motion due to pain and soft tissue contracture. The goal when working on range of motion is to gain a functional amount of movement for the joint. Range of motion exercises are useful to diminish the effects of disuse and immobilization. (Brody 2011). Range-of-motion exercises can be applied actively or passively. True passive range-of-motion exercise is performed without muscle contraction and is facilitated by a therapist, who creates the motion, such as gentle flexion and extension of the elbow. In the active range of motion exercise,

Table 14.1 Range of motion exercises.

Exercise	Description
Hind limb	
Toe extensions	Gently hold each toe individually, with your index finger on top and thumb on the bottom, near the foot. Lightly pull the toe while bending the toe up, away from the paw pads.
Toe curls	Gently hold each toe individually, with your index finger on top and thumb on the bottom, near the foot. Lightly pull the toe while bending it down over your thumb, toward the paw pads.
Tail presses	Place your index finger on one side of the tail and thumb on the other side, between the vertebrae near the base of the tail. Apply gentle pressure for 5 seconds, and then move down the tail to the next space between the vertebrae. Continue to the end of the tail.
Hock extension (170 degrees)	With the dog lying on its side, place on one hand on the distal aspect of the tibia and the other hand on the upper metatarsals. Gently move the paw so that the tarsal joint is straight.
Hock flexion (40 degrees)	With the dog lying on its side, place one hand on the stifle to stabilize and the other hand on the upper the metatarsals or the bottom of the paw. Gentle move the top of the paw toward the knee joint.
Hip joint extension (163 degrees)	With the dog lying on the side, place one hand just above the stifle and the other hand on the pelvis. Gently guide the leg backward.
Hip joint flexion (55 degrees)	With the dog lying on its side, place one hand just behind the stifle and gently guide the stifle toward the ribs/back.
Front limb	
Toe curls	As described for hind limb above.
Carpus hyperextension (195 degrees)	Place one hand on the distal radius and ulna, and the other hand on the front foot. Gently bend the foot out in front of the limb until tension is reached.
Carpus flexion (30 degrees)	Place one hand on the distal radius and ulna, the other on the foot. Gently bend the foot caudally until resistance or the paw pads touch the back of the limb.
Elbow extension (165 degrees)	Place one hand on the distal humerus and the other hand on the distal radius and ulna, the other above the carpus. Straighten the limb until resistance is felt.
Elbow flexion (30 degrees)	Place one hand on the distal humerus and the other hand on the distal radius and ulna, above the carpus. Gently guide the wrist toward the shoulder joint.
Shoulder joint extension (165 degrees)	With the dog lying on its side, place one hand behind elbow, and use the other hand to help hold the limb parallel to the floor. Gently guide the limb forward by pushing behind the elbow.
Shoulder flexion (45 degrees)	With the dog lying on its side, place hand in the front of the elbow and gently guide the elbow toward the ribs/back.
Biscuits to the side	With the dog in a standing position and using a treat as a lure, guide the pet's head around to the shoulders, ribs and rump.

the patient is encouraged to perform exercises that cause the joint to assume the desired range, such as walking over cavalettis.

Complete relaxation is rare in veterinary patients, so most range of motion exercises are active assisted. When applying exercises to increase the range of motion, improvement in active range of motion compared with passive range of motion must be considered. It may not be feasible to reach a normal range of motion, depending upon the lesion(s) affecting the joint, so the focus is on a functional outcome.

It is best to perform passive range of motion exercises in a quiet environment with the patient on a comfortable surface in lateral recumbency. When performing these exercises, it is best to involve only one joint at a time, while keeping the other joints in a neutral position. The movements should start small and increase until the endpoint of the range of motion is reached, and the patient appears to resist slightly. Applying steady pressure for 15–30 seconds at the end of flexion and extension of the joint results in stretching. Ten to fifteen repetitions performed two to three times a day is generally sufficient.

To assess the success of range of motion exercises, a goniometer can be used before and after therapy. The measurements may be recorded in the patient's medical record and followed throughout treatment. It is important to remember that improvements achieved with range of motion exercises will be slow and gradual. These movements can be done to determine if there is a joint that has a limited range of movement, and also as treatment to help stop or slow down any further decrease in the joint's movement. This list is not all inclusive, but is a good general guideline and covers all the major joints. All of the joint movements can be measured with a goniometer (not pictured) to determine the angles of flexion, extension, abduction, adduction, internal and external rotation.

Strengthening and Therapeutic Exercises

Therapeutic exercises are one of the most important tools in the patient maintaining or returning to the best function possible. The intensity of an exercise may be decreased or increased by changing the duration, frequency and speed that the pet performs the task. The best therapeutic exercises for a particular patient will be determined by the problem list, goals, current strength and endurance of that pet. During the rehabilitation program, these exercises will constantly be reevaluated and altered so they continue to be challenging and promote strength. An area of strength training which has received a great deal of interest lately is core strengthening. This is done to help prevent thoracolumbar and lumbosacral injuries, especially in the aging patient, canine athlete, and in chondrodystrophic breeds. Core strengthening exercises include three-leg standing, two-leg standing, and standing on an uneven surface. Care must be taken to avoid excessive work in this kind of strength training, as fatigue occurs rapidly. Some types of therapeutic exercise are shown in Table 14.2.

Balance and Proprioception

Many geriatric patients struggle with body awareness, especially with proprioception. Proprioception is defined as the awareness of body's position. Afferent information from proprioceptors (mechanoreceptors) contributes to conscious sensations, total posture, and segmental posture. Improving proprioception enhances patient neuromuscular

Table 14.2 Strengthening exercises.

Exercise	Description
Fore limb	
Walking downhill	Walk downhill starting with a mild incline and increasing to a steeper hill.
Cavalettis	Walking over cavalettis, mop/broom handles, or PVC pipe. Begin by setting the distance between poles greater than the distance from the top of the pets shoulders to it's feet. Ensure that the pet walks slowly, making sure that each foot is placed individually and there is no bunny hopping. Place the treats on the ground so they are looking at the floor and not at your hand.
Digging	Have the dog dig in the sand or designated area for a treat. One can also hide toy or treat under blanket.
High five or wave	Start by placing a scrunchie on the nose or some masking tape on the head, when the dog paws to get it off, give them a treat as reward for lifting the paw.
Three-leg standing	Start by lifting one leg off the ground. If lifting the rear leg, lift the limb backwards; whereas if lifting the front leg, lift the limb forward. Support the leg lightly, not allowing the pet to compensate by pushing your hand. Try to have the dog hold this position as long as they can, then repeat with the other legs.
Wheelbarrow	Lift the pet's hind legs off the floor by gently holding under the abdomen. Start with standing, and then progress by moving forward then eventually backward.
Stand to down to stand	From a standing position have the pet move to a sphinx lying position then stand again.
Play bow or push-ups	Use a treat to lure the pet from a normal standing position to its nose between its front paws into a bowing position then have it return to normal standing position.
Lateral walking	This is one of the most important exercises for geriatrics that live in homes with slick floors. Stand on one side of the dog, then step toward the dog's side causing, them to move in a side-stepping motion.
Hind limb	
Three-leg standing	As described above.
Sit to stand to sit	Have the pet sit then move to a standing position then return to a sitting position.
Sit to stand on an elevated surface	This technique is helpful for the weaker patient. Have the pet sit on an object that is elevated (box, owner's leg, step). As the patient gets stronger, lower the height of the object gradually.
Cavalettis	As described above.
Front feet on step	Keep the pet's back legs on the floor and place the front limbs on a step or couch cushion or chair.
Dancing	Lift front legs off of the ground, initially just from a standing position, then as the pet gets stronger can move forward and backward.
Walking up stairs	Find some steps with a gentle incline and increase the angle of the incline as the pet gets stronger.
Walking backwards	Make an alleyway using chairs or hallway, walk toward the pet as it is facing you. When the dog takes a step backwards, give reward. Increase the number of steps backwards over time.

Table 14.2 (Continued)

Exercise	Description
Lateral walking	As described above.
Core	
Roll over both directions	From a lying position, have the pet roll over in one direction then roll over in the opposite direction.
Wobble board	Standing on a wobble board, rocker board, balance disc, boogie board on the water.
Beg or sit pretty	Have the pet bring their front feet off of the ground from a sitting position, eventually to a stable position where the back is straight.
Sit ups and side sit ups	From a lying position, either on the side or on the back, lure your dog to follow the treat with its whole upper body off of the floor then return to the normal lying position.
Tummy tickles	Tickle under the abdomen and chest causing you pet to arch or round its back.
Crawling	From the sphinx lying position, use a treat to lure you pet to crawl, staying as low as possible. Consider the use of chairs for the pet to crawl under.
Cross leg standing	Hold diagonal legs up simultaneously while trying to keep the pet from pushing against you for support.

control and functional joint stability. Therapeutic exercise can address this problem through many avenues. In the debilitated patient, proprioception training might be as simple as assisted standing, which progresses to standing with the addition of gentle rocking by the therapist. When the patient is able to resist these movements without losing balance, more challenges can be added, such as performing these exercises with both front feet on a balance disk (or couch cushion), to walking on a disc or cushion, sand, snow, shallow water, tall grass, and other unstable surfaces, as the patient gains strength.

More active proprioception exercises include walking through a 'pile' of PVC rails or over cavaletti poles, set at irregular heights and distances (Figure 14.11). Standing on a small trampoline or bed, as the dog gains skill on this surface, gentle perturbations can be added by gently pushing to knock the dog off balance, but not knock them over. They should be nudged from all directions as this will increase proprioception and increase strength. Balance discs or blocks are another proprioception tool. The dog can be placed upon these blocks and asked to stand. The blocks can then be slid apart, forward, together and so on, requiring the dog to reestablish its balance. Boogie boarding, a small Styrofoam surfboard, can be used in the pool or in the tub. Have the dog stand on top of the boogie board while proving gentle support to keep the pet from jumping or falling. Altering the course on a walk in figure eights or practicing walking on and off a curb in a zigzag pattern also increases active proprioception.

Massage

Most owners can learn how to perform some simple massage techniques that will give their pet companion relief from muscle soreness and joint stiffness (Table 14.3). Therapeutic massage is the manipulation of the soft tissue (skin and muscle) for the

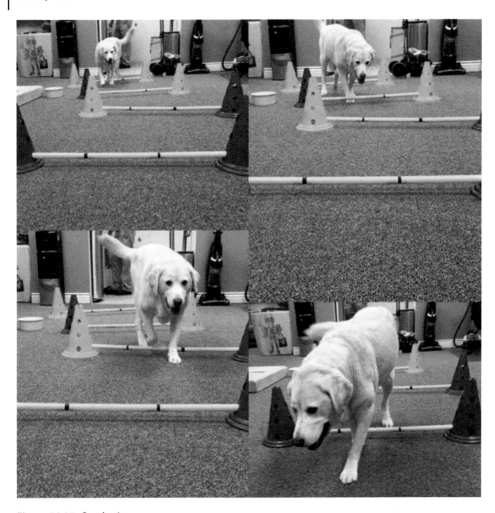

Figure 14.11 Cavalettis.

purpose of increasing blood supply. Effects of massage can include reduction of pain (acute and chronic), decreasing local lactic acidosis and reducing edema, increasing tissue flexibility and breaking down adhesions, reducing stress/cortisol levels and simultaneously strengthening the human–animal bond. Basic techniques of massage are easily applied in the home or clinical setting and are particularly useful for management and comfort of hospice cases (Ballner, 2001).

There are certain situations when a dog should not be massaged at all, or when a specific site should be avoided. These include fever, shock, stroke, broken skin or bleeding wounds, bone fractures, or skin disorders such as ringworm or mange (Hourdebaigt, 2004).

Aquatherapy

Aquatherapy can occur in almost any body of water, bathtub, pool or underwater treadmill (Figure 14.12). Water therapy allows patients with weakness or poor balance to stand without fear of falling. It is beneficial because it allows active muscle contractions

Table 14.3 Massage techniques.

Exercise	Description
Resting touch ("laying on of hands")	This is a starting position, in which hands are simply in contact with the patient, exerting minimal force or pressure. The deliberate application of hands can have a calming effect on the patient, reducing anxiety, reducing cortisol levels, and lessening pain sensations through the gate mechanism.
Petrissage (kneading)	Movements with applied pressure that are deep and compress the underlying muscles. Kneading, wringing, skin rolling, and pick-up-and-squeeze are the petrissage movements. They are all performed with the padded surface of the hand, the surface of the fingers and also the thumbs. During kneading, the hands should be molded to the area, and the movements should be slow and rhythmical.
Effleurage (long flowing stokes)	Soothing, stroking movements used at the beginning and the end of the massage. Effleurage is also used as a linking move between the different strokes and movements. It is a form of massage involving a circular stroking movement made with the palm of the hand. Effleurage can be firm or light without dragging the skin and is performed using either the padded parts of the fingertips or the palmar surface of the hands, and works as a mechanical pump on the body to encourage venous and lymphatic return by starting at the bottom of the limb and pushing back towards the heart.
Compression (gentle squeezing)	This stroke uses a rhythmic pumping movement and is applied using the palmar aspect of the hand. The goal of compression is to spread muscle fibers. When using compression, there should be no gliding over the skin. Compression is most effective when applied to the belly of the muscle, and it is commonly applied proximal to distal.
Friction (focused)	A focused stroke used in a small, localized area. The hands or fingers of the therapist need to maintain a certain amount of stability and consistent pressure to achieve maximum results. This stroke moves superficial layers of tissue against underlying structures. Either circular or transverse movement is used to separate tissue. Keeping firm contact with the skin, the movement is either circular, longitudinal, or across the muscle fibers. The heel of the hand, fingers, braced finger, and thumb(s) may be used to focus on a very specific area. The pressure used should be firm but never too deep.
Tapotement (tapping)	Rhythmic percussion, is most frequently administered with the edge of the hand, a cupped hand, or the tips of the fingers. There are different types of tapotement including beating (closed fist lightly hitting area), slapping (use of fingers to gently slap), tapping (use of fingertips), and cupping (cup the hand and gently tap area). Tapotement is primarily used to "wake up" the nervous system. The strokes are stimulating and can release lymphatic buildup in tissues.
Vibration	Involves oscillatory movements that shake or vibrate the body. These are normally performed at the end of a massage session to stimulate the body with motion.

without as much concussive forces on the joints. Swimming and underwater treadmill therapy can be beneficial not only in patients with injuries, but also in patients with osteoarthritis and obesity. Additionally, it can be used for conditioning healthy canine athletes. Swimming and underwater treadmills can provide cardiovascular conditioning without as much stress on the musculoskeletal system. The temperature, hydrostatic pressure, buoyancy, and resistance properties of water are the reasons that aquatherapy is so valuable in veterinary rehabilitation.

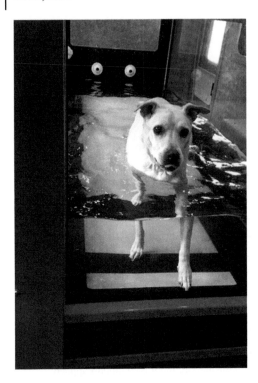

Figure 14.12 Underwater treadmill.

Wheelchairs

Often, in the geriatric patients, the only thing that is really missing is the strength in the hind limbs, or severe arthritis in a joint. Carts come in different configurations. There are carts for hind limb dysfunction, carts for fore limb issues and quad carts help support all four limbs. Every patient should be properly measured before ordering a wheelchair. Each company has different measurement requirements and they are very knowledgeable in fabricating the best possible cart for the pet.

Orthotics

In certain cases, there are orthopedic issues, such as cranial cruciate rupture, where surgery is not an option. Orthotics can be a valuable tool to help maintain mobility in these instances. The company that constructs the orthotic along with the veterinarian can determine if the patient will benefit from the support of the orthotic.

Assistive devices

Knuckling and toe dragging can be a source of frustration for the owner, since it can cause their pet to bleed every time they are out for a walk. There are a few different items to help curtail the toe dragging, knuckling issue. Soft Claws® nail caps can provide another layer of protection for those that are dragging their toenails. The Orthopets Toe-Up® has been developed to assist those dogs who suffer from hind-paw knuckling. The sling prevents knuckling by supporting the two middle digits, and is attached via an adjustable elastic cord to a strap on the hock.

A Ruffwear® boot is also available for those cases where prolonged use of the Toe-up Sciatic Sling is required, or where the dog has delicate or sensitive interdigital skin. Thera-Paw® also produces standard and custom assistive devices for pets with mild to moderate, distal hind limb weakness, the Hindlimb Dorsi-Flex Assist (Thera-Paw) will reduce knuckling, flex the tarsal joint, enhance proprioception, and improve gait. The same company also provides an option for the forelimb (Forelimb Dorsi-Flex Assist) toe dragging and knuckling. There are certain criteria that each pet must meet for these devices to be of benefit. For pets with severe, whole hind limb weakness, a device known as the Biko Progressive Resistance Bands may be more appropriate. This device includes metatarsal cuffs and progressive resistance bands that, when clipped onto the d-ring of a snug-fitting chest harness, will help to advance the whole limb. Note that the paws are not incorporated into this device and the pet may still knuckle. The Help'EmUp™ harness also has a rehabilitation kit that attaches to the harness, which can also help in some of the knuckling, toe dragging instances (Figure 14.11). If fore or hind limbs splaying apart on the floor is a considerable issue, DogLeggs offer hobbles. These hobbles limit the amount of abduction of the limbs. The hobble strap length is adjustable. For dogs or cats with neurologic dysfunction, a more rigid item can be placed around the hobble strap to prevent adduction during supervised rehabilitation therapy, if desired.

Making a Plan

When developing a rehabilitation program for a geriatric patient, one has to look at the whole patient and take into consideration the systems that are affected by aging. In the case of mobility issues, the musculoskeletal and neurologic systems are of primary concern. Common aging conditions likely to affect the musculoskeletal and neurologic systems include neoplasia, sarcopenia, degenerative joint disease, obesity, osteoporosis, intervertebral disc disease, degenerative myelopathy, fibro cartilaginous emboli, lumbosacral disease, geriatric onset laryngeal paralysis polyneuropathy, and cognitive dysfunction.

Physical, neurological and orthopedic exams should be performed to determine the physical limitations that need to be addressed and to have documented baseline information. Appendix 14.1 shows an example of a neurologic exam checklist, and Appendix 14.2 shows an example of an orthopedic exam checklist. During the orthopedic exam, it is helpful to measure the range of motion with a goniometer, as this will provide initial range of motion data for the limbs. These measurements will also be helpful in determining the amount of progress made during the therapy. Appendix 14.3 shows and example mobility checklist.

It is most important to discuss the owner's goals. If in application of a well thought out rehabilitation plan, the patient progressed from barely being able get up from the floor to easily getting up and navigating house, but still being unable to use the doggie door – which is all the owner really wanted – will they see the rehabilitation therapy as a success? The needs or expectations of the owner are paramount to a successful physical therapy plan. The physical, neurological and orthopedic exam will help you, together with the owner, to set reasonable goals. Another key component to developing a therapy plan is determining what the owner is able to do at home, and whether the owner is able to transport the pet to a facility that offers laser, underwater treadmill, or other specialized services. Sometimes getting a large dog in and out of the car several times a week is too much. Box 14.1 shows an example treatment plan for George.

Box 14.1 Example Treatment Plan

The following is an example of a treatment options for a mobile, but weak, geriatric patient, George, a 12-year-old Yellow Labrador Retriever, 70lbs. Please remember that every rehabilitation program should be tailored to the individual patient.

Physical Exam Findings:	Shortened middle hind toenails from dragging the feet; decreased range of motion; muscle atrophy of the hind limbs; swaying gait; tight muscles with trigger points.
Goals:	To maintain limb function, slow further muscle atrophy, and prevent other areas from becoming painful due to overuse.
Medications:	Identify any areas of pain that need to be addressed with medication(s). George is on thyroid medication, NSAID and monthly Adequan® injection.
Lifestyle:	Discuss with the owner as appropriate for the patient.

- George is currently overweight; weight loss may help him to stay mobile longer.
- Make sure that George is getting a minimum of 1g/lb/day protein, so there is enough protein in the diet to support muscle maintenance. (To calculate and compare percentage of nutrients in dog food, use a dog food calculator from, for example Dog Food Advisor: http://www.dogfoodadvisor.com/dog-feeding-tips/dog-food-calculator).
- Please place non-slip runners or yoga mats covering every area to which George has access, and covering the paths he takes to go outside.
- In the house, there should be non-slip runners on every step, including the floor at the bottom and the floor at the top.
- If George prefers to lie on a cool area of the floor instead of on the runners, place a small fan on the floor to encourage him to sleep where he has footing to stand back up.
- If there is an incontinence issue, we could clip the fur away from the areas that may stay damp or soiled.
- Trim the hair off the bottom of George's feet in between the pads.
- If there are areas of the house where the floors are slippery that cannot be covered with runners, apply Dr. Buzby's ToeGrips™ (http://www.orthopets.co.uk/mobility-solutions/ToeGrips).
- Make sure that, when someone is home during the day, George stands up at least every two hours.
- If there is a lot of swaying when George walks, toe dragging, or difficulty getting up off the floor, a Help'em Up harness or sling is recommended.
- Most pets love to have access to a window or glass door, to watch the world outside, since they may be less active.
- Brain games are a very effective way to help relieve some energy since George is not able to burn it off physically.
- George may need a wheelchair down the line; some owners find them scary and you may need time to adjust to the idea. Wait until it is necessary to start using the wheelchair, because ideally we want the muscles to be used as long as possible and to avoid dependence on the wheelchair.

Box 14.1 (Continued)

- Invite human friends or "fur" friends to the home if George is social (he may prefer one over the other).
- You can teach an old dog new tricks! It is very beneficial and fun to teach new tricks or have some fun exercises on therapeutic equipment. If George is too large for you to feel comfortable walking outside away from the house, there are dog-specific treadmills for exercise in the house.

Therapy
- Laser therapy can help to decrease trigger points in the muscles that are being worked harder because of the weakness of the hind limbs.
- Acupuncture will help with overall wellbeing, will address proprioceptive deficits of the hind limbs, and can include dry needling to treat trigger points.
- Chiropractic care helps with neuromodulation, decreasing pain, and assuring proper spinal alignment and mobility, since the gait will be altered.
- Massage is very important to bring increased blood flow to the muscles, alleviate trigger points, and ensure the health of the compensatory muscles.
- Transcutaneous electrical nerve stimulation will help ease pain in specific areas.
- Neuromuscular electrical stimulation will help combat muscle atrophy.
- Therapeutic ultrasound or hot packs should be used to warm muscles prior to exercise.
- Underwater treadmill to maintain muscle strength while minimizing impact to joints.
- Range of motion of each limb joint and massage to be performed by owner every day.

Therapeutic Exercises
- Walk twice every day include figures of eight or zigzags on the walk.
- "High fives" – start with two or three for each front limb and increase the number each week as George gets stronger.
- Sit to stands – start with two or three in a row every day and gradually increase number over time.
- Cavalettis – potentially increasing the height or reducing the distance between the poles as George becomes stronger.

This is not an all-inclusive list but an overview to help better understand the options that are available to aid our geriatric patients. Veterinary rehabilitation is becoming an integral part of managing mobility issues the pet population. Every day, new scientifically based treatments are emerging to give us better therapies to improve the quality of life of our patients.

References

Ballner, M. (2001) *Dog Massage: A Whiskers-to-Tail Guide to Your Dog's Ultimate Petting Experience*. New York, NY: St. Martin's Press.

Brandt, K. D. (2010) *Diagnosis and Nonsurgical Management of Osteoarthritis* (5th ed.) Caddo, OK: Professional Communications Inc.

Brody, L. T. (2011). "Impaired Range of Motion and Joint Mobility." In L. T. Brodie and and C. M. Hall (eds). *Therapeutic Exercise: Moving Toward Function* (3rd ed.), pp. 124–67. Baltimore, MD: Williams and Wilkins.

Bennett, D. and Morton, C. J. (2009) "A Study of Owner Observed Behavioral and Lifestyle Changes in Cats with Musculoskeletal Disease Before and After Analgesic Therapy." *Feline Medicine and Surgery*, 11(12): 997–1004.

Canapp, D. A. (2007) "Select Modalities." *Clinical Techniques in Small Animal Practice*, 22(4):160–5.

Chai, R. J., Vukovic, J., Dunlop, S., Grounds, M. D., Shavlakadze, T. (2011) "Striking Denervation of Neuromuscular Junctions Without Lumbar Motoneuron Loss in Geriatric Mouse Muscle". *PLoS One*, 6: e28090. doi: 10.1371/journal.pone.0028090.

Clarke, S. P., and Bennett, D. (2006) "Feline Osteoarthritis: A Prospective Study of 28 Cases." *Journal of Small Animal Practice*, 47: 439–45.

Crone, C. (1993) "Reciprocal Inhibition in Man." *Danish Medical Bulletin*, 40: 571–81.

Crook, T., McGowan, C., Pead, M. (2007) "Effect of Passive Stretching on the Range of Motion of Osteoarthritic Joints in 10 Labrador Retrievers." *Veterinary Record*, 160: 545–7.

Cruz-Jentoft, A. J., Baeyens, J. P., Bauer, J. M., Boirie, Y., Cederholm, T., Landi, F. (2010) "Sarcopenia: European Consensus on Definition and Diagnosis: Report of the European Working Group on Sarcopenia in Older People." *Age and Ageing*, 39(4): 412–23.

Deschenes, M. R. (2004) "Effects of Aging on Muscle Fibre Type and Size." *Sports Medicine,*. 34(12): 809–24.

Farnfield, M. M., Breen, L., Carey, K. A., Garnham, A., Cameron-Smith, D. (2012) "Activation of mTOR Signalling in Young and Old Human Skeletal Muscle in Response to Combined Resistance Exercise and Whey Protein Ingestion." *Applied Physiology Nutrition and Metabolism*, 37: 21–30.

Freeman, L. M. (2012) "Cachexia and Sarcopenia: Emerging Syndromes of Importance in Dogs and Cats." *Journal of Veterinary Internal Medicine*, 26: 3–17.

Fyfe, M. C. and Bullock, M. I. (1985) "Therapeutic Ultrasound: Some Historical Background and Development in Knowledge of its Effect on Healing." *Australian Journal of Physiotherapy*, 31(6): 220–4.

Ge, H.-Y. and Arendt-Nielsen, L. (2011) "Latent Myofascial Trigger Points." *Current Pain and Headache Reports*, 15(5): 386–92.

Ge, H.-Y., Arendt-Nielsen, L., Madeleine, P. (2012) "Accelerated Muscle Fatigability of Latent Myofascial Trigger Points in Humans." *Pain Medicine*, 13: 957–64.

Ge, H-Y., Fernández-de-las-Peñas, C., Yue, S.-W. (2011) "Myofascial Trigger Points: Spontaneous Electrical Activity and its Consequences for Pain Induction and Propagation." *Chinese Medicine*, 6: 13. doi: 10.1186/1749-8546-6-13.

Hamm, K. and Alexander, C. M. (2010) "Challenging Presumptions: Is Reciprocal Inhibition Truly Reciprocal? A Study of Reciprocal Inhibition Between Knee Extensors and Flexors in Humans." *Manual Therapy*, 15(4): 388–93.

Hardie, E. M., Roe, S. C., Martin, F. R. J. (2002) "Radiographic Evidence of Degenerative Joint Disease in Geriatric Cats: 100 Cases (1994–1997)." *Journal of the American Veterinary Medical Association*, 220(5): 628–32.

Hayes K. W. (1993) "Conductive Heat." In *Manual for Physical Agents* (4th ed.)., pp 9–15. Norwalk, CT: Appleton and Lange.

Hourdebaigt, J. P. (2004) *Canine Massage: A Complete Reference Manual* (2nd ed.). Wenatchee, WA: Dogwise Publishing.

Ibarra, J. M., Ge, H.-Y., Wang, C., Vizcaino, V. M., Graven-Nielsen, T., Arendt-Nielsen, L. (2011) "Latent Myofascial Trigger Points are Associated with an Increased Antagonistic Muscle Activity During Agonist Muscle Contraction." *Journal of Pain*, 12: 1282–8.

Jennett, S. (2008) Churchill Livingstone's Dictionary of Sport and Exercise Science and Medicine. Elsevier Limited.

Johnson, J. and Levine, D. (2004) "Electrical Stimulation." In D. L. Millis, D. Levine and R. A. Taylor, *Canine Rehabilitation and Physical Therapy*, pp. 289–302. St. Louis, MO: W.B. Elsevier Saunders.

Krüger, J. P., Endres, M., Neumann, K., Stuhlmüller, B., Morawietz, L., Häupl, T., Kaps, C. (2012) "Chondrogenic Differentiation of Human Subchondral Progenitor Cells is Affected by Synovial Fluid from Donors with Osteoarthritis or Rheumatoid Arthritis." *Journal of Orthopaedic Surgery and Research*, 7: 10. doi: 10.1186/1749-799X-7-10.

Landi, F., Marzetti, E., Martone, A. M., Bernabei, R., Onder, G. (2014) "Exercise as a Remedy for Sarcopenia." *Current Opinion In Clinical Nutrition and Metabolic Care*, 17: 25–31.

Lascelles, B. D. (2010) "Feline Degenerative Joint Disease." *Veterinary Surgery*, 39(1): 2–13.

Maeda, Y., Lisi, T. L., Vance, C. G. T., and Sluka, K. A. (2007) "Release of GABA and Activation of GABAA in the Spinal Cord Mediates the Effects of TENS in Rats." *Brain Research*, 1136(1): 43–50.

Mannheimer, J. S. and Lampe, G. N. (1984) *Clinical Transcutaneous Electrical Nerve Stimulation*. Philadelphia, PA: Davis.

Mayo Clinic. (2014) "Myofascial pain syndrome." Available at http://www.mayoclinic.org/diseases-conditions/myofascial-pain-syndrome/basics/definition/con-20033195.

Millis, D. L., Tichenor, M., Hecht, S. (2014) "Prevalence of Osteoarthritis in Dogs Undergoing Routine Dental Prophylaxis." Proceedings of the World Small Animal Veterinary Association Meeting, Cape Town, South Africa.

Morley, J. E., Baumgartner, R. N., Roubenoff, R., Mayer, J., Nair, K. S. (2001) "Sarcopenia." *Journal of Laboratory Clinical Medicine*, 137(4): 231–43.

Muir, W. W. III, Wiese, A. J., Wittum, T. E. (2004) "Prevalence and Characteristics of Pain in Dogs and Cats Examined as Outpatients at a Veterinary Teaching Hospital." *Journal of the American Veterinary Medical Association*, 224(9): 1459–63.

Palmer, J. E., and Knight, K. L. (1996) "Ankle and Thigh Skin Surface Temperature Changes with Repeated Ice Pack Application." *Journal of Athletic Training*, 31: 319–23.

Petty, M. C. (2012) "Myofascial Pain Syndrome in Dogs." *DVM360 News Center*. Available at http://veterinarynews.dvm360.com/myofascial-pain-syndrome-dogs.

Scarlett, J. M. and Donoghue, S. (1998) "Associations Between Body Condition and Disease in Cats." *Journal of the American Veterinary Medical Association*, 212: 1725–31.

Shmalberg, J. (2014) "ACVN Nutrition Notes: Canine Performance and Rehabilitative Nutrition. Part 1: Canine Performance Nutrition." *Today's Veterinary Practice*, 4(6): 72–6.

Simons, D. G., Travell, J. G., Simons, L. S. (1999) *Myofascial Pain and Dysfunction: Upper Half of Body. The Trigger Point Manual. Volume 1*. Baltimore, MD: Lippincott Williams and Wilkins.

Sutherland, J. C. (2002) "Biological Effects of Polychromatic Light." *Photochemistry and Photobiology*, 76: 164–70.

Vance, C. T., Dailey, D. L., Rakel, B. A., Sluka, K. A. (2014) "Using TENS for Pain Control: The State of the Evidence." *Pain Management*, 4(3): 197–209.

Veterinary Specialty Care (n.d.) "Hyperbaric Therapy Chamber." Available at http://veterinaryspecialtycare.com/diagnostic/hyperbaric-therapy-chamber.

Wall, P. D. (1994) *Textbook of Pain* (3rd ed.). London, UK: Churchill Livingstone.

Wall, R. (2104) Introduction to Myofascial Trigger Points in Dogs. *Topics in Companion Animal Medicine*, 29: 43–8.

Youssef, A. R., Longino, D., Seerattan, R., Leonard, T., Herzog, W. (2009) "Muscle Weakness Causes Joint Degeneration in Rabbits." *Osteoarthritis and Cartilage*, 17: 1228–35.

Online Resources

Furthering Education in the Area of Mobility Issues

University of Tennessee, Certificate of Canine Rehabilitation Program (CCRP):
http://ccrp.utvetce.com

Canine Rehabilitation Institute, Canine Rehabilitation Therapist Certification (CCRT):
http://www.caninerehabinstitute.com

Healing Oasis (veterinary spinal manipulation therapy, veterinary massage and rehabilitation therapy:
http://healingoasis.edu

Curacore (medical acupuncture for veterinarians):
https://www.onehealthsim.org

Chi Institute (traditional Chinese medicine):
http://www.tcvm.com

Myopain Seminars (canine trigger point therapy):
http://www.myopainseminars.com

Option for Animals, College of Animal Chiropractic:
https://optionsforanimals.com

Chicago School of Canine Massage:
http://www.chicagoschoolofcaninemassage.com

Products

Assisi Loop®: NPAID® (Non-Pharmaceutical Anti-Inflammatory Device), Food and Drug Administration-cleared device which uses targeted pulsed electromagnetic field technology.
http://www.assisianimalhealth.com
http://www.mtavet.com

Balance disc, exercise balls or peanuts:
Useful in animals that have difficulty bearing full weight, as they can straddle the ball or peanut, but still be able to maintain an upright posture and develop their core strength. Useful in stretching and can be used to increase weight bearing in rear limbs and also to flex elbows and shoulders.
https://fitpawsusa.com
www.balancedcanineproducts.com/index.htm www.totofit.com

Canine wheelchairs, carts and rear support harnesses:
http://eddieswheels.com
http://www.handicappedpets.com
http://doggon.com
http://ruffrollin.com

Cavaletti poles, obstacle course and exercise equipment:
Very important in gait retraining and proprioception. Owners can also make their own obstacle course at home using common household items (brooms, hose, PVC pipes, rakes, pillows, etc.).
https://fitpawsusa.com
www.balancedcanineproducts.com/index.htm

Goniometer:
A specialized "ruler" that provides measurement of joint angles (flexion/extension). It is very important to use the correct landmarks when using this tool in order to obtain accurate measurements.
http://www.balancedcanineproducts.com/goniometer.htm

Geriatric supplements:
http://animalnecessity.com

Gulick, Gulick II Plus tape measure:
A specialized tape measure that allows a consistent measurement of muscle girth. When the ball is visible at the end of the tape, 4 ounces of pressure is being exerted, this allows multiple users to obtain roughly the same measurements with minimal interuser variation.
www.fitnessmart.com/fitstore2/products/67020.html

Laser:
Laser therapy alleviates pain and inflammation, reduces swelling, stimulates nerve regeneration and cells involved in tissue repair.
http://www.litecure.com/companion
http://respondsystems.com
http://www.k-laser.com
http://www.celasers.com
http://spectravet.com

Non-slip materials applied to the dog's nails or pads to prevent slipping:
https://www.toegrips.com
http://www.therapaw.com

Orthotics and prosthetic devices:
Based on custom casts made of dog's limb. Useful for numerous pathologies including: brachial plexus injuries, partial calcaneal tendon tears, carpal hyperextension, etc.
www.orthopets.com
http://www.therapaw.com
http://www.animalorthocare.com
http://www.dogleggs.com
https://goherogo.com

PEMF (pulsed electromagnetic field) therapy bed:
PEMF has been used since the 1970s to stimulate cells and energize natural cellular processes.
http://respondsystems.com/pemf

Protective booties:
http://www.therapaw.com
http://pawzdogboots.com

Shockwave:
Sound energy technology for various musculoskeletal injuries causing chronic pain and lameness in horses and dogs.
http://www.pulsevet.com

Support harnesses:
http://helpemup.com

Treadmill, land:
Used most commonly for strengthening and conditioning and to reeducate a dog's balance from front to back as well as normal foot placement. Land treadmills can often be inclined so as to allow more weight to be placed on the rear limbs to help facilitate strengthening.
http://dogtread.com
www.fitfurlife.com/dog-treadmills

Treadmill, underwater:
Allows muscle strengthening with reduced impact on the joints and also helps with gait retraining and proprioception.
http://h2oforfitness.com
www.hudsonaquatic.com

Wobble board:
Used in core strengthening by keeping the animal slightly off balance so they must use their core muscles to maintain balance.
https://fitpaws.com
www.balancedcanineproducts.com/index.htm

Appendix 14.1   Example neurology checklist.

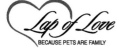

BECAUSE PETS ARE FAMILY

LAP OF LOVE

NEUROLOGY Checklist

PATIENT INFORMATION

Pet Name: _____   Age: _____

Owner
Name: _____   Breed: _____

MEDICAL HISTORY

_____

_____

CRANIAL NERVES

☐ CN I	☐ Olfactory	☐ Smell
☐ CN II	☐ Optic	☐ Menace, vision, PLR
☐ CN III	☐ Oculomotor	☐ PLR, strabismus, nystagmus
☐ CN IV	☐ Trochlear	☐ Strabismus, nystagmus
☐ CN V	☐ Trigeminal	☐ Jawtone, facial sensation temporal muscle mass
☐ CN VI	☐ Abducens	☐ Strabismus, nystagmus
☐ CN VII	☐ Facial	☐ Menace, blink, lip droop, ear movement, facial symmetry
☐ CN VIII	☐ Vestibulocochlear	☐ Nystagmus, head tilt, hearing
☐ CN IX	☐ Glossopharyngeal	☐ Gag reflex, swallowing
☐ CN X	☐ Vagus	☐ Gag reflex, swallowing
☐ CN XI	☐ Accessory	☐ Head and shoulder movement
☐ CN XII	☐ Hypoglossal	☐ Tongue movement

HISTORY

☐ SEIZURES **(Forebrain or Systemic Dz)**	☐ General ☐ Partial	☐ Psychomotor ☐ General
☐ BEHAVIOR **(Cerebrum)**	☐ Abnormal ☐ Vocalizing ☐ Inappropriate elimination	☐ Wandering ☐ Stuck in Corners
(Diencephalon)	☐ Temperature ↑ or ↓ ☐ Appetite ↑ or ↓	☐ Water intatke ↑ or ↓
☐ TREMORS	☐ Intension tremor **(Cerebellum)** ☐ Myotonia **(Myopathy)** ☐ Postural tremor **(Weakness, Sys. Dz)**	☐ Myoclonus **(Demyelination, seizure disorder)**
☐ HEARING **(Brainstem, ears)**	☐ Very deep sleep ☐ Startles easily	☐ Failure to respond to commands

☐ VISION
(Forebrain, CN2, eye)

☐ Bumps into things in full light

☐ Bumps into things in low light

☐ SWALLOWING
(Brainstem)

☐ Regurgitation
☐ Voice change

☐ Dysphagia

☐ BREATHING
(Cervical Spinal Cord)

☐ Abdominal with chest excursions

☐ Abdominal

MENTAL STATUS

☐ Level of Consciousness
(Brainstem >Forebrain)

0-Coma
1-Depressed, stupor
4-Agitated, Aggressive

2-Normal
3-Excited

☐ Dementia
(Forebrain)

EYES

☐ IRIS / PUPIL
(FeLV, active forebrain
edema)

☐ Hippus (Pupils alternating in size)

☐ Hemidilaiton (D shaped)

(Forebrain, brainstem)

☐ PLR Direct ↑ or ↓
☐ PLR Consensual ↑ or ↓
☐ Miosis OS or OD

☐ Mydriasis OS or OD
☐ Anisocoria OS or OD

☐ HORNER'S SYNDROME
(Brainstem, neck, T1-T3,
thorax, ear)

☐ Ptosis OS or OD
☐ Miosis OS or OD

☐ Enopthalmos OS or OD
☐ Nicitans prolapse OS or OD

☐ NYSTAGMUS
(Inner, middle ear, CN8 >brainstem)
(Brainstem>inner, middle ear, CN8)
(Brainstem>inner, middle ear, CN8)
(Brainstem)

☐ Spontaneous Horizontal →
☐ Spontaneous Vertical →
☐ Rotary →
☐ Positional →

☐ Fast phase R or L, OS or OD or OU
☐ Fast phase ↑ or ↓, OS or OD or OU
☐ OS or OD or OU
☐ Horizontal, vertical or rotary

☐ VISION
(Forebrain)

☐ Tracking full light ↑ or ↓
☐ Obstacles full light ↑ or ↓

☐ Tracking low light ↑ or ↓
☐ Obstacles low light ↑ or ↓

☐ MENACE
(Forebrain, brainstem, cerebellum,
too young)

☐ Nasal OS ↑ or ↓
☐ Lateral OS ↑ or ↓

☐ Nasal OD ↑ or ↓
☐ Lateral OD ↑ or ↓

☐ CORNEA
(Brainstem, coma)
(CN3, CN7)

☐ Corneal reflex OS ↑ or ↓
☐ Dry cornea OS or OD

☐ Corneal reflex ↑ or ↓
☐ Dry nose L or R

GAIT

☐ HEAD POSITION
(Forebrain)
(Brainstem, ear, CN8)
(Brainstem)
(Cerebellum, bilateral vestibular)
(Forebrain)

☐ Head turn L
☐ Head tilt L
☐ Strabismus OS
☐ Bobble head
☐ Head pressing

☐ Head turn R
☐ Head tilt R
☐ Strabismus OD

UMN – hyperreflexia, maintenance of strength, increased resting tone of muscle, spasticity of the limbs.
LMN – hyporeflexia, weakness, reduced resting tone of muslces, decreased ability to generate tone with limb movement

☐ POSTURAL REACTIONS   ☐ Proprioceptive Positioning   ☐ Placing non-visual
    (Brain, Spinal cord, peripheral   ☐ Placing visual (+ vision)   ☐ Hemi-walking
    nerves, UMN, LMN)   ☐ Wheelbarrowing

☐ POSTURAL HOPPING   ☐ UMN – wide hops   ☐ LMN – short hops

☐ STRIDE LENGTH
    (Pain or LMN)   ☐ Short L or R front (Cerv/Thoracic SC)   ☐ Short L or R rear (Lumbar SC)
    (UMN or cerebellum)   ☐ Long Stride

☐ ATAXIA
    (Forebrain, brainstem, SC, PN)   ☐ Sensory–CP deficits, wide based, knuckle
    (Cerebellum)   ☐ Cerebelar – hypermetria, intention tremor
    (CN8, inner or middle ear dz)   ☐ Unilateral Vestibular – head tilt, nystagmus
    (Bilateral CN8, ear dz or brainstem)   ☐ Bilateral Vestibular – side to side head
    (Cerebrum)   ☐ Wandering   ☐ Wide circles

REFLEXES

☐ BICEPS REFLEX   ☐ LMN = C6-C8, musculocutaneous n.   ☐ UMN = CNS lesion above C6

☐ TRICEPS REFLEX   ☐ LMN = C7-T2, upper radial nerve   ☐ UMN = CNS lesion above C7

☐ EXTENSOR CARPI RADIALIS   ☐ LMN = C7-T2, upper & lower radial n.   ☐ UMN = CNS lesion above C7

☐ WITHDRAWAL REFLEX   ☐ LMN Thoracic = C6-T2, axillary nerve   ☐ UMN Thoracic (Crossed extensor)
                 musculocutaneous nerve, radial nerve   = CNS above C6
                 median nerve or ulnar nerve
                ☐ LMN Pelvic = L7-S2, sciatic nerve   ☐ UMN Pelvic (Crossed extensor) =
                                                 CNS above L6-L7

☐ PANNICULUS REFLEX   ☐ LMN one side other normal = C8-T1   ☐ Ends cranial to sacral area = spinal
                 brachial plexus, lateral thoracic n.   cord lesion 1 to 4 segments cranial

☐ GASTROCNEMIUS RELEX   ☐ LMN = L6-S2 spinal cord, sciatic nerve   ☐ UMN = CNS above L6

☐ PATELLAR REFLEX   ☐ LMN = L4-L6 Spinal cord, femoral nerve   ☐ UMN = CNS above L4
                ☐ Pseudohyperreflexia-L6-S1 spinal cord

☐ PERINEAL REFLEX   ☐ LMN = S1-Cd spinal cord, perineal and
                pudendal nerve

MYOTOMES

FORELIMB NERVE	Segment	Muscle
☐ SUPRASCAPULAR N.	☐ (C5), C6, C7	☐ Supraspinatus, Infraspinatus
☐ SUBSCAPULAR N.	☐ C6, C7	☐ Subscapularis
☐ MUSCULOCUTANEOUS N.	☐ C6, C7, C8	☐ Biceps brachii, brachialis coracobrachialis
☐ AXILLARY N.	☐ (C6), C7, C8	☐ Deltoid, Teres major/minor, superficial and deep pectoralis
☐ RADIAL N.	☐ C7, C8, T1, (T2)	☐ Triceps brachii, extensors, ulnaris lateralis
☐ MEDIAN N.	☐ C8, T1, (T2)	☐ Flexor carpi radialis, superficial digital flexor
☐ ULNAR N.	☐ C8, T1, (T2)	☐ Flexor carpi ulnaris, deep digital flexor

HINDLIMB

☐ FEMORAL N.	☐ L4, L5, L6	☐ Iliopsoas, quadriceps, sartorius
☐ OBTURATOR N.	☐ (L4), L5, L6	☐ External obturator, pectineus, gracilis adductor
☐ CRANIAL GLUTEAL N.	☐ L6, L7, S1	☐ Middle/deep gluteal, tensor fascia lata
☐ CAUDAL GLUTEAL N.	☐ L7, (S1, S2)	☐ Superficial/middle gluteal
☐ SCIATIC N.	☐ L6, L7, S1, (S2)	☐ Biceps femoris, semimembranosus semitendinosus
☐ COMMON PERONEAL N.	☐ L6, L7	☐ Peroneus longus, lateral/long digital extensor, cranial tibial
☐ TIBIAL N.	☐ L7, S1	☐ Gastrocnemius, popliteus, superficial/ deep digital flexor
☐ PUDENDAL N.	☐ S1, S2, S3	☐ External anal sphincter

NOTES

_____

_____

_____

_____

_____

_____

_____

_____

_____

_____

_____

Dr. Signature   Date

Appendix 14.2   Example orthopedic checklist.

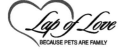

LAP OF LOVE

ORTHOPEDIC Checklist

PATIENT INFORMATION

Pet Name: _____   Age: _____

Owner
Name: _____   Breed: _____

MEDICAL HISTORY

_____

_____

OBSERVATION

☐ Lameness at a Walk

☐ 0 Walks normally
☐ 1 Slight lameness
☐ 2 Obvious weight-bearing lameness

☐ 3 Severe weight-bearing lameness
☐ 4 Intermittent non-weight bearing lameness
☐ 5 Continuous non-weight-bearing lameness

☐ Posture

☐ Topline (kyphotic – lordotic)
☐ Offloading a limb
☐ Sit test

☐ Overall symmetry
☐ Muscle tone
☐ Able to rise from sit or down

☐ Behavior

☐ Neutral
☐ Confident

☐ Shy
☐ Aggressive

RANGE OF MOTION

Pain Assessment Score

0-no pain during palpation of joint
1-mild pain during palpation of joint
4-Would not allow palpation of joint

2-Moderate pain during palpation of joint
3-Severe pain during palpation of joint

☐ Toes (fore & hind limb)

☐ Flexion
☐ Medial deviation
☐ Traction
☐ DJD

☐ Extension
☐ Lateral deviation
☐ Sesamoids
☐ Pain assessment score 0, 1, 2, 3, 4

☐ Tarsus

☐ Flexion (38°)
☐ Medial deviation
☐ Traction at 90°
☐ DJD

☐ Extension (165°)
☐ Lateral deviation
☐ Hyperextension test in standing
☐ Pain assessment score 0, 1, 2, 3, 4

☐ Stifle

☐ Flexion (41°)
☐ Medial deviation
☐ Cranial drawer
☐ DJD

☐ Extension (162°)
☐ Lateral deviation
☐ Meniscal test
☐ Pain assessment score 0, 1, 2, 3, 4

☐ Hip

☐ Flexion (50°)
☐ Internal rotation
☐ Abduction

☐ Extension (162°)
☐ External rotation
☐ Barlow, Barden + Ortolani
☐ Pain assessment score 0, 1, 2, 3, 4

RANGE OF MOTION CONTINUED

☐Carpus	☐Flexion (32°) ☐Medial deviation ☐DJD	☐Extension (196°) ☐Lateral deviation ☐ Pain assessment score 0, 1, 2, 3, 4
☐ Elbow	☐Flexion (36°) ☐Pronation ☐Traction at 90° ☐DJD	☐Extension (166°) ☐Supination ☐Pain assessment score 0, 1, 2, 3, 4
☐ Shoulder	☐Flexion (57°) ☐Internal rotation ☐Abduction ☐DJD	☐Extension (165°) ☐External rotation ☐Pain assessment score 0, 1, 2, 3, 4

PALPATION OF BONES AND MUSCLES

☐ TMJ	☐Lateral deviation ☐Masseter muscles	☐Rostral deviation ☐Temoralis and Frontalis muscles
☐ Spine	☐**Cervical spine** ☐**Thoracic spine** ☐Epaxial muscles ☐Ribs 2-13 ☐Intercostal muscles ☐**Lumbar spine** ☐Multifidus muscles ☐Iliopsoas ☐**Pelvis** ☐Sacrotuberous ligament	☐Adjacent muscles ☐Rib 1 ☐Multifidus muscles ☐Hypaxial muscles ☐Sternum and Xiphoid ☐Epaxial muscles ☐Quadratus lumborum ☐**Sacrum** ☐Coccygeal vertebrae
☐Tarsus	☐Calcaneal process ☐Check for joint effusion	☐Malleoli ☐Calcaneal tendon
☐Stifle	☐Distal femur and epicondyles ☐Patella ☐Fibula ☐Popliteal lymph nodes ☐Quads ☐Cranial tibia muscle	☐Proximal tibia, condyles and tibial crest ☐Patellar tendon ☐Medial buttress ☐Flexor tendons ☐Hamstrings ☐Gastrocnemius
☐Hip	☐Greater trochanter ☐Pectineus ☐Tensor fascia lata ☐Gracilis	☐Gluteals ☐Sartorius ☐Inguinal lymph nodes
☐Carpus	☐Distal radius and ulna ☐Carpals ☐Extensor tendons	☐Styloid processes ☐Metatarsals ☐Flexor tendons
☐Elbow	☐Olecranon ☐Medial Compartment ☐Biceps and brachialis	☐Epicondyles ☐Radial head ☐Triceps

☐Shoulder

☐Scapula
☐Humerus
☐Biceps tendons
☐Infraspinatus
☐Teres minor
☐Teres major

☐Subscapularis
☐Supraspinatus
☐Triceps long head
☐Lattisimus Dorsi
☐Prescapular lymph nodes

NOTES

_____

_____

_____

_____

_____

_____

_____

_____

_____

_____

_____

_____

_____

_____

_____

_____

_____

_____

_____

Dr. Signature   Date

Appendix 14.3   Example mobility checklist.

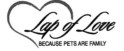

Lap of Love

MOBILITY Checklist

PATIENT INFORMATION

Pet name: _____   Age: _____

Owner
name: _____   Breed: _____

MEDICAL HISTORY

_____

_____

MEDICATIONS

- ☐ NSAID
- ☐ Steroids
- ☐ Fentanyl patch
- ☐ Buprenorphine

- ☐ Amantadine
- ☐ Gabapentin
- ☐ Tramadol
- ☐ Joint injections

- ☐ Adequan
- ☐ Glucosamine supplement
- ☐ Vitamin B12
- ☐ Subcutaneous fluids

LIFESTYLE

- ☐ Weight loss
- ☐ Protein 1 g/lb body weight
- ☐ Runners on the floor
- ☐ Runners on Stairs & landing
- ☐ Small fan on the floor

- ☐ Sanitary clip
- ☐ Trim bottom of feet
- ☐ Dr. Buzby Toe Grips
- ☐ Help up every 2 hours
- ☐ HelpeEmUp harness or sling

- ☐ Can see out of window
- ☐ Brain games
- ☐ Wheelchair or wagon/stroller rides
- ☐ Bring over "Friends"
- ☐ Tricks, FitPAWS or DogTread

THERAPIES

- ☐ Laser therapy
- ☐ Therapeutic ultrasound
- ☐ Underwater treadmill

- ☐ Acupuncture/dry needling
- ☐ TENS/NMES

- ☐ Chiropractic
- ☐ HBOT
- ☐ Massage

RANGE OF MOTION AND THERAPEUTIC EXERCISES

- ☐ Toe curls
- ☐ Tail presses
- ☐ Hock flex/extend
- ☐ Stifle flex/extend
- ☐ Hip flex/extend
- ☐ Scrunchie above hock

- ☐ Toe curls
- ☐ Carpus flex/extend
- ☐ Elbow flex/extend
- ☐ Shoulder flex/extend
- ☐ Biscuit to sides
- ☐ Massage

- ☐ Hot pack 10 minutes
- ☐ Cold pack 10 minutes
- ☐ Cavalettis
- ☐ Balance disk standing
- ☐ Double disk standing
- ☐ Balance shifting

- ☐ Sit to stand
- ☐ Elevated sit to stand
- ☐ Backwards walking
- ☐ Wave/shake paw
- ☐ Weaves/ figure 8s
- ☐ Walking for ____ minutes

Owner goals: _____

_____

Notes: _____

_____

_____

Dr. Signature   Date

15

Age-Related Gastrointestinal Conditions and Considerations for Nutrition

Shea Cox

This chapter discusses morphological and physiological age-related changes that occur to the gastrointestinal system, including considerations for nutrition in our aging patients. Direct evidence and models that study gastrointestinal changes in aging healthy animals are lacking. Because of this, information regarding specific age-related changes is often inferred from human studies and information must be procured from both human and veterinary resources.

Age-Related Gastrointestinal Changes

Normal aging of the gastrointestinal tract is associated with both structural and functional changes. It should be noted that aging accounts for only subtle alterations in overall gastrointestinal structure, and implications regarding function generally remains minimal unless accompanied by comorbid disease processes.

Taste and Smell

As pets age, the number of taste buds begins to decrease and the level of taste bud regeneration declines. Smell is also diminished due to a decrease in olfactory bulb fibers and an increased rate of apoptosis of the olfactory receptors. Mucus, which helps odors stay in the nose long enough to be detected by the nerve endings, has a decreased production in the nasal passages, further contributing to a loss of smell (Fortney, 2008).

Gastrointestinal Motor Function

In human studies, the intestinal myenteric and submucosal plexus demonstrate age-related changes that can heighten over time. These changes primarily involve the cholinergic neurons and concurrent enteric glial cell losses. There also appears to be greater losses in the distal gastrointestinal tract compared with proximal sites (Salles, 2007). Dystrophic axonal swelling occurs in the sympathetic, vagal, dorsal root and enteric nitrergic innervation of the gut; it is these autonomic nervous system changes that may in part explain the age-related decline in motor function that can be seen in geriatric patients (Orr and Chen, 2002).

Treatment and Care of the Geriatric Veterinary Patient, First Edition. Edited by Mary Gardner and Dani McVety.
© 2017 John Wiley & Sons, Inc. Published 2017 by John Wiley & Sons, Inc.
Companion Website: www.wiley.com/go/gardner/geriatric

Although there is an increase in the prevalence of disorders of gastrointestinal function and motility with age, age itself has minimal direct effects. Alterations in motor function are more likely the result of the presence of primary disease such as tumors of the gastrointestinal tract, inflammatory or neurological diseases, systemic disorders, or from the effects of medications.

The Esophagus

Clinically significant esophageal dysfunction does not result solely from age, although mild age-related changes have been described in people. Such alterations include a decrease in the amplitude of contractions, the number of peristaltic waves following a swallow, an increase in disorganized contractions in the body of the esophagus, and an overall weakening of esophageal smooth muscle. Despite these age-related changes, esophageal function is generally well preserved, even in advanced age (Shaker and Staff, 2001).

The Stomach

Gastroparesis and delayed gastric emptying are considerably more common in geriatric human patients. This is generally not due to age itself, but to the presence of other diseases (such as chronic kidney disease or hypothyroid disease), which can contribute to slower rate of gastrointestinal transit time and impaired gastric emptying (O'Mahony *et al.*, 2002). The gastric mucosa undergoes changes with age, including gastric mucosal atrophy and a decrease in the quantity of gastric acid secretion. Although gastric acid output decreases with age, the majority of healthy older populations are able to maintain a normal level of gastric acid secretion (Nakamura *et al.*, 2006). Pepsin secretion does not decline, but there is a decline in gastric bicarbonate, sodium ion and non-parietal fluid secretion with age. Gastric mucosal blood flow also decreases with age, as does the blood flow to most organs, which can lead to a slower healing following mucosal injury (Hall *et al.*, 2005). Gastric prostaglandin synthesis may diminish, increasing susceptibility to the adverse effects of non-steroidal anti-inflammatories (NSAIDs) on the mucosa, which is an important consideration in our geriatric patients. While gastric aging may induce abnormalities of the gastric epithelium, most alterations are generally a result of chronic insults, such as effects of comorbidities or due to medications (for example, NSAID gastritis; Salles, 2009). Mucosal protective mechanisms may also be impaired with age (Newton, 2004).

Small Bowel Motility

Small intestinal motility is responsible for the digestion of food, for nutrient absorption, and for the clearance of cell debris, secretions, and residual undigested materials. Age-related morphological changes that occur in the small intestine in both humans and animals include a reduction in number of neurons in myenteric plexus and a reduction in splanchnic blood flow (Wade and Cowen, 2004). Normal absorptive surface is maintained, and the surface-to-volume ratio in the jejunum and enterocyte height remain unchanged (Nagar and Roberts, 1999). Mucosal regeneration increases with age (Hall *et al.*, 2005). Orocecal transit time does not change significantly with age in healthy populations, but it does become altered in the presence of disease.

Colonic Motility

The role of enteric neurodegeneration in constipation has been noted in animal models. Constipation and colonic motor functional alterations are generally not a direct consequence of aging, but due to the presence of other underlying disease processes.

Immune Function

The gastrointestinal tract surface represents the single largest immunological organ, with much of the body's immunoglobulin-producing cells (Blechman and Gelb, 1999), and aging is accompanied by a decline in the mucosal and secretory immune response. Changes include a decline in regulatory-type cytokine production, T cell compartment, antibody responses to antigens and the composition of the lymphoid tissues (Santiago *et al.*, 2011). The total number of T and B cells generally remains stable (Gomez *et al.*, 2005). Intestinal mucosal immunosenescence (the gradual deterioration of the immune system brought on by natural age advancement) occurs, and may be a consequence of reduced homing of immunoglobulin A plasma cells (Schmucker *et al.*, 2003). Although age does not correlate with surface epithelium and number of intraepithelial lymphocytes, absorption of lipids is somewhat impaired and may result from a decline in blood flow and ischemia (Meier and Sturm, 2009). A better understanding and research of T cell metabolism, hormones and microbiota may provide further insights into the immune responses that are associated with aging.

Hepatobiliary System

In human studies, liver volume and blood flow have been shown to decrease by 20–40% between the third and the tenth decades of life (Wynne *et al.*, 1989). Additionally, hepatocyte proliferative response appears to decline in the elderly, which can have implications in hepatic regeneration after liver disease, and has also been linked to a reduction in hepatocyte telomere length (Takubo *et al.*, 2000). Although overall liver function is minimally altered, there is a general decline in the P450 enzyme system in animals (McLachlan and Pont, 2012). Despite these well-documented age-related changes in hepatic function, age itself is not associated with significant abnormalities in blood tests that are commonly performed to assess liver function (Schmucker, 2005).

The gall bladder experiences minimal age-related changes. The biliary duct does become marginally dilated as a result of an increased amount of connective tissue (Tohno *et al.*, 2004), but gall bladder contractions are generally not affected.

Common Gastrointestinal Conditions

The spectrum of gastrointestinal pathology in the aged pet is diverse and can affect all sites along the gastrointestinal tract.

Malabsorption

Vitamin B12 (cobalamin) deficiency can occur at all ages, with a slight predilection for the geriatric cohort. Deficiency most commonly results from food-cobalamin malabsorption, which will be discussed in greater detail later in this chapter.

Diarrhea

Diarrhea can be a common finding in the older population. Factors that can predispose a geriatric patient to development of diarrhea can include lower protection against enteric organisms, changes in the immune system (for example, decline in B and T cells), decreased antibody and cytokine production and decline in mucosal immunity due to decreased IgA secretion. Aging is also associated with alteration in microflora in the intestine; anaerobic and bifidobacterial colonies decrease with concurrent increase in colonization by enterobacteria. Medication-induced diarrhea is another underlying etiology, and can be a common cause in our older patients, owing to frequent implementation of polypharmacy to control other age-related diseases.

Constipation

Colonic motility plays a role in formation of stool. Constipation is a common syndrome in the geriatric patient, and it is a term that describes difficulties experienced in evacuating feces rather than a specific disease entity (McCrea *et al.*, 2008). Aging is associated with enteric neurodegeneration and a significant decline in both cell number and density throughout the gastrointestinal tract (Phillips *et al.*, 2007). Although smooth muscle relaxation remains normal, cholinergic neurons are reduced in number (Bernard *et al.*, 2009). A study of extrinsic colonic nerves in rodents has shown a dramatic age-related degeneration of sympathetic motor neurons of the myenteric plexus and decline in colonic transit (Bernard *et al.*, 2009). There is also much information on age-related changes of the extrinsic innervation of the human colon regarding the degenerative process of interstitial cells of Cajal (which are the intestinal pacemakers) as potential cause of constipation with age (Wiskur and Greenwood-Van Meerveld, 2010). The functional consequence of such changes is delayed transit in the large bowel because there is less contraction, which leads to inefficient peristalsis (Wiskur and Greenwood-Van Meerveld, 2010). As previously mentioned, unrelated factors can lead to the development of constipation, including comorbidities (such as metabolic or endocrine disease, obstructive lesions), mediations (for example, opioids) and dehydration.

Pancreatitis

Old age is not a risk factor with regards to the development of pancreatitis. However, old age can negatively influence prognosis if there is age-related decline in organ function or if there are comorbid conditions present. In contrast to the effects of age on function, changes in pancreatic structure do occur with aging, and human studies have shown changes in duct proliferation, lobular degeneration, and fatty infiltration, which can resemble the changes of chronic pancreatitis (Ross and Forsmark, 2001).

Gastrointestinal Cancers

Malignant neoplasms can occur with greater frequency with advancing age. Phenomena such as the accumulation of DNA damage and dysfunctional proteins are common to the aging process and cancer. Carcinogenesis and aging similarly involve alterations in metabolism and immunosenescence, hypermethylation of promoters and telomere shortening (Arai *et al.*, 2010).

Pharmacology and Therapeutic Considerations

Aging is an important factor in the biotransformation of drugs, and the changes associated with aging affect both pharmacokinetics and pharmacodynamics of medications. Impaired systems and organ function can further lead to an increased potential of adverse drug effects.

As stated earlier, advancing age leads to changes in overall body composition. With the increase in body fat, a decline in muscle mass, and a larger decline in total body water, the volume of distribution of highly polar, water soluble medications will decrease, while that of lipophilic medications, will increase with advancing age (Rivera and Antognini, 2009). For example, in aging pets where there is a decrease in lean muscle mass and an increase in total body fat, fat-soluble drugs will tend to accumulate in adipose tissues and prolonged effects can occur, as elimination of these drugs is slow and decreased (Howland, 2009). Dosing is an important consideration in cases of chronic administration to help prevent potential adverse or toxic adverse effects.

Although changes are observed in the gastrointestinal tract with age, absorption by passive diffusion remains unchanged for most drugs (Sostress *et al.*, 2009). However, pre-systemic elimination by the intestinal mucosal and the first pass through the liver must be taken into account when evaluating oral bioavailability. Plasma concentrations of highly cleared medications may be higher, as liver mass and hepatic perfusion decline with aging. The dosage regimen for the geriatric population needs to be based on age-related changes in pharmacokinetics, which may be difficult, as dosing for safety and efficacy is guided by few clinical trials in the geriatric population (Rivera and Antognini, 2009).

In addition to the gastrointestinal tract (namely the small bowel), age-related pharmacokinetic changes result from reduced hepatic clearance and prolonged elimination half-life. Most drugs are absorbed from the gastrointestinal tract and pass through the liver. Additionally, most medications need to be biotransformed to more polar metabolites by several cytochrome P450-dependent phase I and phase II pathways (for example, acetylation, glucuronidation, or sulfonation) before their final excretion. Hepatic blood flow and mass generally decline with age and high-extraction drugs may be affected by these changes. Liver blood flow declines with age causing impaired biotransformation (Rosenthal and Nussinovitch, 2008).

Although direct drug absorption is generally not affected, drug effects can vary, owing to interactions with other medications, nutrients and comorbidities. Polypharmacy in the geriatric patient is frequent, and clinicians should be aware of drugs that may result in adverse gastrointestinal effects.

Nutrition and Digestion

Two major effects of aging include a decreased ability to adapt to changes in nutrition and a decrease in the reserve capacity to handle large nutritional excesses or deficiencies. Older patients often have subclinical diseases that further affect their nutritional status and health. Because of this, the role of nutrition becomes an increasingly important consideration not only in the prevention of disease, but in addition helping to maintain the aging pet's quality of life (Figure 15.1).

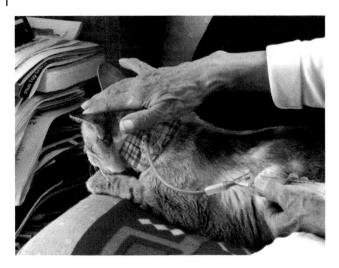

Figure 15.1 Lily, tube feeding.

Effects of Aging on Nutritional Requirements

Energy requirements

Maintenance energy requirements decrease as a pet ages. This is due primarily to changes in body composition, mainly a decrease in lean body mass (muscle) and an increase in fat tissue, which in turn leads to a fall in the overall basal metabolic rate. Many pets become less active as they age, further reducing their overall energy needs. There is also an age-related reduction in the digestibility of nutrients, especially that of fat and protein. This reduction further impacts both body and muscle condition, and subsequently, the energy requirements needed by the pet (Perez-Camargo, 2004).

In dogs, a decrease of approximately 20% in maintenance energy requirements has been documented, with the greatest decrease occurring in dogs greater than seven years of age when compared with young adult dogs (Harper, 1998). However, in another study evaluating Papillons, Labradors, and Great Danes, it was found that the smaller breeds of dog had a higher maintenance energy requirement than larger breeds, associated with an increase in lean body mass but a decrease in fat mass (Speakman, 2003). Many cats appear to have a decrease in requirement similar to other species (Laflamme and Ballam, 2002); however, after 11 years of age, maintenance energy requirement per unit body weight increases (Cupp, 2004).

Obesity may result if the requirement for energy decreases but energy intake does not; however, the prevalence of obesity decreases as dogs and cats age, and a greater proportion of dogs and cats over 12 years of age are underweight compared with other age groups (Lund *et al.*, 2006).

Protein

Aging is associated with a loss of lean muscle mass, and as discussed, maintenance energy requirement is related to the amount of lean muscle mass (Figures 15.2 and 15.3). Because of this, dietary protein intake is an important nutritional requirement to

Figure 15.2 Benny, showing gastrointestinal weight loss.

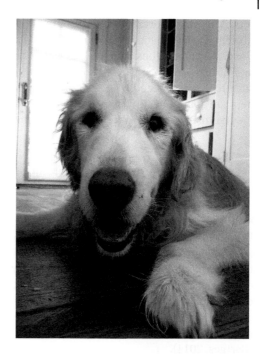

Figure 15.3 Meli, showing gastrointestinal weight loss.

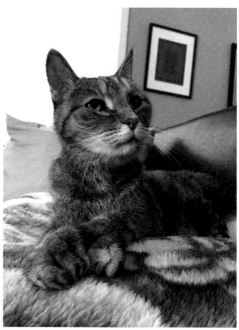

meet in the aging pet; for example, adequate protein intake will slow the loss of lean muscle mass, while inadequate protein intake will increases the rate of this loss (Kealy, 1999). In healthy older pets, protein restriction is unnecessary (and may actually be detrimental), and restriction can result in further loss of lean muscle mass leading to increased morbidity and mortality (Cupp *et al.*, 2004). If dietary protein becomes insufficient, protein will then become mobilized from lean body mass to help support essential functional protein synthesis. While a geriatric pet can adapt to a decreased protein intake and still maintain nitrogen balance, it will ultimately progress to a protein-depleted state that is associated with the gradual but continued loss of lean muscle mass. These pets can appear healthy, but they can have a decreased ability to respond to environmental insults such as infections (Wannemacher and McCoy, 1966).

Fat

Fat digestibility may decrease with age. In patients that require increased energy intake, however, increased dietary fat may be required.

Fiber

Dogs and cats do not have a specific dietary fiber requirement, although fiber affects not only nutrient availability, but both gastrointestinal function and the microbiota of the gastrointestinal tract. Increasing dietary fiber may also help those pets prone to developing constipation due to decreased intestinal motility. An increased dietary fiber content may help with this. However, care does need to be taken, as diets with increased dietary fiber are often formulated to contain less fat and be less calorically dense. This may result in decreased energy intake and a loss of both body weight and condition (Bartges, 2014).

Other Nutrients

Oxidative damage plays an important role in the aging process, which can lead to a deficiency of antioxidant nutrients. This can in turn adversely affect antioxidant function, immune function and markers of health (Freeman, 2005). Omega-3 fatty acids may play an important role in geriatric patients, as they work to decrease inflammation, which can be beneficial with age-related comorbidities such as osteoarthritis and renal disease.

Aging patients that have a decreased intestinal fat digestibility may also have a decrease in the availability of vitamins, minerals, and electrolytes.

Water intake is an important nutrient to monitor because glomerular filtration rate and urine concentrating ability declines as a pet ages, predisposing the geriatric population to dehydration. Geriatric pets may also have a decreased thirst response. The aging process alters important physiological control systems associated with thirst and satiety. In human studies, evidence suggests that the reason for this is that the elderly have a higher baseline osmolality and thus a higher osmotic operating point for thirst sensation (with little or no change in sensitivity), and also exhibit diminished thirst and satiety in response to the unloading (hypovolemia) and loading (hypervolemia) of baroreceptors (Kenney and Chiu, 2001).

Weight loss

The regulation of body composition is dynamic over time, and as a pet ages, there is a propensity for weight loss. Weight loss can occur from a variety of reasons, including:

- the body's regulation of energy intake
- ingestion of inadequate calories

- a normal, age-related decrease in appetite, which may in part be due to a decreased energy expenditure as well as a diminished sense of taste and smell
- disuse atrophy
- changes in hormonal regulation and/or hormonal deficiencies
- effects of disease or comorbidities, such as chronic renal disease
- any combination of these factors.

Therapeutic Considerations

Diet

The optimal diet for the geriatric pet depends mainly upon that particular pet's overall health. Box 15.1 gives generalized recommendations with regards to diet considerations in the geriatric pet.

Appetite stimulants

Cyproheptadine and mirtazapine are two common appetite stimulants used in geriatric hospice patients. Cyproheptadine has anecdotal efficacy in many patients, but its efficacy has never been scientifically evaluated, and twice daily administration is generally necessary, which can prove challenging for owners. Mirtazapine has become more commonly used, and this medication demonstrates anti-nausea properties in addition to its appetite-stimulating properties, owing to its action as the 5HT3 receptor. Exploration of its pharmacodynamics and pharmacokinetics has also provided information that has allowed for more effective use in cats. Because higher doses are more commonly associated with adverse effects in cats (including hyperexcitability, vocalization, and tremors), smaller, more frequent doses (1.875 mg daily, or every other day in patients with chronic kidney disease) are recommended (Quimby, 2015). Owners should be aware that mirtazapine and cyproheptadine cannot be administered concurrently, because mirtazapine is a serotonin agonist while cyproheptadine is a non-selective serotonin antagonist; cyproheptadine is in fact used as an antidote for serotonin effects of a mirtazapine overdose.

Box 15.1 Recommendations for Dietary Considerations for the Geriatric Pet

- In aged patients that are metabolically efficient, healthy, and continue to maintain their body condition, a continuation of their regular diet is very reasonable.
- In aged patients that are metabolically efficient, healthy, but gaining body weight and increasing their body condition, then caloric restriction and/or possibly feeding a diet that is higher in fiber should be considered.
- In aged patients that are metabolically inefficient, but otherwise healthy and losing weight and body and/or muscle condition, feeding a more calorically dense and higher protein diet is indicated.
- In aged patients that are metabolically inefficient and not clinically healthy, dietary recommendations are directed towards modifying nutrients that impact upon the underlying disease.
- Restriction of other nutrients in the healthy aged pet, such as protein, is not warranted at this time.

Cobalamin supplementation

Cobalamin (vitamin B12) is an essential cofactor for several enzyme systems and plays a major role in the metabolism of several amino acids. Because of the important metabolic role of cobalamin, deficiency of this vitamin can lead to a variety of clinical signs, including gastrointestinal, hematological, immunological, and neurological, and therefore must be corrected.

Cobalamin absorption is a complex system that relies on a multitude of factors and processes. Cobalamin is initially bound to dietary protein and is then released in the stomach and duodenum by the action of gastric acid and proteinases. R-protein, a carrier protein, binds any free cobalamin until transit to the duodenum. Here, cobalamin is transferred to yet another protein, an intrinsic factor, and in humans and dogs, it is released by the stomach and pancreas, while in cats, it is released only by the pancreas. Enterocytes in the ileum then absorb cobalamin/intrinsic factor complexes, and following absorption, the cobalamin is released from the intrinsic factor and transferred to another group of carrier proteins, the transcobalamins, which allow entry of the vitamin into cells (Steiner, 2014).

A definitive diagnosis of cobalamin deficiency can be challenging, as signs can be nonspecific and can vary depending on the age when it occurs, the severity of deficiency and the duration of the condition. For example, patients with cobalamin deficiency may only present with mild signs of gastrointestinal disease, which could either be the cause or the effect of the cobalamin deficiency.

With regards to the gastrointestinal tract, cobalamin deficiency can impair intestinal mucosal regeneration and can, in turn, cause mucosal atrophy, further exacerbating diarrhea and making the patient refractory to the usual therapies. It is often found that patients with underlying gastrointestinal disorders due to cobalamin deficiency will not respond to therapy until cobalamin is supplemented. The only routinely available diagnostic tool to assess cobalamin status in dogs and cats is a serum cobalamin concentration, although it is acceptable to treat our geriatric hospice patients empirically when diagnostics have been declined in lieu of palliative care.

Cobalamin deficiency is usually secondary to reduced cobalamin absorptive capacity, so the use of dietary cobalamin supplementation is generally ineffective in the restoration of cobalamin stores. Because of this, the route of choice for supplementation is by parenteral injection. Cobalamin should be used, as it is a non-irritant that can be given subcutaneously. The author empirically uses the following dosing schedule: 250 µg per injection in cats, 500–1500 µg per injection in dogs, subcutaneously, once weekly for six weeks, then every two weeks for six weeks, then once monthly. It should be noted that one should not use injectable multivitamin preparations because the cobalamin concentration is too low and they often cause pain at the injection site (Ruaux, 2002).

Palliative Care Considerations

Palliative care is especially important when there are concurrent multiple medical comorbidities, such as cancer or renal failure, that conspire to weaken the geriatric patient with a predominant GI problem. The goals of palliative care treatments for older animals with gastrointestinal issues focus more on suppressing morbidity and enhancing quality of life aspects. In our geriatric pets with gastrointestinal symptoms, palliative care generally includes pharmacologic approaches to managing anorexia, nausea, vomiting, diarrhea, constipation, diarrhea, dehydration, and any discomfort that may be associated with symptoms or disease.

Conclusion

Gastrointestinal changes can occur in our geriatric patients, but age itself has minimal direct effects, and alterations in gastrointestinal function are generally the result of other primary disease processes that are also present. Proper management, in addition to an understanding of the interplay of comorbidity in addition to these gastrointestinal changes, will ensure that we meet the needs of our patients, helping them to maintain a high quality of life through their advancing years.

References

Arai, T., Kasahara, I., Sawabe, M., Honma, N., Aida, J., Tabubo, K. (2010) "Role of Methylation of the hMLH1 Gene Promoter in the Development of Gastric and Colorectal Carcinoma in the Elderly." *Geriatrics and Gerontology International*, **10**(Suppl 1): S207–12.

Bartges, J. (2014) "Feeding Geriatric Patients: What is the Best Nutritional Approach?" Paper presented at the American College of Veterinary Internal Medicine, Knoxville, TN.

Bernard, C. E., Gibbons, S. J., Gomez-Pinilla, P. J., Lurken, M. S., Schmalz, P. F., Roeder, J. L., *et al.* (2009) "Effect of Age on the Enteric Nervous System of the Human Colon." *Neurogastroenterology and Motility*, **21**: 746–e46.

Blechman, M. B., and Gelb, A. M. (1999) "Aging and Gastrointestinal Physiology." *Clinical Geriatric Medicine*, **15**: 429–38.

Cupp, C., Perez-Camargo, G., Patil, A., Kerr, W. (2004) "Long-Term Food Consumption and Body Weight Changes in a Controlled Population of Geriatric Cats." *Compendium for Continuing Education for the Practicing Veterinarian*, **26**(Suppl2A): 60.

Freeman, L. M., Rush, J. E., Milbury, P. E., Blumberg, J. B. (2005) "Antioxidant Status and Biomarkers of Oxidative Stress in Dogs with Congestive Heart Failure." *Journal of Veterinary Internal Medicine*, **19**: 537–41.

Fortney, W. (2008) Aging Process: Why Pets Age and How We Can Influence the Process. Atlantic Coast Veterinary Conference, Manhattan, KS. *DVM360*. Available at http://veterinarycalendar.dvm360.com/aging-process-why-pets-age-and-how-we-can-influence-process-proceedings.

Gomez, C. R., Boehmer, E. D., Kovacs, E. J. (2005) "The Aging Innate Immune System." *Current Opinion in Immunology*, **17**(5): 457–62.

Hall, K. E., Proctor, D. D., Fisher, L., Rose, S. (2005) "American Gastroenterology Future Trends Committee Report: Effects of Aging of the Population on Gastroenterology Practice, Education and Research." *Gastroenterology*, **129**:1305–38.

Harper, E. J. (1998) "Changing Perspectives on Aging and Energy Requirements: Aging and Energy Intakes in Humans, Dogs and Cats." *Journal of Nutrition*, **128** : 2623–6S.

Howland, R. (2009) "Effects of Aging on Pharmacokinetic and Pharmacodynamic Drug Processes." *Journal of Psychosocial Nursing and Mental Health Services*, **47**:15–18.

Kealy, R. D. (1999) "Factors Influencing Lean Body Mass in Aging Dogs." *Compendium for Continuing Education for the Practicing Veterinarian*, **21**: 34–7.

Kenney, W. L., and Chiu P. (2001) "Influence of Age on Thirst and Fluid Intake." *Medicine and Science in Sports and Exercise*, **33**(9): 1524–32.

Laflamme, D. P., and Ballam, J. M. (2002) "Effect of Age on Maintenance Energy Requirements of Adult Cats." *Compendium for Continuing Education for the Practicing Veterinarian*, **24**(Suppl9A): 82.

Lund, E. M., Armstrong, P. J., Kirk, C. A., Klausner, J. S. (2006) "Prevalence and Risk Factors for Obesity in Adult Dogs from Private Veterinary Practices." *International Journal of Applied Research in Veterinary Medicine*, **4**: 177–86.

McCrea, G. L., Miaskowski, C., Stotts, N. A., et al. (2008) "Pathophysiology of Constipation in the Older Adult." *World Journal of Gastroenterology*, **14**: 2631–8.

McLachlan, A. J., Pont, L. G. (2012) "Drug Metabolism in Older People: A Key Consideration in Achieving Optimal Outcomes with Medicines." *Journal of Gerontololology A Biological Sciences and Medical Sciences*, **67**(2): 175–80.

Meier, J., and Sturm, A. (2009) "The Intestinal Epithelial Barrier: Does it Become Impaired with Age?" *Digestive Diseases*, **27**(3): 240–5.

Nagar, A., and Roberts, I. M. (1999) "Small Bowel Diseases in the Elderly." *Clinical Geriatric Medicine*, **15**(3):473–86.

Nakamura K, Ogoshi K, Makuuchi H. (2006) "Influence of Aging, Gastric Mucosal Atrophy and Dietary Habits on Gastric Secretion." *Hepatogastroenterology*, **53**(70): 624–8.

Newton, J. L. (2004) "Changes in Upper Gastrointestinal Physiology with Age." *Mechanisms of Ageing and Developement*, **125**(12): 867–70.

O'Mahony, D., O'Leary, P., Quigley, E. M. (2002) "Aging and Intestinal Motility: A Review of Factors that Affect Intestinal Motility in the Aged." *Drugs and Aging*, **19**: 515–27.

Orr, W. C., and Chen, C. L. (2002) "Aging and Neural Control of the GI Tract: IV. Clinical and Physiological Aspects of Gastrointestinal Motility and Aging." *American Journal of Physiology Gastrointestinal and Liver Physiology*, **283**(6): G1226–31.

Perez-Camargo, G. (2004) "Cat Nutrition: What's New in the Old?" *Compendium for Continuing Education for the Practicing Veterinarian*, **26**(Suppl2A): 5–10.

Phillips, R. J., Pairitz, J. C., Powley, T. L. (2007) "Age-Related Neuronal Loss in the Submucosal Plexus of the Colon of Fischer 344 Rats." *Neurobiolical Aging*, **28**: 1124–37.

Quimby, J. (2015) "Evidence-Based Treatment of Chronic Renal Disease in Cats." In American College of Veterinary Internal Medicine (ACVIM) Forum, Indianapolis, IN, 3–6 June 2015, pp. 184–6. Lakewood, CO: ACVIM; 2015.

Rivera, R., and Antognini, J. (2009) "Perioperative Drug Therapy in Elderly Patients." *Anesthesiology*, **110**: 1176–81.

Rosenthal, T., and Nussinovitch, N. (2008) "Managing Hypertension in the Elderly in Light of the Changes During Aging." *Blood Pressure*, **17**: 186–94.

Ross, S. O., and Forsmark, C. E. (2001) "Pancreatic and Biliary Disorders in the Elderly." *Gastroenterology Clinics of North America*, **30**(2): 531–45.

Ruaux, C. (2002) "Cobalamin and Gastrointestinal Disease." In *Proceedings of the 20th ACVIM Congress, Dallas, TX, May–June 2002*, pp. 500–503.

Salles, N. (2007) "Basic Mechanisms of the Aging Gastrointestinal Tract." *Digestive Diseases*, **25**(2): 112–17.

Salles, N. (2009) "Is Stomach Spontaneously Ageing? Pathophysiology of the Aging Stomach." *Best Practice and Research Clinical Gastroenterology*, **23**(6): 805–19.

Santiago, A. F., Alves, A.C., Oliveira, R. P., Fernandes, R. M., Paula-Silva, J., Assis, F. A., Carvalho, C. R., Weiner, H. L., Faria, A. M. (2011) "Aging correlates with reduction in regulatory-type cytokines and T cells in the gut. *Immunobiology*, **216**(10): 1085–93.

Schmucker, D. L. (2005) "Age-Related Changes in Liver Structure and Function: Implications for Disease?" *Experimental Gerontology*, **40**(8–9): 650–9.

Schmucker, D. L., Owen, R. L., Outenreath, R., Thoreux, K. (2003) "Basis for the Age-Related Decline in Intestinal Mucosal Immunity." *Clinical and Developmental Immunology*, **10**(2–4): 167–72.

Shaker, R., and Staff, D. (2001) "Esophageal Disorders in the Elderly." *Gastroenterology Clinics of North AmErica*, **30**: 335–61.

Sostress, C., Gargallo, C., Lanas, A. (2009) "Drug-Related Damage of the Ageing Gastrointestinal Tract." *Best Practice and Research Clinical Gastroenterology*, **23**: 849–60.

Speakman, J. R., van Acker, A., Harper, E. J. (2003) "Age-Related Changes in the Metabolism and Body Composition of Three Dog Breeds and their Relationship to Life Expectancy." *Aging Cell*, **2**: 265–75.

Steiner, J. M. (2014) "Why Measure Vitamin B12?" In *The Great African Adventure, 39th World Small Animal Veterinary Association Congress, Cape Town, South Africa Proceedings*, pp. 383–386. Geneva: Kenes International.

Takubo, K., Nakamura, K., Izumiyama, N., Furugori, E., Sawabe, M., Arai, T., *et al.* (2000) "Telomere Shortening with Aging in Human Liver." *Journal of Gerontology A Biological Sciences and Medical Sciences*, **55**(11): B533–6.

Tamura J, Kubota K, Murakami H, et al. Immunomodulation by vitamin B12: augmentation of CD8+ T lymphocytes and NK cell activity in vitamin B12 deficient patients by methyl B12 treat- ment. *Clin Exp Immunol.* 1999;**116** : 28–32.

Tohno, Y., Tohno, S., Yamada, M. O., Azuma, C., Moriwake, Y., Minami, T. *et al.* (2004) "Age-related changes of elements and relationships among elements in the common bile and pancreatic ducts. *Biological Trace Element Research*, **101**(1): 47–60.

Wade, P. R., and Cowen, T. (2004) "Neurodegeneration: A Key Factor in the Ageing Gut." *Neurogastroenterology and Motility*, **16**(Suppl 1): 19–23.

Wannemacher, R. W. Jr., and McCoy, J. R. (1996) "Determination of Optimal Dietary Protein Requirements of Young and Old Dogs." *Journal of Nutrition*, **88**: 66–74.

Wiskur, B., and Greenwood-Van Meerveld, B. (2010) "The Aging Colon: The Role of Enteric Neurodegeneration in Constipation." *Current Gastroenterology Reports*, **12**: 507–12.

Wurtman JJ, Lieberman H, Tsay R et al. Calorie and nutri- ent intakes of elderly and young subjects measured under identical conditions. *J Gerontol* 1988;**43**:B174–80.

Wynne, H. A., Cope, L. H., Mutch, E., Rawlins, M. D., Woodhouse, K. W., James, O. F. (1989) "The Effect of Age upon Liver Volume and Apparent Liver Blood Flow in Healthy Man." *Hepatology*, **9**(2): 297–301.

16

Urinary and Fecal Incontinence
Faith Banks

Urinary Incontinence

Urinary incontinence is defined as the involuntary leakage of urine. It can occur from bladder storage dysfunction, urethral dysfunction or structural anomalies (Rothrock, 2015). With urinary incontinence, the pet does not have conscious control of urination. Thus, it needs to be differentiated from behavioral urinary issues (submissive urination), simple lack of housetraining, territorial marking of anxious cats or of unneutered males, or the senile loss of housetraining from cognitive dysfunction syndrome (Brooks, 2012). Urge incontinence may mimic urinary incontinence and can be seen in cats with severe feline lower urinary tract disease, or in dogs with severe cystitis or calculi. Although the amount of urine in their bladders may be small, the sensation may be overwhelming and the pet feels the need to void, perhaps in inappropriate locations. With true urinary incontinence, owners may see urine dribbling out of the pet; they may see wet fur around their pet's vulva or prepuce, or a they may find a wet spot on the pet's bed where they sleep.

Proper micturition comprises a urine storage phase and a urine voiding phase (Rothrock, 2015). A breakdown in this simple-sounding yet complex neurological system may result in incontinence. Urinary incontinence can be divided into neurogenic or non-neurogenic causes. Neurogenic causes can be further classified based on upper motor neuron (UMN) and lower motor neuron (LMN) causes, depending on the location of the lesion within the nervous system.

Causes of incontinence

There are two causes of neurogenic urinary incontinence. A lesion cranial to the sacral spinal cord segment at L7 causes disruption of the inhibitory control by the higher centers, so that sympathetic tone remains inappropriately high during the micturition reflex. This would produce "a UMN bladder" – a spastic or reflex bladder, whereas an LMN lesion (caudal to L7) would produce a flaccid or atonic bladder. In pets with this condition, a poor urine stream and incomplete emptying of the urinary bladder will ensue. With chronicity, this distention will lead to atonia of the detrusor muscle and the bladder will not be able to contract or empty properly (Rothrock, 2015). Lesions of the sacral spinal cord segments, pelvic nerve, and/or pudendal nerve cause reduced or absent pelvic sensation and loss of detrusor contraction. The bladder muscle will be flaccid and overdistended, which will lead to permanent bladder atony and subsequent overflow incontinence (Rothrock, 2015).

Non-neurogenic causes of urinary incontinence are either congenital or acquired abnormalities. In this chapter, we focus on acquired causes, as congenital causes are usually addressed prior to the geriatric stage of life. Acquired abnormalities may be inflammatory or infiltrative diseases (neoplasia) of the bladder or urethra, which would prevent normal voiding of urine. These underlying causes can usually be differentiated with a thorough medical history, physical exam and minimum database, including a urinalysis and urine culture. Diagnostic imaging may be needed to assist in ruling out urolithiasis or neoplasia.

The most common causes of urinary incontinence in geriatric dogs are urethral sphincter mechanism incontinence (USMI), urinary tract infections and disorders that cause polyuria and polydipsia (thus overloading the storage phase). Loss of house training, as seen in cognitive dysfunction syndrome, may be seen in geriatric dogs and cats. These pets will typically posture to urinate (or defecate), in contrast to true USMI, in which the urine may be seen leaking from them as they sleep.

Bladder tumors are more common in geriatric dogs compared with younger dogs, but they are not a common type of cancer in dogs. The most common type of bladder tumor is the transitional cell carcinoma (Krawiec, 1989). Treatment of this tumor is usually palliative, owing to its aggressive nature to metastasize and the location at the neck of the bladder which makes surgical excision difficult (Krawiec, 1989). Chemotherapy drugs are being evaluated, but at the moment, piroxicam is the anti-inflammatory drug of choice to ameliorate symptoms associated with this disease.

USMI is most commonly seen in large-breed, spayed, female dogs, but it can also be seen in male dogs. It is the most commonly diagnosed cause of urinary incontinence in dogs (Figure 16.1). The onset may be seen as early as three years after spaying, but it is more common in geriatric dogs.

Approximately 20% of spayed females develop urinary incontinence because of sphincter mechanism incontinence. Dogs weighing less than 44 lbs show a lower occurrence rate of 10%, and dogs weighing more than 44 lbs have a 30% rate of occurrence. Doberman Pinschers, Boxers, and Giant Schnauzers are at greatest risk for sphincter mechanism incontinence (Chew and Brown, 2004).

The hallmark sign of urinary incontinence seen by the owner is urine leakage while at rest, or the wet spot left in the pet's place. This may happen consistently or intermittently. Enuresis is the term given to the passage or leaking of urine while an animal is resting or asleep. These dogs may void normally during waking hours; thus, the voiding phase is normal, but the filling phase is altered, due to a faulty sphincter holding in the urine. Causes are multifactorial, but individual anatomy, a pelvic location of the internal urethral sphincter owing to removal of the broad ligaments during spay, and lack of estrogen stimulating the receptors in the internal sphincter are all possible contributing factors (Rothrock, 2015). Obesity may also play a role.

USMI is a very manageable condition. Ensuring proper diagnosis and treatment is paramount, so owners do not get too frustrated with a constant mess, thus tearing at the human–animal bond.

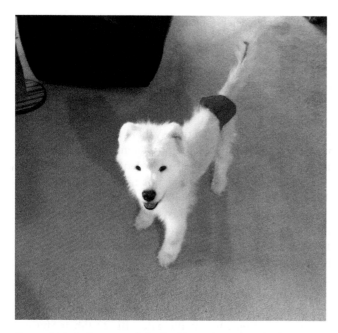

Figure 16.1 Serissa not only had sphincter laxity but also had diabetes and Cushing's disease, which led to constant urinating in the house (on rugs). Her owners used a doggy diaper, but used female sanitary napkins as they were easier to use and more economical.

Medical Treatment for USMI

Estrogen is a commonly used medication for the treatment of dogs with hormone responsive urinary incontinence. It enhances the urethral closure primarily by increasing the number and responsiveness of alpha receptors in urethral smooth muscle (Lane, 2013). Diethylstilbestrol is a synthetic estrogen and is the most widely used drug for USMI (0.1–1 mg/dog every 24 hours for five to seven days, followed by once- or twice-weekly administration). Estrogens effectively relieve incontinence in 60–80% of dogs with USMI (Chew, 2004).

Estriol (Incurin™, Merck) is a drug available in Europe and the USA. Product information for Incurin reports improvement or continence in 99% of treated dogs by six weeks of treatment. The starting dose is 2 mg/dog/day for one week, then the dose is reduced at weekly intervals to the minimum effective dose (Lane, 2013).

The alpha-adrenergic agonist, phenylpropanolamine (PPA, 1.5 mg/kg orally every 8–24 hours) is also used, with 90% or greater responding in small studies. This drug stimulates receptors within the internal urethral sphincter, increasing resting urethral sphincter tone (Rothrock, 2015). It may be used in conjunction with estrogens in resistant cases and is often needed from one to three times a day.

Ephedrine is also an alpha-adrenergic agonist that is similar to PPA (2–4 mg/kg orally twice daily), although it may have more adverse effects, such as tachycardia (Rothrock, 2015).

Another class of drug that works in dogs with USMI are the anticholinergic drugs. These medications do not work on the sphincter but on the body of the bladder, by relaxing the muscle fibers and allowing easier storage of urine (Rothrock, 2015). Imipramine, an anti-anxiety medication, falls into this class of drug. This option can be used if the combination of diethylstilbestrol and PPA do not work.

In male dogs, testosterones have a target action on the prostate and seem to be more effective than estrogens in controlling USMI. Adverse effects may include associated negative male behaviors.

Surgical intervention is not a typical route taken in geriatric patients, especially because medical management is usually quite effective. When necessary, surgical options for treatment of urinary incontinence include colposuspension and cystoure-thropexy. Colposuspension involves tacking the vagina to the ventral abdomen, thus entrapping and compressing the urethra. Cystourethropexy is a modification of the above procedure, which can also can be performed on males. Fibers from urethral muscles are tacked down and compressed to the urethra (Rothrock, 2015). The above medications would be used in conjunction with these procedures.

The newest therapy to treat USMI is one that uses injections of collagen into the urethra via endoscope. It is showing promise, especially when used with the medications listed above. Several injections would be used. It is not a common form of treatment at this time.

Acupuncture may be helpful in dealing with urinary incontinence. The most common set of points used by veterinary acupuncturists is called the kidney tiara and is composed of a series of four points: GV-4 (Ming Men or life gate), BL-23 (Shen Shu or Kidney Association point), BL-52 (Zhi Shi or room of will) and GB-25 (Jing Men or capital gate and Mu Point of the Kidney).

Veterinary chiropractic adjustments may also be used to help increase bladder function in older dogs. If a subluxation in the area of T12 to L7 is found, restoring normal range of motion within the TL vertebral segments may improve the incontinence by increasing sympathetic tone to the bladder (Lowell, 2003).

Routine follow-up, including examination, blood pressure, and minimum database (including full blood count, chemistry panel, urinalysis, and culture and sensitivity) should be done in dogs after initiating medical management.

Although urinary incontinence may press the limits of the human–animal bond, it is a very treatable disorder. With early intervention, education and medical management, this problem can be successfully treated, leading to a significant reduction in the pet's accidents within the home, and thus maintaining a pet's spot, not wet spot, on an owner's bed and in their heart.

Fecal Incontinence

What goes in, must come out. Unfortunately, as our pets age, many of them will lose the ability to control when and where this latter part occurs. Fecal incontinence is the inability to control defecation, which results in the involuntary passage of feces (Katherman and Shell, 2014). Pets with fecal incontinence, therefore may not posture to have a bowel movement and they may not be conscious of the fact they are passing stool. The problem often begins with an occasional rogue fecal ball found in a corner of the room where a dog was sleeping. Sometimes feces can be seen coming out of the pet as they cough, climb stairs, or struggle to stand from a recumbent position. If the fecal incontinence is neurologic in origin, there may also be associated urinary incontinence.

Fecal incontinence may be seen in pets of any age, but as they age, certain diseases with associated fecal incontinence become more common. Diagnosis is usually based on a thorough history, physical exam and neurological exam (Figure 16.2). Subsequent x-rays and magnetic resonance imaging may be indicated to help localize a lesion along the spinal cord. Referral to a neurologist may even be necessary to help localize the lesion and decide whether surgery is indicated. There is no sex predilection with fecal incontinence and generally half are more than 11 years old (Guilford, 1990).

Fecal incontinence is a very challenging issue for owners to deal with as it is unpleasant and unhygienic to live with a pet with this problem. On top of this, fecal incontinence is often seen in large-breed dogs with their associated large amounts of stool. This is not good for the human–animal bond and many pets are euthanized when urinary or fecal incontinence (or both) become the new norm. Doggy or kitty diapers may work for small dogs (Figure 16.3) and cats, but putting a diaper on a fecally incontinent large dog may not be manageable or desirable. Diapers to contain urine, on the other hand, may be easier to maintain for an owner.

All causes of fecal incontinence are not discussed here, as we are assuming that the pet was continent until it reached its geriatric years. With this assumption, fecal incontinence can be grouped into two broad categories: reservoir incontinence and anal sphincter incontinence. Anal sphincter incontinence can be further subdivided into non-neurologic and neurologic related.

With reservoir incontinence, conscious control is overwhelmed, leading the pet to posture to defecate while not being able to stop the passage of the feces. This category of incontinence is caused by the colon or rectum's ability, or rather, inability to contain the feces, and is characterized by frequent conscious defecation. Owing to the pet's awareness of the passage of stool, it cannot be classifed as true fecal incontinence. Reservoir incontinence may be seen in geriatric pets with diseases of their colon or rectum, as seen in colitis or cancer. If the colon is not able to process ingesta properly by absorbing water and storing the feces, large amounts of feces may be expressed. Otherwise healthy geriatric pets with severe diarrhea may develop a temporary or transient fecal incontinence if they are not able to control the urge to defecate.

Adenocarcinoma of the colon and rectum is seen in dogs and has a high curative rate with surgery. Anal sac adenocarcinoma is also seen in dogs over 10 years of age and with equal prevalence in males and females. The median survival time of dogs with anal sac adenocarcinoma with surgery and chemotherapy is about 18 months (Thomson, 2005).

The anal sphincter is a ring of muscle that opens and closes the opening of the anus (Smith and Tilley, 2015). Non-neurologic-related anal sphincter incontinence occurs when there is a failure of the muscles or nerves supplying the anal sphincter to contain the feces adequately, which results in involuntary dribbling of feces from the anus (Guilford, 1990). This type of fecal incontinence may be seen in geriatric pets with perianal fistulas or trauma to the sphincter from a previous anal sacculectomy, or from neoplasia affecting the sphincter. Fortunately, anal neoplasia is uncommon in dogs and rare in cats. The most common anal neoplasms are anal sac adenocarcinoma and benign perianal adenomas, but perianal adenocarcinomas, squamous cell carcinomas, and melanomas can also occur (Rothrock, 2011).

Neurologic-related anal sphincter incontinence is further divided into LMN and UMN causes. In dogs with LMN disease, they will often have decreased anal tone, decreased perineal and pudendal–anal reflexes, decreased anal and rectal sensation,

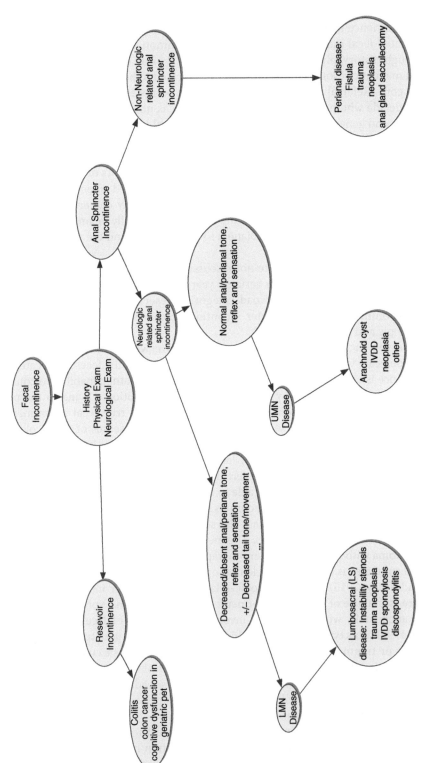

Figure 16.2 Algorithm to aid in diagnosis of fecal incontinence.

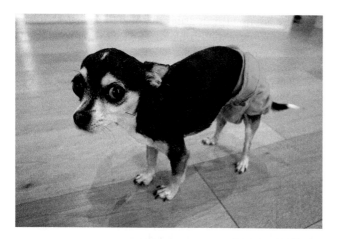

Figure 16.3 B.D is a fussy, senior chihuahua with a very small bladder. Choosing a soft carpet to urinate on was preferred over the outside cold or rainy weather. Wearing a doggie diaper helps her to 'hold it' and prevents 'accidents' in the house, thus maintaining the human animal bond.

and sometimes decreased tail tone and movement. In cases where there is concurrent paraparesis and proprioceptive deficits, the lesion has extended cranially to involve the sciatic nerve. These dogs will often have lumbosacral instability/stenosis, discospondylitis, severe spondylosis, intervertebral disk disease, neoplasia or have evidence of trauma (Katherman and Shell, 2014). Degenerative myelopathy and cauda equina syndrome, often seen in large-breed, geriatric dogs, can also cause fecal incontinence.

The degree of clinical signs will depend on the extent of the compression of the L7, sacral and caudal nerve roots. Pudendal nerve root involvement causes fecal or urinary incontinence, while caudal nerve root involvement causes a weak or paralyzed tail. Sciatic nerve root involvement causes lameness, pelvic limb weakness, proprioceptive deficits and muscle wasting (Davies and Shell, 2001).

UMN incontinence is not as common as LMN incontinence. In this type of condition, anal and perianal tone, reflexes and sensation are all normal. These dogs may still have signs of paraparesis or quadriparesis (Katherman and Shell, 2014). Depending on where the lesion is located, there may be urinary incontinence as well, with a bladder that is difficult to express. The presence of urinary and fecal incontinence strongly suggests neurologic-related anal sphincter incontinence. Arachnoid cysts are common causes of UMN fecal incontinence. The prognosis for amelioration of UMN fecal incontinence is fair to good after surgical correction but poor with LMN disease (Katherman and Shell, 2014). This is the reason localization of the lesion is useful, as the prognosis for repairing the underlying problem and the associated incontinence is quite different with UMN compared with LMN disease. Diagnosis may be made with lateral and ventral/dorsal radiographs, myelogram, computed tomography or magnetic resonance imaging of the affected area.

Treatment for fecal incontinence should be focused on addressing the underlying issue causing the incontinence, as there is no specific cure to treat fecal incontinence in and of itself. At the present time, there are no proven drugs that will reverse the incontinence, but several may be tried to ameliorate the problem. The following have been proposed to aid in fecal incontinence (Katherman and Shell, 2014):

- Phenylpropanolamine at 1.5–2 mg/kg orally every 8–12 hours may help to increase the resting tone of the internal anal sphincter.
- Diphenoxylate (Lomotil®) at 0.05–0.2 mg/kg orally every 6–8 hours in dogs and 0.05–0.1 mg/kg orally every 12 hours in cats may help to slow the passage of stool. Constipation, bloating and sedation are possible side effects. This is an off-label recommendation.
- Loperamide (Immodium®) at 0.04–0.2 mg/kg PO q 8–12 hours may be given initially then decreased to the lowest effective dose. This may cause constipation and is off label and not recommended in cats. This drug is contraindicated for Collies, Shelties and Old English Sheepdogs, as these breeds may carry a mutant form of the MDR1gene, which can limit their ability to metabolize this drug.

Geriatric pets may have increased toileting needs when compared with their younger counterparts. They may require more frequent trips outdoors, or more litter boxes around the home to allow easier access when they get the urge to eliminate. Doggie doors or indoor pee pads may be helpful by allowing increased access to areas where defecation is acceptable. Arthritis or degenerative joint disease will make posturing to urinate and defecate more difficult, so a pet may not fully evacuate their rectum or bladder when taking the opportunity to void. Muscle loss and weakness further complicate the issue. Managing a pet's pain may improve fecal incontinence by ameliorating mobility limitations associated with getting up and out to eliminate. Nonsteroidal anti-inflammatory drugs, gabapentin, neutraceuticals and opioids may all be used (singly or in combination) for analgesia. Reduced awareness, as seen in cognitive dysfunction syndrome, may result in the pet being less aware of its external environment and possibly less able to signal to the owner that they need to "go" (Hunthausen, 2008). Addressing cognitive dysfunction syndrome may be a useful path for aiding in house soiling issues. With aging comes degeneration. Multiple factors are likely involved, including muscular atrophy of the hind end, with subsequent weakness and senility as well.

While medications may be needed, changes in a pet's daily routine can also be quite helpful when managing fecal incontinence. Scheduled feeding will help owners to monitor timing of food going in and subsequent feces coming out. Changing diets to a highly digestible food, thus producing a low amount of stool, or conversely, increasing the fiber to produce a firmer stool may stimulate the rectum of the dog to allow them to be more aware of the signs of rectal distention and the need to evacuate.

Taking dogs out 15–20 minutes after feeding to void may be helpful. Confining incontinent pets to areas of the house that allow for easier clean up will decrease the stress on the owner. Removing valuable carpets will prevent further damage. Baby gates or playpens may also be used to limit the access of an incontinent pet to all areas of the house. As previously mentioned, pet diapers may be used in certain pets that tolerate wearing them and the subsequent clean up. Special care must be taken in outdoor pets that have fecal incontinence, as maggots may become an issue.

Other Help for Pet Owners

Encourage pet owners to not get angry or discipline their elderly pet, as the house soiling may not be intentional or controllable. Some examples of incontinence products that can help keep pets and their environments dry include:

- doggy diapers (Figure 16.3)
- belly bands
- diaper pads
- waterproof bed pads
- throw rugs
- rubber mats.

These items can be purchased at local pets stores or online at specialty pet websites.

Unfortunately, fecal and urinary incontinence are issues that press the limits of the human–animal bond and many pets are euthanized when these issues become commonplace. Understanding the underlying reason for the incontinence and making some changes to the environment, diet, and medical treatment may help pet owners and their fecally incontinent pets live peacefully together.

References

Brooks, W. C. (2012) "Urinary Incontinence." Pet Health Library, Veterinary Information Network. Available at http://www.veterinarypartner.com/Content. plx?P=A&S=0&C=0&A=1724.

Chew, D. C., and Brown, S. A. (2004) "Fixing the Dripping in Senior Female Dogs." IAMS Senior Care 2004. Veterinary Information Network. Available at http://www.vin.com/members/cms/project/defaultadv1.aspx?id=3853279&pid=11171&catid=&.

Davies, C. and Shell, L. (2001) "Fecal Incontinence." In *Common Small Animal Diagnoses: An Algorithmic Approach, Section 7*. Philadelphia, PA: Saunders.

Guilford, W.G. (1990) "Fecal Incontinence in Dogs and Cats." *Compendium of Continuing Education for Veterinarians*, **12**(3): 313–26.

Hunthausen, W. L. (2008) "Canine House Soiling Proceedings." Available at http://veterinarycalendar.dvm360.com/canine-housesoiling-proceedings?id=&sk=&date=&pageID=6.

Katherman, A. E., and Shell, L. (2014) "Fecal Incontinence." Veterinary Information Network. Available at http://www.vin.com/Members/Associate/Associate.plx?from=GetDzInfo&DiseaseId=2712.

Krawiec, D. R. (1989) "Urologic Disorders of the Geriatric Dog." *Veterinary Clinics of North America Small Animal Practice*, **19**(1): 75–85.

Lane, I. F. (2013) "Medical Management of Canine Incontinence." University of Tennessee, Knoxville at Central Veterinary Conference 2013, Washington DC. Veterinary Information Network. Available at http://www.vin.com/members/cms/project/defaultadv1.aspx?id=6566212&pid=11377&catid=&

Lowell, D. N. (2003) "Use of Acupuncture and Chiropractic for Urinary Incontinence." Presented at the Western Veterinary Conference 2003.

Rothrock, K. (2015) "Urinary Incontinence." Veterinary Information Network. Available at http://www.vin.com/Members/Associate/Associate.plx?from=GetDzInfo& DiseaseId=1108.

Rothrock, K. (2011) "Anal Neoplasia." Veterinary Information Network. Available at http://www.vin.com/Members/Associate/Associate.plx?DiseaseId=709.

Smith, F. and Tilley, L. (2015) "Incontinence, Fecal." In *Blackwell's Five-Minute Veterinary Consult: Canine and Feline*, (6th ed.), pp. 745–6. Ames IA: Wiley Blackwell.

Thomson, M. (2005) "The Rear-End of the Dog." Presented at the Australian College of Veterinary Scientists Science Week 2005.

17

Thermoregulation

Brad Bates

As pets age, their ability to regulate body temperature decreases, making them less adaptable to changes in environmental temperature (Doctors Foster and Smith Inc., 2016). Geriatric pets have multiple changes that contribute to this loss of body temperature regulation, predisposing them to hypo- or hyperthermia. This chapter reviews general body temperature regulation, specific changes that occur as pets age and how these changes affect body temperature regulation, and outlines management efforts to help protect geriatric pets from hypo- or hyperthermia.

Body Temperature Physiology: A Brief Review

The anterior hypothalamus regulates and maintains body temperature within a narrow limit, often referred to as the hypothalamic "set point" (Cunningham and Klein, 2007; Reineke, 2009). Table 17.1 shows the normal rectal temperatures of various domestic animals. Information from central and peripheral body receptors and other inputs are integrated within the hypothalamus, which then influences heat-losing or heat-conserving processes in the body. Some of these processes remain the same as pets age, but certain specific changes occur in geriatric patients. These changes can contribute to body heat loss or impaired ability to maintain body temperature, leading to hypothermia. Conversely, some diseases of old age can predispose a geriatric pet to hyperthermia and subsequent heat stroke (Cunningham and Klein, 2007).

Body temperature depends on a tightly regulated balance between heat input and heat output. The ability to regulate this balance is often impaired in geriatric pets (Cunningham and Klein, 2007). Heat input to the body comes from external sources such as ambient temperature, as well as internal sources including the generation of body heat through metabolism and oxidation of nutrients. General muscle function also contributes to internal sources of heat (Reineke, 2009). Heat produced at every stage of food metabolism is eventually dissipated from the body through evaporation, conduction, convection, and radiation (Cunningham and Klein, 2007). A specific discussion of these mechanisms is beyond the scope of this chapter. Changes in the geriatric patient, including loss of subcutaneous fat, can affect these heat-losing and heat-conserving processes (Cunningham and Klein, 2007).

Treatment and Care of the Geriatric Veterinary Patient, First Edition. Edited by Mary Gardner and Dani McVety.
© 2017 John Wiley & Sons, Inc. Published 2017 by John Wiley & Sons, Inc.
Companion Website: www.wiley.com/go/gardner/geriatric

Table 17.1 Normal rectal temperatures of various domestic mammals.

Species	Temperature (°C)	
	Average	Range
Dog	38.9	37.9–39.9
Cat	38.6	38.1–39.2
Horse	37.7	37.2–38.2
Cattle (beef)	38.3	36.7–39.1
Cattle (dairy)	38.6	38.0–39.3
Goat	39.1	38.5–39.7
Donkey	37.4	36.4–38.4
Pig	39.2	38.7–39.8
Sheep	39.1	38.5–39.9
Chicken	41.8	40.6–43.0
Rabbit	39.4	38.6–40.1

Source: Adapted from Cunningham and Klein (2007) and Aiello and Moses (2012).

Animals can gain heat from the environment in one of two ways: when the ambient temperature exceeds body temperature and when a radiant heat source is applied to or near the body (Cunningham and Klein, 2007). Managing environmental temperature is even more important for the general care of geriatric pets. It is important to know the ideal ambient temperature ranges for your pet, which varies by species. Later in this chapter, we review some management efforts that can be used to provide radiant heat or to help insulate a pet.

Changes in body temperature away from the hypothalamic "set point" leads to the activation of physiologic processes to elevate or decrease body temperature. For example, the hypothalamus regulates and initiates cooling mechanisms when core body temperature rises above this point. Unlike cats and humans, dogs will begin panting, which initiates evaporative cooling as the first process initiated in response to increases in body temperature (Reineke, 2009). The next process in dogs, and usually the first process in cats and other animals, is dilation of peripheral veins (vasodilation), as well as increased cardiac output. Together, these processes lead to evaporation, conduction, convection, and radiation, all of which contribute to body cooling (Reineke, 2009). Hyperthermia and potential heat stroke results from the failure of this normal thermoregulation (Reineke. 2009). See below for a brief description of heat stroke.

Decreases in body temperature initiates shivering and heat-seeking behaviors. Although shivering can be effective in restoring body temperature, it is associated with a significant increase in metabolic oxygen demand. This may result in an "oxygen debt", and may be significant for patients suffering from cardiac and/or respiratory diseases (Reuss-Lamky, 2015). Heat-seeking behaviors can include hovering around heating vents and furnaces, and even laying on warm surfaces such as computers, a common behavior seen in cats (Figure 17.1).

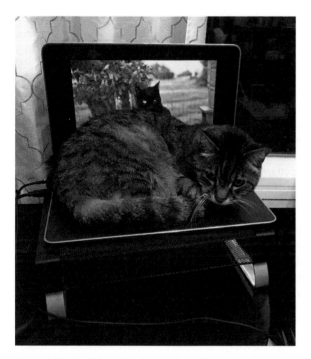

Figure 17.1 Bodhi, an 18-year-old cat in kidney failure, started to lay on his owner's laptop.

Hypothermia

Hypothermia is defined as a body temperature below the normal hypothalamic "set point" (Reineke, 2009; Palmer, 2012). The normal temperature range for canines and felines is 100–102.5 °F (37.8–39.2 °C) (Table 17.1). Decreases in body temperature of just one degree from this normal value can have adverse effects on health, especially for those that are already geriatric and compromised. Smaller geriatric pets are more susceptible to hypothermia because they have a higher surface area to body mass ratio, which compounds their decreased thermoregulatory ability (Palmer, 2012). Extra care, in regards to ambient temperature, should be taken when caring for geriatric pets that are small in body size. See below for management techniques to ensure appropriate body temperature in geriatric pets. Box 17.1 describes the case of Bodhi, a geriatric cat.

Altered Thermoregulation in Geriatric Patients

Physiologic changes in response to a lowered body temperature, such as vasoconstriction and shivering, occur in geriatric animals but at relatively lower body temperatures than those in younger patients (Glowaski, 2002). Additionally, the ability to vasoconstrict and reduce skin blood flow is decreased with advanced age, leading to greater heat loss in geriatric pets exposed to a cold environment, as compared with younger pets. These alterations in the geriatric patient's ability to regulate body temperature predisposes them to hypothermia (Glowaski, 2002). Many pets will therefore seek out warmer spots to sleep or lay in. A dog that used to love the cold tile floor may now prefer a bed or blankets. Or a cat may lay on the sunny window sill more or even steal a spot on a warm laptop (Figure 17.1).

Box 17.1 Thermoregulation Case Study

Patient: Bodhi (15-year-old male Domestic Shorthair)

History

Bodhi was adopted from a rescue at the age of 13 years. He came to his owner in Iris stage 2 kidney failure. No pertinent history was given to the rescue and it was unknown why he was sent there. Bodhi's diet is a veterinary prescription kidney diet, which he loves.

 Bodhi takes amlodipine for high blood pressure, receives 100 ml subcutaneous fluids every other day and a subcutaneous vitamin B12 injection weekly.

Discussion

Bodhi's family always keeps the house at 72 degrees, year round. Despite this, Bodhi will always get on his mother's laptop for a heat source (Figure 17.1). His family has also discovered that he would lay in a sunny spot in one area of their house. After discussion with his veterinarian, his mother purchased a heating bed for Bodhi (Figure 17.2). As a result, his family has noticed that he is less likely to sit on the warm computers and even seems a bit happier and more comfortable. He does like to lay in the sunny spot too from the French doors.

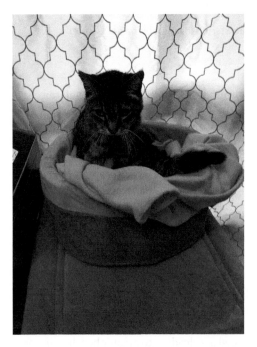

Figure 17.2 Bodhi's family purchased him a cat bed containing a warming pad.

Predisposition for Hypothermia in the Elderly

Human studies have shown that elderly people have reduced ability to maintain body temperature regulation and defend their core temperature during cold exposure, thus increasing the risk of hypothermia as compared to younger individuals (Young, 1991).

Age-related changes in the elderly, including lowered ability to increase metabolic heat production in response to cold exposure and a slower cutaneous vasoconstrictor response, appear to be factors (Young, 1991). These findings have also been shown in geriatric pets and similar changes can be expected.

Similar human studies exhibit some gender differences which may or may not exist to the same extent in animal species. Also, some studies show that age-related effects to cold exposure may be more related to age-associated changes in body condition and physical fitness, rather than to age directly (Young, 1991). Other studies aimed at separating the effects of age from concurrent factors, such as fitness level, body composition, and the effects of chronic disease, have shown that temperature tolerance appears to be minimally compromised by age and much more associated with these physical changes (Kenney and Munce, 2003). It is possible that this same correlation is found in animal species. The significance of these findings relates to the potential to focus on preventing and managing age-associated physical changes and diseases (such as weight/body condition loss or gain, physical fitness/stamina, and drug therapy for underlying diseases) as a means of preventing body temperature aberrations.

Changes in Metabolic Rate with Age

Metabolic rate affects heat production by the body, and as metabolic rate decreases, so does the ability to internally produce heat. As pets age, their basal metabolic rate decreases over time. This plays a major factor in the diminished ability for geriatric pets to regulate their body temperatures, especially with changes and extremes in ambient temperatures (Cunningham and Klein, 2007). Preventing decreases in metabolic rate may not be possible as pets age, but ensuring adequate caloric intake and providing a balanced diet may allow for adequate or improved generation of body heat through nutrient metabolism and maintenance of body condition.

Loss of Body Condition and Subcutaneous Fat with Age

As pets age and enter the geriatric stage, weight loss from fat and muscle deterioration are major concerns and common occurrences. Sarcopenia, an age-related loss of muscle mass, is a common clinical sign in the geriatric pet population (Kenney and Munce, 2003; Cunningham and Klein, 2007). As discussed earlier, aging in humans and animals is associated with a diminished vasoconstriction response during exposure to cold. This phenomenon is exacerbated by sarcopenia when a patient is exposed to cold environments. This loss of muscle also contributes to diminished heat production from less muscle activity and lower metabolism (Kenney and Munce, 2003). Thus, loss of body condition and subcutaneous fat can predispose a pet to hypothermia.

Although body surface area may not change considerably during adult life, body surface does often increase during the geriatric years. Smaller animals have a relatively greater surface area per kilogram of body weight versus larger animals. As pets age and enter the geriatric years, their body condition and overall body size often decreases, owing to muscle and fat loss. The resulting increase in body surface area provides a larger area for heat loss (Cunningham and Klein, 2007) Additionally, fat metabolism is a very effective way to produce heat in the body. As the percentage of body fat decreases with age, so does the heat production from fat metabolism. The loss of body fat affects overall body heat production and can lead to a hypothermic state in a geriatric pet (Cunningham and Klein, 2007).

Hyperthermia

Hyperthermia is defined as an elevation in body temperature, which occurs when heat production and/or input exceed heat loss. The term hyperthermia incorporates fevers (pyrogenic), as well as non-pyrogenic disease processes. With fevers, chemical mediators called pyrogens act on the anterior hypothalamus to raise the hypothalamic "set point" (Reineke, 2009). This leads to internal mechanisms and processes, as well as behavioral changes, that can increase body temperature, mostly assisting with controlling the underlying disease process. Owing to certain protective physiologic mechanisms, fevers rarely cause complications often seen with non-pyrogenic hyperthermia and subsequent heat stroke. It is important to note that most studies have shown that a true fever will actually benefit the patient, and can reduce the morbidity and mortality associated with infectious diseases (Reineke, 2009). Heat stroke, however, is a condition of non-pyrogenic hyperthermia, severe enough to cause multi-organ dysfunction, often including central nervous system damage (Reineke, 2009).

Heat Stroke

Heat stroke is an extreme increase in body temperature and can be caused by exertional and non-exertional factors, or a mix of the two. Most episodes of heat stroke seen in geriatric pets are due to exertional factors and are typically seen as the warm seasons approach, before pets have a chance to acclimate to the change in ambient temperature. Certain internal factors can predispose to heat stroke by impairing the geriatric pet's ability to dissipate heat, including obesity, laryngeal paralysis, tracheal collapse, and the extreme anatomical characteristics of brachycephalic breeds. Exogenous factors, such as extreme ambient temperature and humidity, poorly ventilated housing, and inadequate water consumption contribute to the development of hyperthermia and subsequent heat stroke (Reineke, 2009).

Heat stroke is classified as an emergency, with clinical signs that often include profound and excessive panting, collapse, alterations in mentation, and gastrointestinal signs, including decreased appetite, vomiting, and diarrhea. Usually, a combination of external factors, such as high ambient temperatures, and internal factors including diseases like obesity and/or laryngeal paralysis are seen with episodes of heat stroke. An elevated rectal temperature with the above classic clinical signs support the diagnosis of heat stroke. It is important to remember that severe dehydration leading to poor (rectal) tissue perfusion (hypovolemia) and measures initiated to help cool the pet may lead to a normal or low rectal temperature, making the diagnosis a bit more elusive (Reineke, 2009). While true heat stroke can occur in the geriatric patient, it is rare, as their aging biology lends more readily to hypothermic conditions.

Complications of heat stroke are common, and include several temporary and permanent changes to the patient. These result from poor tissue perfusion, secondary to hypovolemia and severe vasodilation, as well as loss of fluids from excessive panting, vomiting, diarrhea, and even hemorrhage resulting from disseminated intravascular coagulation (DIC). The development of DIC is common with heat stroke, and leads to a very poor prognosis. DIC is a state of hemostatic imbalance where, initially, coagulation is triggered, leading to a hypercoagulable state and the potential for thrombi formation throughout small vessels. Coagulation can quickly become uncontrolled, and eventually platelets and coagulation factors are depleted leading to a hypocoagulable state (Stokol, 2014). Cortical blindness is common with heat stroke and can resolve if the patient improves with treatment (Reineke, 2009).

Prognosis for pets with heat stroke is often guarded. Treatment can be expensive and challenging, owing to the many systemic complications. Overall mortality rate can be as high as 50%, and with delayed presentation for emergency treatment, the prognosis can be even worse (Reineke, 2009).

Geriatric Diseases That Affect Temperature Regulation

Since body tissues are poor heat conductors, heat is transferred around the body from metabolic heat sources (for example, the liver, heart, or limb muscles) via convection in the circulation. Thus, any disease process that affects circulation will also affect the ability for heat to be dispersed through the body. Diseases that may cause profound dehydration can therefore also affect the ability to maintain a normal body temperature. These diseases include, but are not limited to, Diabetes Mellitus, Hyperthyroidism, Cushing's disease, and kidney disease (Cunningham and Klein, 2007).

Elderly people and pets with heart failure are commonly on diuretics. In people, it has been shown that diuretics can increase the risk for thermoregulatory failure and hyperthermia, because of reduced cardiac output and resulting impaired heat dissipation related to hypovolemia (Szakacs, 2015). Similar findings would be expected in geriatric pets treated with diuretics.

Some diseases in elderly people increase heat production, and therefore can predispose to hyperthermia. These include Hyperthyroidism, Pheochromocytoma and Obesity (Szakacs, 2015). A similar predisposition for hyperthermia can be expected in geriatric pets suffering from similar conditions. Additionally, certain age- and breed-related diseases in animals can predispose to hyperthermia due to impaired heat-dissipating mechanisms as stated previously, namely Laryngeal Paralysis and Tracheal Collapse (Reineke, 2009). Age related factors, including obesity and progressive tracheal cartilage dysfunction, will compound the anatomic changes seen in brachycephalic breeds and cause progressive dyspnea as these pets enter their geriatric years. The impairment of normal respiration and panting can predispose these pets to hyperthermia and heat stroke.

Effects of Hypo- and Hyperthermia

Nearly all major organ systems are adversely affected by excessive and prolonged hypothermia and hyperthermia. Hypothermia can cause decreased cardiac output, resulting in an increased risk of arrhythmias and subsequent reduced tissue perfusion and oxygenation. Poor tissue circulation may increase the risk of drug-related adverse effects owing to delayed drug metabolism, and impaired clearance of medications from decreased hepatic metabolism and/or impaired excretion from kidney function (Glowaski, 2002; Reuss-Lamky, 2015). Decreased intestinal motility associated with poor tissue oxygenation may enhance time for absorption of drugs, leading to higher blood concentrations and potential adverse effects (Glowaski, 2002). These changes can contribute to an increase in adverse effects seen in geriatric pets on medications. Additionally, poor cardiac output and subsequent impaired tissue perfusion and oxygenation will lead to and contribute to organ dysfunction, including that seen with chronic kidney disease and other ailments. Additionally, hypothermia can lead to suppressed immune function, resulting in increased risk of infection and delayed wound healing (Reuss-Lamky, 2015). Bleeding may also be seen, owing to impaired platelet function and effects on the coagulation cascade. The vasoconstriction that accompanies hypothermia causes relative tissue hypoxia and the hypoxia results in decreased wound healing, potentially predisposing geriatric pets to skin inflammation, infections and decubital sores. The decreased clearance of drugs may result in severe and irreversible organ damage related to medication use (Glowaski, 2002).

The effects of hyperthermia are most severe when they lead to heat stroke. It can be expected that prolonged hyperthermia can lead to dehydration from respiratory fluid loss, especially with panting in dogs. As discussed earlier, dehydration related to elevated body temperature can confound diseases often seen in geriatric pets, and can predispose them to hyperthermia.

Geriatric Pet Management: Preventing Hypo- and Hyperthermia

Preventing hypothermia is easier and more efficient than treating it once it occurs. Simple measures to prevent and treat hypothermia include: providing a warm environment, towels, blankets, or clothing (such as sweaters), and using heating devices/sources (Reuss-Lamky. 2015).

Heating devices include heating blankets and beds (Figure 17.2), radiant heat lamps, heated rice bags, and heated water containers. These heat sources rely on the ability to transfer heat into the body core. The ability to enhance core body temperature depends on skin temperature, the patient's body condition, and the ability to circulate heat (the patient's state of circulation, thus level of hydration) (Reuss-Lamky, 2015). The efficacy of warming devices can be unpredictable, since the body core is isolated from distal skin surfaces. Nonetheless, skin temperature is an important consideration in providing effective heat transfer to the core (Reuss-Lamky, 2015). Focusing on increasing heat supplied to a geriatric pet and increasing skin temperature can therefore be effective in increasing core body temperature and preventing hypothermia. It is important to note that at least 60% of the body surface area must be in contact with the external heat source for effective rewarming (Reuss-Lamky, 2015).

Convection-type warm air devices such as the BAIR Hugger® and electric fabric warmers such as the HotDog® Warmer (Augustine Biomedical + Design) are mostly used during periods of anesthesia and post-anesthesia in hospitals. These tend to be the most effective means of preventing and treating anesthesia-induced hypothermia (Reuss-Lamky 2015). Use of these devices may not be feasible or necessary in the home environment.

Care must be taken with commercially available wire-electric heating pads and heat lamps since they have been associated with overheating, thermal injury, and electrocution (Kenney and Munce, 2003; Reuss-Lamky, 2015). When an external heat source is used, a thermometer should be placed at the pet's level to monitor actual applied heat (Glowaski 2002). Additionally, a proper barrier (towels or blankets) should be placed between the heat source and the patient. Electrocution is also a possibility with electric heating pads if they come in contact with liquids (Palmer, 2012). This can be of concern in pets with urinary incontinence, vomiting and/or diarrhea.

If warm water containers are used, it is important to warm them to a temperature of 107 degrees F or lower, to avoid skin burns and uneven heating. It is also important to remove them once they cool to the temperature of the patient because at that point they begin to contribute to heat loss, predisposing the pet to hypothermia (Reuss-Lamky, 2015).

Cooling devices can be a simple fan placed near or on the pet, and air conditioning to maintain a comfortable temperature. This is particularly important for diseases associated with brachycephalic breeds and pets with laryngeal paralysis or tracheal collapse, because of impaired heat dissipation from impaired respiratory function and increased effort seen with these conditions. Alcohol spray bottles can be placed near the pet, to allow for quick administration to the paw pads and ear pinnas when overheating is suspected, or heat stroke begins. Subcutaneous fluids, especially if cooled, can also be given in times of distress or when heat stroke is apparent. It is important to not cool a pet with ice water, as very cold fluids will constrict peripheral vessels and impair heat dissipation. There are some products available that help cool pets, including Kool Collar® (Figure 17.3). This product is worn around the neck like a collar and has tube inserts that can be cooled and placed within the collar, providing a cooling sensation to the pet.

Quality of Life Assessment for Geriatric Pets as it Pertains to Thermoregulation

Often, the effects of hypothermia and hyperthermia are overlooked as part of the overall quality of life assessment of geriatric pets. Our pets cannot communicate their feelings, but we can easily relate how it feels to be chronically cold or hot. These are common complaints of geriatric people, and often a frustration because of the inability to manage these changes effectively. Although poor thermoregulation can affect comfort and therefore quality of life of a pet, this will rarely be the determining factor for humane euthanasia. More than likely, the inability to maintain normal body condition will either be overlooked or will be seen as a contributing factor to more evident changes leading to the decision for euthanasia.

Care should be taken to mediate changes in body temperature and allow for greater comfort of geriatric pets. Simple management efforts and awareness can go a long way in keeping our geriatric pets more comfortable. As discussed above, maintaining a

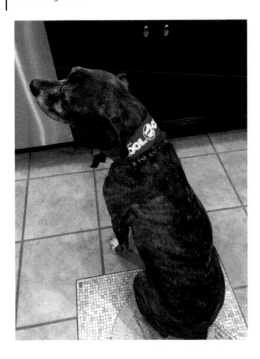

Figure 17.3 Geriatric dog wearing a Kool Collar® to help keep him cooler in the warmer months.

normal temperature can help maintain tissue/organ perfusion and oxygenation, and potentially limit side effects to medications. The inability for these management techniques to either help normalize body temperature of a pet, or the inability for a family or caretaker to provide these necessary steps should play an important role in the decision for humane euthanasia, especially when other important quality of life concerns become apparent.

References

Cunningham, J. and Klein B. (2007) "Thermoregulation." In: *Textbook of Veterinary Physiology* (4th ed.), pp. 639–50. St Louis, MO: Elsevier Saunders.

Doctors Foster and Smith Inc. (n.d.) "Normal Aging and Expected Changes in Older (Senior, Geriatric) Dogs." Available at http://www.peteducation.com/article.cfm?c=2+2110&aid=614.

Glowaski, M. (2002) "Anesthesia for the Geriatric Patient." Presented at Tufts Animal Expo, Tufts University, North Grafton, MA. North Grafton, MA, USA

Kenney, W. L. and Munce T. A. (2003) "Aging and Human Temperature Regulation." *Journal of Applied Physiology*, **95**(6): 2598–603.

Merck Veterinary Manual (2016). "Normal Rectal Temperature Ranges." Kenilworth, NJ: Merck Sharp and Dohme Corp. Available at https://www.msdvetmanual.com/appendixes/reference-guides/normal-rectal-temperature-ranges.

Palmer, D. (2012) "The Hype About Hypos - Part 2: Hypotension, Hypovolemia and Hypothermia." Presented at International Veterinary Emergency and Critical Care Symposium 2012. Auburn University College of Veterinary Medicine, Auburn, AL.

Reineke, E. (2009) "Heatstroke and Hyperthermia." Presented at International Veterinary Emergency and Critical Care Symposium. University of Pennsylvania, Philadelphia, PA.

Reuss-Lamky, H. (2015) "Hypothermia: What's the Hype?" Presented at 37th Annual OAVT Conference and Trade Show. Oakland Veterinary Referral Services, Bloomfield Hills, MI.

Stokol, T. (2014) "Disseminated Intravascular Coagulation: Past, Present and Future." Conference Proceedings, American College of Veterinary Internal Medicine Forum: ACVIM 2014, Ithaca, NY.

Szakacs, J. (2015) "Disorders of Thermoregulation." Universitas Scientiarum Szegediensis. Available at http://web.med.u-szeged.hu/patph/Thermoregulation.

Young, A. J. (1991) "Effects of Aging on Human Cold Tolerance." *Aging Research*, **17**(3): 205–13.

18

Managing Pain in Geriatric Patients

Michael Petty and Sheilah Robertson

Many practitioners are hesitant to treat geriatric animals with analgesic agents or with sedatives and anesthetics. Unfortunately, this means that many older patients needlessly suffer from the pain associated with chronic conditions or are denied the benefit of procedures that require sedation or anesthesia. Pain is a complex multidimensional experience with both sensory and emotional components, and it can have a significant and negative impact on an animal's quality of life and the human–animal bond. This chapter is designed to give the practitioner the confidence to treat their older patients effectively and safely.

General Considerations

Although geriatric patients may belong in a specific "age bracket", there is a wide variation in their health status. A subclassification of the geriatric population has been suggested (KuKanich, 2012). This includes healthy patients, those with subclinical organ dysfunction and those with overt conditions. Age- and disease-related changes in organ function and body composition can impact on the pharmacokinetics (absorption, distribution, metabolism and elimination) of drugs, and dose and dosing intervals may require adjustment in geriatric patients. Organ dysfunction may or may not be measurable. In many cases, significant decreases in renal and hepatic function can exist yet this will not be reflected by running routine hematology and chemistry tests. Cardiac disease can also have a silent presence; a patient may have no detectable heart murmur or history of exercise intolerance yet echocardiography may show evidence of decreased cardiac function; not enough to cause overt disease, but enough to cause concern with some of the agents used for anesthesia and sedation.

When we give a drug we are looking for a pharmacodynamic effect and in geriatric patients this may be different, owing to changes in body composition (such as decreased lean body mass), drug receptors and neurotransmitters (Landsberg *et al.*, 2010). Age- and disease-related changes in pharmacokinetics and pharmacodynamics can result in adverse effects unless the clinician individualizes each treatment plan.

Treatment and Care of the Geriatric Veterinary Patient, First Edition. Edited by Mary Gardner and Dani McVety.
© 2017 John Wiley & Sons, Inc. Published 2017 by John Wiley & Sons, Inc.
Companion Website: www.wiley.com/go/gardner/geriatric

Decrease in Resilience

It is not unusual for geriatric dogs and cats to have noticeably slower recovery times when they are anesthetized or sedated, or not "bounce back" from physiological disturbances the way they did when younger. These physiologic changes will be described later in this chapter. Additionally, many older animals seem to have a heightened response to painful stimuli, events, and conditions that might not affect a younger patient.

Concurrent Treatments

Many caregivers do not disclose that they are giving over-the-counter drugs, supplements, or botanicals to their pets. Some caregivers might not consider the information important, while others may be embarrassed to reveal they are giving medications that their veterinarian did not prescribe. Whatever the reason, it is important to ask if they are giving any drugs (for example aspirin, which many people do not consider a "drug") or supplements and to make them understand that it is out of concern for drug interactions. One supplement that is of concern is St John's wort, because many drugs used to alleviate chronic pain will also have an effect on serotonin and may put the patient at risk for serotonin syndrome (Mohammad-Zadeh *et al.*, 2008; KuKanich, 2013).

Another concern, more common in the referral situation, is to ascertain whether an animal is under the care of another veterinarian who might also be prescribing medications. The same reasons for looking at over-the-counter supplements for possible interactions hold true for pharmaceuticals. Pertinent questions are included in Box 18.1.

Box 18.1 Example Patient History Form

At [insert name of facility here] it is important that we understand our patient's history, especially in regard to medications. Medications include pharmaceutical drugs that were dispensed by us or any other veterinarian, over-the-counter drugs or preparations including human medications or supplements, and botanical/herbal supplements. Some pet foods, such as those intended for arthritis, may also contain supplements and it is important to list those as well. This is very important because medications we might dispense could cause an unwanted adverse event when combined with some of these items. Please complete the form below.

1) If your pet is seen at more than one veterinary facility, please list the name and contact number in order for us to share your pet's history.
2) If your pet gets any prescription medications, whether prescribed for your pet or not, please list the drug, the strength and the frequency at which you are administering it.
3) If your pet gets any over-the-counter medications or supplements, please list them by name, strength and frequency you are administering them.
4) If your pet gets any botanical/herbal supplements, please list them by name, strength and frequency you are administering them.
5) What is the name of the food(s) you feed your dog or cat?

Behavioral Considerations

Geriatric animals may respond poorly to changes in their environment and many have clinical signs suggestive of cognitive dysfunction (Benaryeh, 2015). Faced with a hospitalization, or extensive inpatient treatments, some of these animals seem to "give up" within moments of being in a strange environment. This might be something as mild as refusing to interact with caretakers, but could also result in more serious issues such as refusal to eat, or drink water. Encourage caregivers to bring in and leave familiar toys or blankets, which are often a comfort to any animal, but especially to the aged animals (Figure 18.1). Keeping the hospital stay as short as possible will be beneficial; when possible schedule these patients first thing in the morning so that they can be discharged on the same day.

Nursing care is especially important in aging animals. Special attention should be paid to important functions like food (for example, hand feeding) and fluid intake. Padded bedding in the cage should be used for all geriatric animals as most suffer from some degree of degenerative joint disease (Figure 18.1). Time should be taken to socialize with hospitalized animals (at a separate time from visits to perform medical procedures such as administering medications or taking a rectal temperature), to make them feel more relaxed, to prevent anticipation of what they may perceive as "something bad", and to give the opportunity to look for signs of pain that might not be immediately evident from distant observation or during treatments.

Diagnostics

Since the possibility of concomitant disease increases with an aging population, it becomes very important to run appropriate diagnostic tests prior to starting any kind of treatment. Radiographs, blood chemistry, complete blood count, and urinalysis should not be looked at as a thorough work-up but as a minimum work up. When anesthesia or sedation is needed, taking steps to minimize risk of adverse events is paramount. Increasing age, independent from physical status has been identified as a risk factor for anesthetic death in dogs and cats (Brodbelt, 2009). Remember that you are not just trying to diagnose pain, but comorbidities that might not be readily apparent but could impact the chosen treatments and their outcomes.

Treatment

General Principles

Treatment of long-term pain can be challenging and in most cases will involve trial and error, success and failure. Since many diseases that result in chronic pain are not curable, it is important for the client to understand that the goal is to make their pet comfortable not cure the underlying disease. It should also be clear that keeping a pet comfortable requires both a time and financial commitment. In general, a multimodal approach will be required – this may involve several different drugs (including trial and

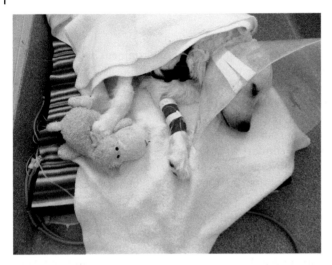

Figure 18.1 Appropriate recovery cage for a geriatric patient. Warmth is provided by a circulating water blanket, absorbable bedding allows urine to drain in case of an accident, soft padding is present as many of these patients will have joint pain, a blanket provides additional warmth and the dog's own toy provides comfort. The dog is also wearing a harness to assist with helping the dog to rise.

error with drugs within a specific class, such as non-steroidal anti-inflammatory drugs, NSAIDs) and non-pharmacologic therapies. Treatment will not be static and will require adjustment based on progression of the underlying disease and the patient's response to therapy.

It is usually easy, in most cases, to give additional drugs, but almost impossible to take them back. It is best to start with lower doses and gradually increase the dose until the desired effect is achieved, while monitoring for adverse events. This is true for both "immediately" acting drugs such as anesthetic agents (for example, titrate injectable anesthetic agents very slowly intravenously), but also for those drugs administered on a long-term basis such as NSAIDs.

An additional approach is to use drugs that are reversible when possible. These include the μ-opioid agonists (such as methadone and morphine), the alpha-2 adrenergic agonist drugs (such as dexmedetomidine) and benzodiazepines (for example, midazolam). These drugs are, however, mostly used short term for acute pain management and when sedation is required. Below are some specific recommendations, but as a general rule of thumb, the authors recommend that you consider starting with half the dose of medication that you would prescribe for healthy adult animals.

Cardiopulmonary

There are many hemodynamic and cardiac changes in the geriatric animal. For example, the most common heart disease in dogs is mitral regurgitation, the incidence of which increases with age (Hamlin 2005), together with widespread changes in the pulmonary system of both dogs and cats, such as decreased alveolar elasticity (Baetge and Matthews, 2012). These changes sets up the scenario of a decrease in oxygen delivery and subsequent risk to those body tissues for which a steady supply of oxygen is vital.

Central Nervous System

Mean alveolar concentration, which is a measure of the requirement for inhalant anesthesia, declines with age. The exact mechanisms are not known; however, it is known that aging brings with it decreases in brain mass and nerve myelination, neuronal apoptosis, and a depletion of neurotransmitters coupled with a decrease in the receptor affinity for those neurotransmitters.

Hepatic

As animals age, their ability to metabolize drugs can be unpredictable. Decreased hepatic blood flow (for example, in cardiac disease) and altered hepatic function will impact on drug metabolism. Unfortunately, there are no reliable tests of liver function and few data available to guide dose adjustments in geriatric animals (KuKanich, 2012).

Metabolism

For most geriatric patients, there is a steady decrease in body muscle mass, together with an increase in body fat. This can cause a change in the effects of both fat and water soluble drugs. A higher percentage of geriatric dogs are also hypothyroid, further decreasing the basal metabolic rate.

Renal

Decreases in renal function, which is more common in geriatric animals, coupled with decreased cardiovascular function, as discussed above, can impair the kidney's abilities to either excrete (for example, ketamine in cats) or clear (for example, gabapentin) in geriatric patients.

Drugs for Treatment of Long-Term Pain

Degenerative joint disease is the most common cause of chronic pain in dogs and cats. One of the most efficacious treatments is the administration of NSAIDs.

Non-Steroidal Anti-Inflammatory Drugs

Adverse effects of NSAIDs (Monteiro-Steagall *et al.*, 2013) in the geriatric population are similar to other age groups, so there is no particular reason for withholding them when indicated for the treatment of pain in older animals. Of course, the usual contraindications must be considered. One particular area of concern revolves around appetite; the loss of which can be an indicator of gastric ulcers secondary to NSAID use. Many older pets eat sporadically, making it difficult for the caregiver to decide if this might be a normal cycle of appetite waxing and waning or if their pet has inappetence secondary to the formation of an ulcer. Caregivers must be especially vigilant for other signs of gastric ulcers, such as melena and blood in the vomitus. As a rule, the owner should not administer an NSAID unless the pet has voluntarily eaten that day.

Use of NSAIDs in Cats with Renal Disease
Many cats with degenerative joint disease also have chronic kidney disease (Marino *et al.*, 2014). Unlike dogs, renal disease in cats has an inflammatory component. Most cats can be given NSAIDs on a long-term basis, as long as the general precautions listed above are followed and the dosing is appropriate for chronic administration; meloxicam is approved for long-term use in cats in many countries, but not in the United States. Indeed, in some cats there is a slowing of the progression of their renal disease while on NSAIDs, and there is no evidence that NSAIDs decrease their longevity (Gowan *et al.*, 2011, 2012).

Amantadine

There are several pathways by which nociceptive signals can reach the brain. One of these involves the N-methyl-D-aspartate receptor (NMDA), a type of glutamate receptor in the dorsal horn of the spinal cord. Activation of this receptor plays a role in both the transmission of nociceptive signals and the development of chronic pain states such as hyperalgesia (a decreased threshold for normally painful stimuli) and allodynia (response to stimuli that are not normally noxious). Amantadine, originally developed as an influenza medication, decreases the activation of the NMDA receptors and normalizes transmission of sensory information. A study in dogs that were refractory to NSAIDs alone, showed the benefit of combining amantadine and meloxicam for the treatment of chronic pain related to osteoarthritis (Lascelles *et al.*, 2008).

Gabapentin and Pregabalin

The exact mechanism of action of gabapentin and pregabalin is unknown, but they are effective in reducing hyperalgesia in several animal models. Their favorable adverse-effect profile has led to these drugs being embraced for the treatment of a wide range of painful conditions in humans, including elderly patients (Rose and Kam, 2002). Although no large appropriately designed veterinary clinical studies evaluating the efficacy of gabapentin in chronic pain states have been published, there are encouraging case reports and support for its use from pain practitioners.

As mentioned previously, animals may have reduced renal function that is not detectable by routine blood chemistry. Gabapentin is not metabolized, but instead is eliminated unchanged in urine (Rose and Kam, 2002). Any reduction in renal function can result in reduced elimination of gabapentin; significantly increasing its duration of action and plasma concentration. For this reason, it is always a good idea to start at about half the normal starting dose of gabapentin with any older animal, and increase to the desired effect. It is common for most dogs (usually not cats) starting gabapentin therapy to go through an initial period of somnolence, and for that reason it is a good idea to start all animals on a single bedtime dose, so that they are sleepy at an appropriate time of day. If the somnolence continues after seven days, be suspicious of subclinical renal disease, and consider lowering the dose.

Maropitant

The use of maropitant citrate for the control of pain has been both confusing and controversial. Although there are studies showing that maropitant had a pain-relieving effect similar to morphine in dogs undergoing ovariohysterectomy (Marquez *et al.*, 2015), it is not consistent in its efficacy and should not be used as a morphine substitute.

Perhaps its more beneficial effect is the one for which it was intended, as an anti-vomiting medication. Its ability to prevent opioid and chronic kidney disease-related vomiting is robust. It seems that across many species, vomiting and nausea are unpleasant experiences that are often less tolerable than pain. Maropitant should be primarily considered for its anti-emetic effect, and if it helps to reduce visceral pain, that should be considered a bonus side effect. Maropitant is not, however, an effective anti-nausea drug, and if nausea (salivation, lip licking) is present ondansetron is more likely to be effective.

Acetaminophen (Paracetamol)

Acetaminophen (paracetamol) is a drug that should never be considered for use in cats, as even a single dose can be fatal. However, acetaminophen with or without codeine can be safely given to dogs. One study with no placebo control showed that acetaminophen with codeine was not effective over baseline measurements of pain (KuKanich, 2016). Other studies show that acetaminophen has a very short plasma half-life of the order of one hour. Although acetaminophen, with or without codeine, can be safely given to dogs, because of its uncertain pharmacodynamics, it should not be relied on as the sole source of pain relief.

Grapiprant

Grapiprant is a drug in a new class of drugs called piprants. This drug is a non-cyclooxy-genase (COX)-inhibiting NSAID which only blocks the prostaglandin E_2 EP4 receptor. Because it is non-COX-inhibiting, it holds the promise of pain relief similar to COX-inhibiting NSAIDs but without their renal and gastric adverse effects. This drug received Food and Drug Administration approval in 2016 for use in dogs in the United States.

Other Drugs

There is no scientific evidence supporting the use of oral tramadol, hydrocodone and oxycodone for consistent and reliable chronic pain relief in dogs. There are significant species differences in the uptake and metabolism of these drugs; for example, dogs produce very little of the O-desmethyltramadol M1 metabolite after the administration of tramadol; this is an active metabolite required for the opioid actions of this drug (Kogel *et al.*, 2014). Cats, however, do produce high concentrations of M1 metabolite, with resultant opioid and analgesic effects (KuKanich, 2013).

Tramadol, hydrocodone, and oxycodone come with risk, and there is little, if any, evidence of their efficacy in dogs. Tramadol can cause serotonin syndrome (KuKanich, 2013). Unless new evidence comes to light supporting the use of these drugs, the authors recommend that they should not be used for the relief of chronic pain.

Emerging and Future Therapies for Chronic Pain

Targeting Novel Mediators of Pain

Nerve growth factor has been identified as an important mediator of inflammatory and neuropathic pain and is therefore a potential therapeutic target. Nerve growth factor levels are increased in many naturally occurring acute and chronic pain conditions and in animal models of pain. In dogs, a fully caninized anti-nerve growth factor (NGF) monoclonal antibody (NV-01) has been developed; treatment must be species specific to avoid an immune response (Gearing *et al.*, 2013). In a preclinical trial using a kaolin model of inflammatory pain, NV-01 reduced the signs of lameness, had a serum half-life of nine days and was well tolerated. The target population for this drug is dogs with osteoarthritis. In one clinical trial, Canine Brief Pain Inventory scores decreased in dogs for up to four weeks following intravenous administration of NV-01 (Webster *et al.*, 2014). A feline specific anti-NGF monoclonal antibody(NV-02) has also been developed.

Selective Neurotoxins

Inhibition or destruction of specific nociceptive neurons without altering other sensory or motor functions is an attractive option for the control of severe pain. The vanilloid receptor present in the nociceptive neurons of the dorsal root and trigeminal ganglia has been targeted by resiniferatoxin administered intrathecally in dogs with painful and debilitating bone cancers and osteoarthritis (Brown *et al.*, 2005, Karai *et al.*, 2004). In dogs with bone cancer, pain relief was excellent.

Substance P-saporin (SP-SAP) is a chemical conjugate of substance P and a recombinant version of a ribosome-inactivating protein (saporin), which acts as a targeted neurotoxin, selectively destroying cells in the dorsal horn of the spinal cord that bear natural killer-1 receptors. SP-SAP is given by intrathecal injection. In a prospective blinded controlled study of dogs with naturally occurring bone cancer, results during the first two weeks after treatment were equivocal, but after two weeks the dogs that received SP-SAP had lower pain scores compared with dogs that received "standard of care" analgesic therapies (NSAIDs, tramadol and gabapentin); however, some dogs in the SP-SAP group developed ataxia (Brown and Agnello, 2013).

Palliative Stereotactic Radiosurgery

Palliative stereotactic radiosurgery involves the precise delivery of a large, single dose of radiation to a tumor target. This technique has been applied to dogs with appendicular osteosarcoma with good outcomes compared with alternative treatments; pain was reduced and limb function was good to excellent after treatment (Farese *et al.*, 2004). The major limitations of this treatment is cost and availability.

Physical Modalities

Non-pharmaceutical treatments gain extra importance in treating pain in geriatric patients. Most animals can tolerate the majority of physical modalities, with a few exceptions, as noted in Chapter 14. The following are several physical modalities that should be considered for the treatment of pain.

Rehabilitation

As animals age, it is common to lose muscle mass; a condition called sarcopenia. Loss of muscle mass occurs in many older patients but it is a poorly understood condition.

As animals age skeletal muscle atrophy is often observed, which is thought to be the result of a process called autophagy (Pagano *et al.*, 2015), a mechanism for degradation and recycling of cellular constituents that is potentially involved in sarcopenia. Loss of muscle mass can also be secondary to localized or generalized degenerative joint disease. In the case of degenerative joint disease, this often becomes an insidious cycle; painful joints result in a decrease in movement, which causes muscle mass to decrease, which takes support away from painful joints, which makes it even more painful to exercise, and so on (see Chapter 14). Eventually, this can impact the animal's ability to move around, resulting in decreased social interaction, which may contribute to cognition issues (see Chapter 8). Box 18.2 describes the assessment of joint condition by observing a dog's stance.

Loss of muscle mass, if severe enough, can result in the animal's inability to perform basic body functions, including eating and drinking, while posturing to urinate and defecate becomes difficult. Rehabilitation is capable of halting or reversing these changes. It is also used to treat pain via several methods including but not limited to increased joint mobility, stimulation of neuromuscular input and reduction of inflammation.

Cardiovascular disease is a concern for some rehabilitation exercises, and a complete cardiovascular exam should be performed before starting any new physical activity, especially rigorous ones such as the use of a treadmill. Even in the absence of cardiac disease, the presence of partial or complete laryngeal paralysis, a disease of older dogs, in particular the Labrador Retriever, can impact the ability to exercise and pose a respiratory and cardiac health risk to a dog trying to perform even moderate levels of exercise.

Rehabilitation exercises must be matched to the animal's age, body type, and existing conditions. Strenuous exercises often have no place when working with a geriatric patient. Instead, a slower pace of conditioning should be considered, including balance exercises, neuromuscular stimulation and core strengthening. The core of animal rehabilitation involves interactions between the animal and the therapist. Additionally, there are exercises that can be safely taught to animal caregivers, allowing for more frequent therapy in the home setting and reduced clinical visits (Petty, 2016a). There are many other tools at the therapist's disposal. These include laser therapy, pulsed electromagnetic field therapy, and shock wave therapy. It is beyond the scope of this chapter to explore each of these modalities. If you are not trained in these techniques you should consult with a therapist who is certified in animal rehabilitation to discover what treatments might be appropriate for your patient.

Acupuncture

Acupuncture is an evidence-based modality that has many known benefits, especially in the area of pain management. Many organizations, including the National Institutes of Health (National Center for Complementary and Integrative Health, 2016), now consider acupuncture to be beneficial for the treatment of pain, both as an adjunct therapy and, in certain cases, a stand-alone therapy. In common with other physical modalities, it works well in the presence of organ dysfunction, and can be used in conjunction with pharmaceutical agents, including chemotherapy and analgesic drugs. There are several certifying organizations and training centers for veterinarians in the United States (see Box 18.3).

Box 18.2 Posture Evaluation

Dog with healthy joints

Dogs with healthy joints will usually stand with their front legs directly under their shoulders and with their hind legs directly under their hips, or extended rearward in a "show dog' stance, as seen here.

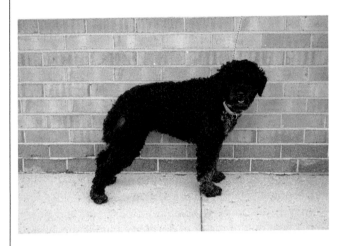

Dog with osteoarthritis

Dogs with arthritis will usually stand with one or more front legs caudal to their shoulder, with the hind legs directly under or slightly cranial to their hips. The caudal position of the front legs is used to take weight off of the pelvic limbs by shifting weight forward, and the forward position of the rear legs is usually a result of myofascial pain in the flexor muscles of the hind legs, making it painful to extend them.

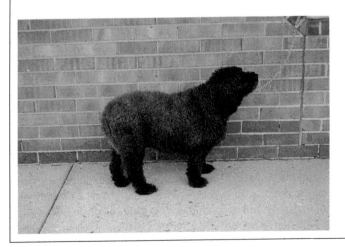

Box 18.3 List of Acupuncture Certifying Organizations and Training Centers in the United States

---

International Veterinary Acupuncture Society: www.ivas.org
CuraCore Integrative Medicine and Education Center (formerly One Health SIM)
Chi Institute of Traditional Chinese Veterinary Medicine: tcvm.com

---

Massage

Massage is often overlooked as a treatment for pain. It has many known benefits, including the relief of myofascial pain, neuromuscular stimulation, and inducing a sense of wellbeing in the animal. Additionally, it can increase blood flow in areas of disease and promote lymphatic drainage where it is present. Although in certain disease states, for example such as in the presence of cancer, a fracture or severe cardiac disease, it might be best to have someone trained in massage therapy to perform the massage, most caregivers can be readily trained in rudimentary massage techniques; often strengthening the bond with their pet (Petty, 2016b).

Weight Loss

Weight gain can and often does happen in the geriatric patient. This often takes the form of increase in total body fat while muscle mass decreases, making extra weight an additional burden to geriatric animals. Extra weight in animals may result in an increase in the levels of circulating inflammatory agents although the evidence for this is not as clear-cut as it is in humans (Greenberg and Obin, 2006). Being overweight or obese also puts extra demands on the cardiovascular and respiratory systems. Another important factor is the additional weight that is carried by the diseased joints of obese animals. Several studies have shown the benefit of weight loss. In one study, a 10% loss of weight had the same pain-reducing benefit of taking an NSAID and had a positive effect on lameness and kinetic gait analysis (Impellizeri *et al.*, 2000; Marshall *et al.*, 2010). Owners may need guidance on calorie intake and nutrition for their ageing cat or dog and they should be discouraged from overfeeding their pet – in many cases, low-calorie treats can be used to satisfy their need to spoil their aged pet.

Myofascial Pain

Myofascial pain remains a poorly understood syndrome, despite it being described in medical texts for hundreds of years (Dommerholt *et al.*, 2011a). A complete explanation of myofascial pain is too lengthy for this chapter; however, a brief explanation follows. Whenever an area of muscle is held in contraction for an extended period of time, that muscle develops something called a taut band: a region of muscle fibers that remain in a state of contraction even when the muscle itself is relaxed. In the case of degenerative joint disease, a leg might develop a taut band because it is held in contraction for lengthy periods to take the weight off an arthritic joint (Dommerholt *et al.*, 2011a). These taut bands are painful in and of themselves, but they also cause additional damage to the joints that they cross. The constant tension in these taut bands causes a decrease in the joint width space that not only reduces the functionality of the joint but can also hasten damage to the compressed articular surfaces.

Treatment of these taut bands usually involves either massage or something called trigger point therapy in which a taut band is found by palpation, then an acupuncture needle is placed into it, causing a spinal reflex that results in a release of the contracted muscle fibers (Dommerholt, 2011b). Unless the perpetuating cause can be completely treated, the taut bands will eventually return requiring periodic treatment. Since osteoarthritis cannot be cured, re-treatment will be required at variable intervals.

Heat and Cold Therapy

Heating and cooling of tissue can be used for pain control, with the additional benefits of reducing edema and swelling, and promotion of healing. Used before and after the directed exercises of rehabilitation, heating and cooling can improve performance and shorten recovery. This modality, like the others in this section, has the advantage of very few contraindications, even in old and debilitated patients.

Cryotherapy is the use of cold, usually to reduce pain and inflammation in acute situations such as injury or surgery. Chronic applications are most commonly confined to reducing chronic and acute-on-chronic pain of conditions such as degenerative joint disease prior to initiating rehabilitation exercises. Penetration of tissue rarely goes deeper than 2–4 cm (Nadler *et al.*, 2004) unless it is combined with compression, for example with an elastic bandage or a Game Ready™ compression system. This should be kept in mind when selecting the target tissue.

Cryotherapy can be applied as direct ice over the desired area, submerging the affected limb in iced water or by using a cold pack. Cold packs are made specifically for rehabilitation applications and are different from the cold packs used for shipping. A homemade cold pack can be made by mixing three parts water to one part 90% isopropyl alcohol, putting it in a sealed plastic bag and then freezing it. Depending on the size of and depth of the area to be treated, 15 minutes is usually adequate for most applications. This can be repeated, but wait until the tissue has become normothermic.

Precautions include using cryotherapy on an animal with a small body or already compromised body temperature, sometimes seen in the post-surgical setting. A layer of protection between the icing agent and the skin, such as a thin cotton towel, should be used to diffuse the cold and prevent frostbite to areas of skin. Finally, prolonged application of cryotherapy to a superficial nerve can cause damage to the nerve resulting in Wallerian degeneration of the nerve. This is especially important when treating the coxofemoral joint because of the close proximity of the sciatic nerve.

Heat therapy can also be used to reduce pain, with the additional benefits of improved joint mobility and increased blood flow. Unlike with cryotherapy, heat therapy is best reserved for chronic or subacute situations. This can include not only chronic issues like osteoarthritis, but also subacute issues such as surgery, after about one week of healing has taken place. The same commercial gel packs that are used for cryotherapy can also be heated in the microwave for heat therapy. Therapy usually involves application of heat for 15–20 minutes to the affected area.

Precautions include applying heat that is too hot, risking damage to the skin and underlying tissues. Never, ever apply heat from a source that is uncomfortable in the operator's hand. Using a thin cotton towel between the source of the heat and the patient's skin can also lower the risk for injury. Every few minutes, the operator should remove the heat source and touch the skin, checking for excessive heat.

End of Life Decisions

It is the wish of most caregivers that their pet will die in their sleep, taking the decision out of their hands. This is seldom the case, and instead difficult decisions must be made. Even with the help of quality-of-life scales, many people find an additional reason to put off the inevitable. Box 18.4 lists some tools available online. See also Chapter 24 for more information on quality-of-life tools.

Frequent evaluations of pain by the veterinary team with input by the caregiver, using structured tools is important not only in measuring treatment outcomes, but also in making end-of-life decisions. It can be helpful to keep track of an animal by taking and storing photographs and videos (with the date taken), so the owner can look back and see the progression of their pet's problems. Guidance as to the effectiveness of pain treatments will usually assist decision making by the caregiver. Pain is important to assess, but is not the only component to consider when making a quality of life assessment; nausea is extremely aversive and may be an adverse effect of treatment or a result of an underlying disease, such a renal failure.

Box 18.4 Some Examples of Online Quality of Life and Pain Measurement Tools

Association for Pet Loss and Bereavement
Quality of Life Scale: http://www.aplb.org/resources/quality-of-life_scale.php

NewMetrica
VetMetrica: Health Related Quality of Life instruments and Acute Pain Measurement for dogs and cats): http://www.newmetrica.com

University of Tennessee, Knoxville Veterinary Social Work
Quality of Life Scale (HHHHMM Scale): http://vetsocialwork.utk.edu/quality-of-life_resources

University of Helsinki Faculty of Veterinary Medicine
Helsinki Chronic Pain Index – versions available for owners and veterinarians: http://www.vetmed.helsinki.fi/english/animalpain/hcpi

University of Pennsylvania PennVet
Canine Brief Pain Inventory (Canine BPI): http://www.vet.upenn.edu/research/clinical-trials/vcic/pennchart/cbpi-tool

North Carolina State College of Veterinary Medicine
Feline Musculoskeletal Pain Index: https://cvm.ncsu.edu/research/labs/clinical-sciences/comparative-pain-research/clinical-metrology-instruments

Sedation and Anesthesia

There may be occasions when an older cat or dog requires sedation or anesthesia for a procedure; for example, diagnostic imaging (radiographs, computed tomography), placement of a nasogastric or esophageal feeding tube, endoscopy, and to obtain biopsies. Because veterinarians are usually more worried about sedation and anesthesia of cats than dogs, this discussion focuses on the cat. A full overview of geriatric anesthesia is not possible in this chapter but some guidelines and general principles are discussed.

As with all medical procedures, a thorough history is important, together with a physical examination and relevant blood work. Geriatric animals usually have some cardiac, hepatic, and renal impairment that will alter distribution, metabolism, and excretion of sedative and anesthetic drugs. Because of this, many people mistakenly think that inhalant agents alone are suitable, since they are minimally metabolized. This approach is not advised, since the inhalant agents are the most cardiovascular and respiratory depressant anesthetic drugs. In addition, masking or box induction are very stressful for the cat.

Low stress and feline-friendly handling are essential. Tachycardia resulting from stress and fear will increase the heart rate, which increases myocardial oxygen consumption and decreases ventricular filling time in cats with hypertrophic cardiomyopathy. The use of a synthetic fraction of feline facial pheromones (Feliway®) can calm cats in unfamiliar surroundings and may facilitate intravenous catheter placement (Kronen *et al.*, 2006). Applying a topical anesthetic cream (a eutectic mix of lidocaine and prilocaine) increases the percentage of catheters that can be placed on the first try.

The approach to sedation and anesthesia is to use either reversible or short-acting agents. Butorphanol is short acting, and opioids such as methadone are reversible. Midazolam is a useful drug in older animals as it can produce sedation and can be given by the intramuscular route (diazepam cannot); it is reversible with flumazenil. Dexmedetomidine can be given at low doses ($2-3 \mu g/kg$ intramuscularly), with additional doses if needed and can be reversed with atipamezole. Recommended induction agents include alfaxalone and propofol; ketamine is best avoided because of the tachycardia it produces. Sedatives and analgesics are anesthetic sparing and significantly reduce inhalant agent requirements, resulting in less cardiorespiratory depression. Whenever possible, a local anesthetic should be used, as they block noxious stimuli and decrease anesthetic requirements. For example, intranasal lidocaine will greatly facilitate nasogastric tube placement, and lacerations can often be repaired with sedation and local anesthetic infiltration. A sample protocol is given in Box 18.5.

Case Studies

Case Study 1: Canine

Sarah is a 13-year-old, 31.7 kg (70 lbs), spayed female Golden Retriever, with a body condition score of 6/9 that was presented with difficulty going up stairs. The client had noticed her difficulty for some time, but it was not until Sarah fell on the stairs that she decided to have Sarah looked at by a veterinarian. On physical exam, Sarah was easy to work with but seemed disconnected with her owner and surroundings. Myofascial

---

Box 18.5 Sample Sedation Protocol for an Aged Cat

Isabella, a 17-year-old spayed female DSH, body weight 3.2 kg, body condition score 3/9, for placement of a temporary nasogastric feeding tube.

Butorphanol 0.2 mg/kg intramuscularly (IM) plus midazolam 0.3 mg/kg IM

This did not provide sufficient sedation after 10 minutes, so dexmedetomidine 2 μg/kg was added (IM). Within 3 minutes, sedation was adequate.

Lidocaine 2% 0.3 ml (6 mg, approximately 2 mg/kg) was placed intranasally and the procedure completed.

No reversal was required.

---

palpation revealed some tender spots in her triceps, her iliopsoas, and the rectus femoris muscles. Extension of her thighs resulted in a painful reaction; licking her lips and trying to withdraw both legs as they were extended. It was also noted that the nails on her left hind foot were worn down. No neurological deficits were found. Based on the exam, it was recommended that radiographs, blood work, and urinalysis be performed.

Radiographs of her pelvis and lower back showed hip dysplasia with severe degenerative joint disease in both hips (Figure 18.2a,b,c). There was one area of spondylosis at L2–3. No other notable changes were observed on the radiographs. The blood work was mostly unremarkable, with the exception of an alanine amino transferase (ALT) of 185 u/l (reference range 20–98 u/l), a blood glucose of 140 mg/dl (reference range 63–118 mg/dl), a blood urea nitrogen (BUN) of 39 mg/dl (reference range 10–32 mg/dl) and a creatinine of 1.9 mg/dl (reference range 0.6–1.4 mg/dl). The urine was isosthenuric, but otherwise normal.

After discussing treatment options with the client, it was decided to start Sarah on several modalities and a weight loss program. Sarah has diarrhea issues with switching dog foods in the past, and had been eating an over-the-counter senior diet for some time. The client opted for cutting back Sarah's food intake by 15% and cutting the frequency and quantity of treats she was receiving. Sarah was put on 150 mg carprofen once daily, and 100 mg gabapentin, starting at once daily at night time and increasing the frequency to three times daily. Sarah underwent trigger-point therapy to treat the myofascial pain and was discharged later that day. A return in three weeks for a recheck and blood work was recommended.

Upon recheck, Sarah weighed 30.8 kg (68 lbs) and the client had noticed some improvement in her confidence while climbing stairs. She stated that Sarah still seemed a bit sleepy after getting the gabapentin. Physical exam showed a decrease in the amount of myofascial pain, and an improvement in extending the rear legs and without resistance from Sarah. Blood was drawn and the BUN was now at 49 mg/dl and the ALT was at 168 u/l. The decision was made to discontinue the carprofen, to reduce the gabapentin to twice daily and to start acupuncture therapy.

After three once-weekly sessions of acupuncture, Sarah was again using stairs with confidence. She was not sleepy on the lower daily dose of gabapentin and her blood values had returned to her pre-NSAID treatment values. It was also noted by the caregiver that Sarah seemed more interested in her surroundings both at home and on excursions, including her trips to the clinic.

(a)

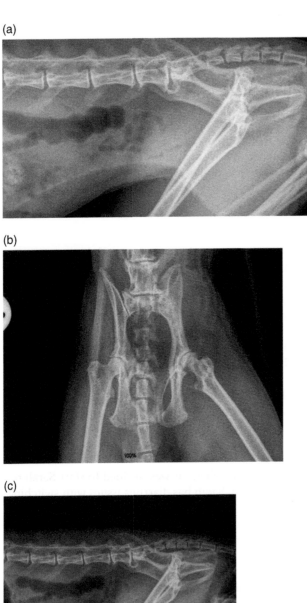

(b)

(c)

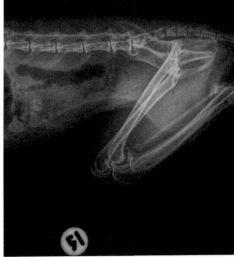

Figure 18.2a,b,c Radiographs of pelvis and lower back showing hip dysplasia with severe degenerative joint disease in both hips.

Discussion

Although Sarah is a fictional dog, she is made up of a conglomerate of patients seen by the authors on a weekly basis. It is common for us to see aged dogs like her, with both osteoarthritis and mild organ dysfunction. This does not stop us from treating with drugs like NSAIDs and gabapentin, but we do so with an abundance of caution and rechecks.

Cognitive dysfunction is often seen in chronic pain cases. The case study mentioned that, "Sarah was easy to work with but seemed disconnected with her owner and surroundings." This type of observation is easy to overlook in a busy exam room; history taking, physical exam, cell phones going off, and kids running around are not conducive to quiet observation. The same brain centers that process pain are closely associated with the "emotional" center. This might result in aggressive behavior (in our experience more commonly associated with acutely painful episodes) but more often than not it seems to be involved with a disconnect. Sometimes the animal acts like it is not even aware of where it is, or stands staring at the hinge side of the door in the exam room, or maybe even just staring off into space. Many of these cognitive issues improve with pain treatment. It may be that, after intervention, the animal's ability to do more things (such as increased exercise leading to a more enriched life) and focus less on their pain helps "reengage" their brain and give them a brighter outlook on things. Increased exercise in itself may promote release of endogenous endorphins and enkephalins which decrease pain and improve mood.

Weight loss was recommended, although Sarah's weight was not outrageous – every little bit helps and we are always looking to the future when certain pharmaceutical options may be taken off the list of possible treatments, perhaps because of adverse reactions or organ decline, and when owners understand the importance of weight loss and strive to achieve this in their pets.

NSAID therapy can be used in dogs with mild renal and hepatic dysfunction. However, this highlights the importance of pretreatment blood work. Had we waited until after starting treatment to do the first blood work, we would have had no idea as to whether or not it was better, the same or worse than before NSAID administration. In Sarah's case, we saw a worsening of the renal values, so the decision was made to stop the NSAID in favor of other therapies. If the client was reluctant to pursue alternative treatments, we might have considered continuing NSAID therapy but insisting on biweekly testing.

Gabapentin has few adverse effects and often has a great benefit in treating long-standing pain, as it can reduce the neuropathic component of pain. However, as it is cleared by the kidneys, we put Sarah on a low dose of gabapentin, and in this case it was the right thing to do; persistent somnolence in older dogs usually means that the gabapentin is not being cleared fast enough prior to the next dose. In this case, we decreased the dose by making it a twice daily treatment, but if there had been no somnolence, we probably would have pushed the daily dosage upward to get the maximum benefit.

Polysulfated glycosaminoglycan (Adequan®) is almost always a great choice for osteoarthritis, but we did not choose to put Sarah on Adequan therapy, as her blood glucose level was high enough that it was flirting with diabetes mellitus. Adequan can elevate glucose levels, so it was left out of the treatment regimen.

Acupuncture and other alternative and complementary treatments are underused. The biggest mistake we see many veterinarians make is to give up when their pharmaceutical regimen does not work. They may not have the skill set to perform acupuncture (we also could have put Sarah through rehabilitation, massage therapy, and so on), and they are reluctant to refer for whatever reason, be it embarrassment at not having the skill, reluctance to lose income, or perhaps other reasons. We owe it to all of our clients and patients to offer the next step in diagnostics and therapy; even if it means a treatment we cannot perform.

Case Study 2: Feline

Sasha is a 13-year-old spayed female Persian cat that was presented with an acute onset of pain. Sasha weighed 3.2 kg (7.0 lbs) and has a body condition score of 5/9. The chief complaint was anorexia, vocalization and lying with the right hind leg out in a splayed position.

Physical examination revealed pain upon palpation of the lower lumbar spine. Sasha was in sternal recumbency with her right hind leg abducted away from her body. Both legs were warm to the touch and had normal pulses. There was a painful response, including growling and resistance when the hind legs were extended.

Sasha was given an injection of buprenorphine because of her acute pain. When relaxed, radiographs of her lower spine and pelvis were taken. She was found to have severe spondylosis at the lumbosacral junction, as well as degenerative joint disease of both coxofemoral joints. A blood panel showed that Sasha had normal laboratory values. After a discussion with the owner, we decided to start Sasha on acupuncture, on a weekly basis, with the immediate goal of reducing pain and the long-term goal of monthly to bimonthly acupuncture for maintenance, and long-term meloxicam therapy at 0.025 mg/kg orally every 24 hours. A follow-up phone call was made five days later, and Sasha's owner reported that she was no longer acting painful, and had started jumping up on window ledges – something she had not done for a few years.

Discussion

It is not uncommon for animals in chronic pain to have an acutely painful episode, bringing the problem to the attention of the owner and hence the veterinarian. Although the owner had not reported Sasha as having a problem previously, it is not uncommon for changes in behavior (no longer jumping to heights) to go unnoticed or to be blamed on advancing years and not pain. Had it not been for the acute pain (probably neurological in origin, possibly cauda equina syndrome), the chronic pain might have gone unnoticed for some time. In these cases, the acute pain needs to be treated in the short term and the chronic pain needs to be treated in the long term.

Showing owners pictures of normal cats versus those with degenerative joint disease can help you with your diagnosis, as these postures may not be exhibited in the examination room (Figure 18.3a,b). Looking at images or videos taken at home can also be helpful in diagnosis cats with degenerative joint disease.

Although, in the United States, meloxicam is only licensed for single use (by injection), it has market authorization for long-term use in many European countries and in Australasia, where it has been used safely and successfully; the label dose is 0.05 mg/kg/day

(a)

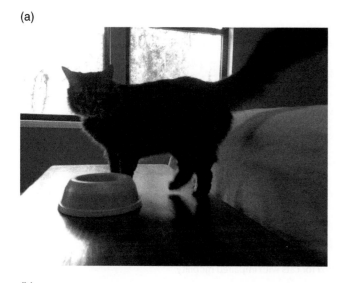

(b)

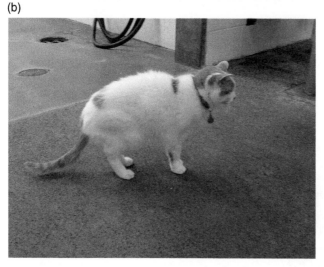

Figure 18.3 Diagnosing degenerative joint disease: (a) Stance of a normal cat. (b) Stance of a cat with hip osteoarthritis.

but most cats can be successfully managed on lower doses (0.01–0.03 mg/kg/day; Gunew *et al.*, 2008). For this reason, meloxicam should be considered in all chronic feline pain issues, especially if other therapies have failed to give pain relief.

Making life easier for these cats can play an important role in treatment; for example, litter boxes should be "easy entry" (Figure 18.4), and raised food bowls are more comfortable when eating (Figure 18.5). Easy access to favorite resting places maintains quality of life and allows cats to live in the 3-dimansional space that is so important to them (Figure 18.6).

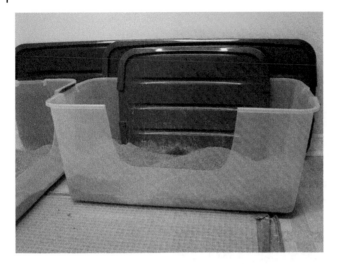

Figure 18.4 An easy-access litter box for cats with impaired mobility.

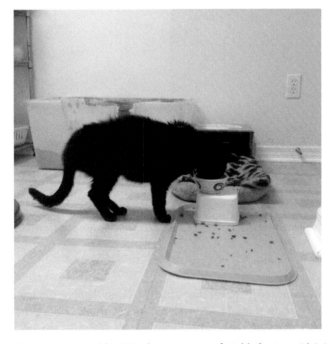

Figure 18.5 Raised food bowls are more comfortable for cats with joint disease.

Figure 18.6 Facilitating access to favorite resting places is important for quality of life.

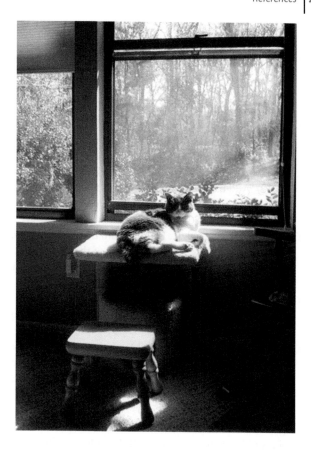

References

Baetge, C. L. and Matthews, N. S. (2012) "Anesthesia and Analgesia for Geriatric Veterinary Patients." *Veterinary Clinics of North America Small Animal Practice*, 42: 643–53.

Benaryeh, B. (2015) "Cognitive Dysfunction: Overview." *Veterinary Team Brief*, Nov/Dec: 25. Available at http://www.veterinaryteambrief.com/clinical-suite/cognitive-dysfunction/overview.

Brodbelt, D. (2009) "Perioperative Mortality in Small Animal Anaesthesia." *Veterinary Journal*, 182: 152–61.

Brown, D. C. and Agnello, K. (2013) "Intrathecal Substance P-Saporin in the Dog: Efficacy in Bone Cancer Pain." *Anesthesiology*, 119: 1178–85.

Brown, D. C., Ladarola, M. J., Perkowski, S. Z., Erin, H., Shofer, F., Laszlo, K. J., Olah, Z., Mannes, A. J. (2005) "Physiologic and Antinociceptive Effects of Intrathecal Resiniferatoxin in a Canine Bone Cancer Model." *Anesthesiology*, 103: 1052–9.

Dommerholt, J., Bron, C., Franssen, J. (2011a) "Myofascial Trigger Points: An Evidence-Informed Review." In Dommerholt, J. and Huijbregts, P. (eds), *Myofacial Trigger Points: Pathophysiology and Evidence-Informed Diagnosis and Management*, pp. 17–50. Sudbury, MA: Jones and Bartlett.

Dommerholt, J., Mayoral del Moral, O., Gröbli, C. (2011b) "Trigger Point Dry Needling." In Dommerholt, J. and Huijbregts, P. (eds), *Myofacial Trigger Points: Pathophysiology and Evidence-Informed Diagnosis and Management*, pp. 159–90. Sudbury, MA: Jones and Bartlett.

Farese, J. P., Milner, R., Thompson, M. S., Lester, N., Cooke, K., Fox, L., Hester, J., Bova, F. J. (2004) "Stereotactic Radiosurgery for Treatment of Osteosarcomas Involving the Distal Portions of the Limbs in Dogs." *Journal of the American Veterinary Medical Association*, 225: 1567–72, 1548.

Gearing, D. P., Virtue, E. R., Gearing, R. P., Drew, A. C. (2013) "A Fully Caninised Anti-NGF Monoclonal Antibody for Pain Relief in Dogs." *BMC Veterinary Research*, 9: 226. doi: 10.1186/1746-6148-9-226.

Gowan, R. A., Baral, R. M., Lingard, A. E., Catt, M. J., Stansen, W., Johnston, L., Malik, R. (2012) "A Retrospective Analysis of the Effects of Meloxicam on the Longevity of Aged Cats with and Without Overt Chronic Kidney Disease." *Journal of Feline Medicine and Surgery*, 14(12): 876–81.

Gowan, R. A., Lingard, A. E., Johnston, L., Stansen, W., Brown, S. A., Malik, R. (2011) "Retrospective Case–Control Study of the Effects of Long-Term Dosing with Meloxicam on Renal Function in Aged Cats with Degenerative Joint Disease." *Journal of Feline Medicine and Surgery*, 13: 752–61.

Greenberg, A. S. and Obin, M. S. (2006) "Obesity and the Role of Adipose Tissue in Inflammation and Metabolism." *American Journal of Clinical Nutrition*, 83: 461S–5S.

Gunew, M. N., Menrath, V. H., Marshall, R. D. (2008) "Long-Term Safety, Efficacy and Palatability of Oral Meloxicam at 0.01–0.03 mg/Kg for Treatment of Osteoarthritic Pain in Cats." *Journal of Feline Medicine and Surgery*, 10: 235–41.

Hamlin, R. L. (2005) "Geriatric Heart Disease in Dogs." *Veterinary Clinics of North America Small Animal Practice*, 35: 597–615.

Impellizeri, J. A., Tetrick, M. A., Muir, P. (2000) "Effect of Weight Reduction on Clinical Signs of Lameness in Dogs with Hip Osteoarthritis." *Journal of the American Veterinary Medical Association*, 216: 1089–91.

Karai, L., Brown, D. C., Mannes, A. J., Connelly, S. T., Brown, J., Gandal, M., Wellisch, O. M., Neubert, J. K., Olah, Z., Iadarola, M. J. (2004) "Deletion of Vanilloid Receptor 1-Expressing Primary Afferent Neurons for Pain Control." *Journal of Clinical Investigation*, 113: 1344–52.

Kogel, B., Terlinden, R., Schneider, J. (2014) "Characterisation of Tramadol, Morphine and Tapentadol in an Acute Pain Model in Beagle Dogs." *Veterinary Anaesthesia and Analgesia*, 41: 297–304.

Kronen, P. W., Ludders, J. W., Erb, H. N., Moon, P. F., Gleed, R. D., Koski, S. (2006) "A Synthetic Fraction of Feline Facial Pheromones Calms but does not Reduce Struggling in Cats Before Venous Catheterization." *Veterinary Anaesthesia and Analgesia*, 33: 258–65.

KuKanich, B. (2016) "Pharmacokinetics and Pharmacodynamics of Oral Acetaminophen in Combination with Codeine in Healthy Greyhound Dogs." *Journal of Veterinary Pharmacology and Therapeutics*, 39(5): 514–17.

KuKanich, B. (2013) "Outpatient Oral Analgesics in Dogs and Cats Beyond Nonsteroidal Antiinflammatory Drugs: An Evidence-Based Approach." *Veterinary Clinics of North America Small Animal Practice*, 43: 1109–25.

KuKanich, B. (2012) "Geriatric Veterinary Pharmacology." *Veterinary Clinics of North America Small Animal Practice*, 42: 631–42.

Landsberg, G. M., Denenberg, S. & Araujo, J. A. (2010) "Cognitive dysfunction in cats: a syndrome we used to dismiss as 'old age'." *Journal of Feline Medicine and Surgery*, 12: 837–48.

Lascelles, B. D., Gaynor, J. S., Smith, E. S., Roe, S. C., Marcellin-Little, D. J., Davidson, G., Boland, E., Carr, J. (2008) "Amantadine in a Multimodal Analgesic Regimen for Alleviation of Refractory Osteoarthritis Pain in Dogs." *Journal of Veterinary Internal Medicine*, 22: 53–9.

Marino, C. L., Lascelles, B. D., Vaden, S. L., Gruen, M. E., Marks, S. L. (2014) "Prevalence and Classification of Chronic Kidney Disease in Cats Randomly Selected from Four Age Groups and in Cats Recruited for Degenerative Joint Disease Studies." *Journal of Feline Medicine and Surgery*, 16: 465–72.

Marquez, M., Boscan, P., Weir, H., Vogel, P., Twedt, D. C. (2015) "Comparison of NK-1 Receptor Antagonist (Maropitant) to Morphine as a Pre-Anaesthetic Agent for Canine Ovariohysterectomy." *PLoS One*, 10: e0140734. doi: 10.1371/journal.pone. 0140734.

Marshall, W. G., Hazewinkel, H. A., Mullen, D., De Meyer, G., Baert, K., Carmichael, S. (2010) "The Effect of Weight Loss on Lameness in Obese Dogs with Osteoarthritis." *Veterinary Research Communications*, 34: 241–53.

Mohammad-Zadeh, L. F., Moses, L., Gwaltney-Brant, S. M. (2008) "Serotonin: A Review." *Journal of Veterinary Pharmacology and Therapeutics*, 31: 187–99.

Monteiro-Steagall, B. P., Steagall, P. V., Lascelles, B. D. (2013) "Systematic Review of Nonsteroidal Anti-Inflammatory Drug-Induced Adverse Effects in Dogs." *Journal of Veterinary Internal Medicine*, 27: 1011–19.

Nadler, S. F., Weingand, K., Kruse, R. J. (2004) "The Physiologic Basis and Clinical Applications of Cryotherapy and Thermotherapy for the Pain Practitioner." *Pain Physician*, 7: 395–9.

National Center for Complementary and Integrative Health (2016) "Acupuncture." Available at https://nccih.nih.gov/health/acupuncture.

Pagano, T. B., Wojcik, S., Costagliola, A., De Biase, D., Iovino, S., Iovane, V., Russo, V., Papparella, S., Paciello, O. (2015) "Age Related Skeletal Muscle Atrophy and Upregulation of Autophagy in Dogs." *Veterinary Journal*, 206: 54–60.

Petty, M. (2016a) "Home Exercises." In: M. Petty, *Dr. Petty's Pain Relief for Dogs*, pp. 190–211. New York, NY: Countryman Press,.

Petty, M. (2016b) "Massage." In: M. Petty, *Dr. Petty's Pain Relief for Dogs*, pp. 212–16. New York, NY: Countryman Press.

Rose, M. A. and Kam, P. C. (2002) "Gabapentin: Pharmacology and its Use in Pain Management." *Anaesthesia*, 57: 451–62.

Webster, R. P., Anderson, G. I., Gearing, D. P. (2014) "Canine Brief Pain Inventory Scores for Dogs with Osteoarthritis Before and after Administration of a Monoclonal Antibody Against Nerve Growth Factor." *American Journal of Veterinary Research*, 75: 532–5.

Further Reading

Epstein, M., Rodan, I., Griffenhagen, G., Kadrlik, J., Petty, M. C., Robertson, S., Simpson, W. (2015). "2015 AAHA/AAFP Pain Management Guidelines for Dogs and Cats." *Journal of the American Animal Hospital Association*, 51: 67–84.

Epstein, M. E., Rodan, I., Griffenhagen, G., Kadrlik, J., Petty, M. C., Robertson, S. A., Simpson, W. (2015). 2015 "AAHA/AAFP Pain Management Guidelines for Dogs and Cats." *Journal of Feline Medicine and Surgery*, 17: 251–72.

Pittari, J., Rodan, I., Beekman G., Gunn-Moore, D., Plozin, D., Taboada, J., Tuzlo, H., Zoran, D. (2009) "American Association of Feline Practitioners. Senior Care Guidelines." *Journal of Feline Medicine and Surgery*, 11: 763–78.

Rigott, C.F. and Brearly, J.C. (2016) "Anaesthesia for Paediatric and Geriatric Patients." In T. Duke-Novakovski, M. deVries, and C. Seymour (eds), *BSAVA Manual of Canine and Feline Anaesthesia and Analgesia* (3rd ed.), pp. 418–27. Quedgeley, UK: British Small Animal Association.

Sparkes, A. H., Heiene, R., Lascelles, B. D., Malik, R., Sampietro, L. R., Robertson, S., Scherk, M., Taylor, P. (2010). "ISFM and AAFP Consensus Guidelines: Long-Term Use of NSAIDs in Cats." *Journal of Feline Medicine and Surgery*, 12: 521–38.

19

Exotic Animal Geriatrics
Amanda Grant

Introduction

Households with an "exotic" pet (that is, a pet other than a cat or dog) have grown exponentially in number over the last decade. Animal Planet estimates that one in ten families with pets have an exotic pet. Some of the most common exotic mammals presented to veterinary practice are the rabbit, guinea pig, rat, and ferret. Many of these species have very short lifespans compared with cats and dogs, and because of this, often present to the veterinarian for the first time at an already advanced age or in geriatric condition. Even though these pets are often smaller in stature and may live in a caged environment, the emotion, time, and financial investment of their owners should not be underestimated. It is the responsibility of the veterinarian to communicate realistic life expectancies of these unique pets, identify geriatric conditions, and help pet parents determine quality of life and treatment options for their aging exotic pet.

This section will help to identify common geriatric conditions in rabbits, guinea pigs, and ferrets. There are many excellent resources available that describe the patho-physiology, diagnostics and detailed treatments of common diseases in these species. Several of the more common diseases processes are highlighted and treatment options specific to managing the exotic pet in a "geriatric" condition are offered.

Veterinary professionals do not have to be experts in exotic animal medicine to measure the quality of life of these special patients. The small-animal quality of life (QoL) scales, such as Dr Alice Villalobos' (2008) HHHHHMM scale, is easily adapted to exotic species. The specific break down is hurt, hunger, hydration, hygiene, happiness, mobility and more good days than bad, and each factor is assigned a value from one to ten, with ten as the highest. Implementing a QoL scale with pet parents, while taking into consideration species-specific nuances, can help to guide the conversation about their pet's condition, allowing for a better patient assessment. Often, the geriatric exotic is the children's pet or classroom pet, and asking questions relating back to the topics from the QoL scale can help to give a clearer clinical picture.

Rabbits and guinea pigs are prey species so they will "hide" signs of illness, making it difficult to determine whether they are in pain. Ferrets can also mask pain, and will

Treatment and Care of the Geriatric Veterinary Patient, First Edition. Edited by Mary Gardner and Dani McVety.
© 2017 John Wiley & Sons, Inc. Published 2017 by John Wiley & Sons, Inc.
Companion Website: www.wiley.com/go/gardner/geriatric

Table 19.1 Some behaviors associated with pain and illness, by species (adapted from Bays *et al.*, 2006).

	Ferret	Rabbit	Guinea Pig
Eyes	Dull, half closed	Dull, half closed/squinting	Dull, unfocused, excessive tearing
Body posture	Head elevated and extended, won't curl up in normal sleeping posture	Head elevated and extended, hunched	Strained expression with bulging eyes, head extended
Mentation	Lethargic, strained facial expressions, separate from group/family	Abnormal aggression/ grouchiness, isolating	Aggression/biting in a normally docile pig, lethargy
Oral/dental	Teeth grinding	Teeth grinding	Pale mucous membranes
Mobility	Hunched up, walking with arched back, rear legs sinking, stiff gait, or completely immobile	Ataxia, stiff movements, lameness, reluctance to move, not getting into litter box	Immobile or very reluctant to move, squealing when handled
Hygiene/ grooming	Stop grooming, urine staining, piloerection	Overgrooming, hair pulling at painful site, or complete lack of grooming	Chewing the painful area, mutilating
Elimination behaviors	Eliminating in unusual spots, straining	Smaller, fewer, or no fecal pellets, polyuria/polydipsia	Smaller, fewer or no fecal pellets, polydipsia
Appetite	Diminished	Anorexia	Anorexia
Abdomen	Tucked, painful on palpation	Pressing abdomen on floor, flinching on palpation, bloating, fever or hypothermia	Flinching on palpation, hypothermia, ears and limbs abnormally cool

often hide and sleep more than usual, but then still come out to eat and play for short bouts, thus appearing "normal." Table 19.1 identifies some behaviors associated with pain and illness by species.

Geriatric Conditions of Ferrets

Ferrets have one of the highest tumor rates of any of our domestic pets, thus making neoplasia the most common presenting underlying geriatric problem. Neurologic conditions often present second to neoplasia, and less commonly from disk disease or osteoarthritis. Cardiomyopathies, dental disease, and cataracts are also routinely found in the senior ferret. Below, each of these conditions is discussed separately, with an emphasis on the therapies, husbandry considerations, and supportive care guidelines for pet parents, as well as prognostic indicators for the "when it's time" discussion.

Neoplasia

Ferrets from American bloodlines are sadly "little tumor factories" and the large majority will be diagnosed with some form of neoplasia between four and years of age, commonly as young as two years. Adrenal disease (adrenocortical), insulinoma, lymphoma, and lymphosarcoma have the highest incidence, with skin, bone, and other neoplasms being in the minority. Adrenal disease is a neoplasia of the adrenal cortex, which results in overproduction of sex steroid hormones and thus causing a cascade of clinical signs affecting many systems. Ferrets with adrenal disease are extraordinarily pruritic and have progressive alopecia. Alopecia can be diffuse, but often starts by thinning of the tail and progresses to the trunk. These animals may be more aggressive than normal and have an even stronger body odor than the typical ferret "musk." The high levels of estrogen lead to vulvar swelling in females and also prostatic hypertrophy causing dysuria in males. Laboratory diagnosis is by adrenal sex hormone panel, for which the author recommends the University of Tennessee Endocrinology Laboratory. Studies have shown this panel to be 95% predictive in diagnosing adrenal disease in ferrets. Abdominal ultrasound looking for gland enlargement can also be performed, as well as surgical excision and biopsy. If pet parents do not wish to pursue surgery or specialty referral, or if the pet is not stable for invasive procedures, or is in geriatric condition, there are several medical management options to help alleviate the discomfort in these itchy, grouchy, often hairless ferrets. Gonadotropin-releasing hormone analogs (GNRH) are widely used to treat the symptoms of adrenal disease, but will not offer a cure. Leuprolide acetate (Lupron®) is often given in a once four-weekly depot injection, with doses and storage recommendations in the exotic animal formulary (Morrissey, 2013). Deslorelin acetate (Suprelorin® F implant) is a small implant placed under the skin that can help alleviate clinical signs for 10–30 months. The author has used these implants for several years, in older and geriatric ferrets, and has not only noted relief from pruritus within days of implantation, but also hair regrowth within a few weeks. Within one month, there is an appreciable decrease in vulvar swelling and the ferrets seem happier and more energized. Another implant option is Ferretonin®. This is also a subcutaneously placed implant with melatonin. It has been reported to help with hair regrowth, pruritus, vulva swelling, and prostate swelling for approximately four months. Melatonin implants are inexpensive and available to pet parents without a prescription. In time, adrenal tumors will grow in size and become cumbersome for the active ferret, but they do have a low metastatic rate. The long-term prognosis is affected by progressive prostatic disease, bone marrow suppression from hyperestrogenism, carcinoma metastasis, and/or development of a concurrent neoplasm or other condition (Quesenberry and Carpenter, 2012).

Insulinoma is a neoplasia of the beta cells in the islets of Langerhans in the pancreas, which causes excessive insulin secretion and thus hypoglycemia. Ferrets with insulinoma can present with clinical signs that range from ataxia, dullness, and hypersalivating, to recumbency, seizures, and a comatose state. They will often be nauseous, retch, and paw at their mouths. Additionally, they can develop muscle wasting, especially in the rear limbs, and walk with a "dropped" gait. Diagnosis is most commonly based on history, and a fasting glucose level of less than 60 mg/dl. In the geriatric ferret, with likely a chronic state of this condition, medical treatment is based on managing clinical signs and avoiding hypoglycemic crisis. These ferrets will need a diet that is high in protein and fat and low in glycemic carbohydrates. Pet parents must be advised not to give any high sugar treats, and to ensure that food is always fresh and available, and that the ferret eats regularly. If the ferret does not eat regularly, it will need to be hand fed. Carnivore Care™ (Oxbow Animal Health) is a great powdered feeding formula that is high in protein, easily digestible, and palatable for the sick ferret. Canned Hills® a/d® diet and chicken or turkey baby food can also be used for hand feeding. Most geriatric ferrets with insulinoma will need glucocorticoid medications, in addition to their dietary changes. Prednisone and prednisolone can be made into a palatable suspension by a compounding pharmacy, but the pharmacist must be advised to avoid flavorings that contain alcohol or sugar. The author has compounded with fish oil, and has found that most ferrets love the taste. The dose of prednisone/prednisolone, and the need for blood sugar monitoring when using oral steroids, is well described in Quesenberry's and Carpenter's (2012) *Ferrets, Rabbits, and Rodents.* This resource also offers additional therapies, including less available medications.

The mainstay of managing a geriatric insulinoma ferret is consistent dosing of oral steroids and frequent meals or hand feeding with easily digestible high-protein food. Insulinoma in ferrets has a low metastatic rate compared with dogs, but unlike in dogs, many nodules can spread throughout the pancreas in the ferret. This results in a progressive neoplasia, so doses of prednisone and frequency of meals will often need to be increased. The long-term prognosis is affected by increase in hypoglycemic episodes, morbidity from high doses of steroids, and metastasis (Quesenberry and Carpenter, 2012). Pet parents of geriatric ferrets with insulinoma should use the QoL scale regularly, to help to determine when it is time to consider euthanasia, before the ferret ends up in crisis or organ failure.

Lymphoma/lymphosarcoma is the third most common neoplasia of ferrets. These animals present with swollen, firm lymph nodes, either in one area or generalized. Not all present with lymphadenopathy. Many will exhibit general malaise, anorexia, diarrhea, or weight loss. This neoplasia in ferrets is diagnosed as with cats and dogs, through blood work, radiographs, biopsy, and histopathology. There are many chemotherapy protocols and radiation treatments available for ferret lymphoma, and specialty referral is recommended if a pet parent wants to explore that option. A palliative option involves shrinking the tumors and restoring some quality of life with the use of oral steroids. Prednisone can be compounded to a palatable liquid form and given once daily. As with insulinoma, providing a high protein and fat, and low carbohydrate diet, or formula is vital. Fish oils, antioxidants, and free-radical scavenger-type products are available. Ferrets with lymphoma can decline quite quickly as disease progresses, and pet parents must be coached (educated) with regards to which clinical signs to monitor. Ferrets can become dyspneic with cervical or thoracic lymphadenopathy. They can develop chronic diarrhea or tenesmus from mesenteric lymphadenopathy and diffuse infiltration into the intestinal wall. Multiple organ failure is also common, owing to metastasis and leukemia, so pet parents should watch for pale gums, weakness, and changes in the ferret's breath odor (Quesenberry and Carpenter, 2012).

Cardiomyopathy

Heart disease is common in older ferrets with dilated cardiomyopathy and congestive heart failure being the most prevalent presentations. Clinical signs are similar for both conditions, and include lethargy, anorexia, hind-end weakness, lack of playing, sleeping more than usual, loss of muscle mass, collapse and dyspnea. Ferrets with cardiomyopathy can also develop pleural and/or abdominal effusions. Diagnosis in ferrets is congruent with that in small animal medicine, with cardiomegaly evident on radiographs, electrocardiography, and echocardiography. Treatment involves diuretics, angiotensin-converting-enzyme inhibitors, pimobendan and close monitoring of kidney function. If the ferret responds well to medications and pleural/abdominal effusion resolves, they can live an additional 6–18 months, provided that another disease does not arise (Oglesbee, 2006). If patients do not respond well, or if they need multiple thoracocentesis treatments, or develop renal failure, then the pet parent should be advised toward euthanasia. The author also advises these ferret parents of the necessity for regular medication dosing, close monitoring, and providing good nutrition, often by hand feeding. Pain medications should also be used in the end stage of disease, while the pet parents are being advised that the time is near.

Dental Disease

Many ferrets over the age of three years have some form of dental disease. They eat a predominantly hard kibble diet and like to chew on cage bars and anything else they can get their mouths on, resulting in a lot of broken canines. The enamel starts to resorb as the ferret ages, and the teeth take on a yellowish color, lose opacity, and become more fragile. Dental tartar, gingivitis, and dental abscess can develop, similar to other companion animals. Ferrets with one or more of these conditions may be found chewing only on one side of the mouth, grinding their teeth, hypersalivating, and they may exhibit foul breath. Teeth can be scaled and polished under anesthesia, and ferret parents can be taught how to brush their pets teeth with a finger brush and feline toothpaste. The author has used clindamycin pulse therapy and over-the-counter dental rinses when anesthetic dental cleaning is not possible, to try to improve dental health palliatively. Many ferrets with advanced dental disease will require soft foods, such as baby food or cooked diets, to maintain their nutrition (Johnson-Delaney, 2010).

Cataracts

Cataracts are a common finding in the older ferret. As in other species, cataracts in ferrets are diagnosed by the classic white eye appearance, ophthalmic exam and tonometry. One study showed diets high in fat and low in protein and vitamin E, can lead to cataract development. Cataracts usually do not cause a problem with the ferret, given there is no secondary glaucoma or lens luxation. Cataract surgery can be done via phacofragmentation, but no artificial lenses are available in a suitable size for a ferret (Quesenberry and Carpenter, 2012). Blind ferrets can do remarkably well, as they are highly adaptable, by memorizing their surroundings and using their excellent sense of smell.

With any geriatric condition in the ferret, the veterinarian's recommendations will depend on the severity of the case, age of the patient, and the ability and willingness of the pet parent to take on labor and time intensive treatments. Many ferrets with neoplasia and cardiomyopathy present in an "end-stage" or inoperable state, and in these situations, treatments are generally focused on medical management and nursing care to maintain a good quality of life. Often, these geriatric ferrets are sleeping more, eating and playing less, or not at all. Pain control and adequate nutrition via hand feeding are critical in any of these conditions. Adapting the cage environment to one level and helping with bathroom hygiene may improve quality of life for the less mobile ferret. Continuing to offer the ferret opportunities to interact and play maintains happiness in these inquisitive critters. When a ferret is no longer "full of life," or finds no joy in interactions with people or other ferrets, then the time to consider euthanasia is near.

Geriatric Conditions of Rabbits

Rabbits have a projected life expectancy of 6–12 years, depending on the breed. Often, the rabbit patient is presenting to the veterinarian for the first time in an older, geriatric state. Rabbits are prey species, and as such they are good at hiding pain and other signs of illness. Therefore, they may progress to an advanced state of disease before any abnormalities are noted and before any veterinary care is sought. Geriatric rabbits frequently present with orthopedic problems, renal disease, neoplasia, and head tilt. Some of these conditions can be medically managed to restore quality of life while others are best addressed with palliative and nursing care. As with ferrets, using the QoL scale will assist the veterinarian and rabbit parent in developing a plan together for the aging rabbit.

Neoplasia

There are several reported forms of neoplasia in pet rabbits. The most common form in female rabbits is uterine adenocarcinoma. This reproductive neoplasia has an incidence of greater than 60% in unspayed female rabbits over three years of age, and up to 80% in specific breeds. As the rabbit ages, the endometrium undergoes cellular changes that predispose it to growth of carcinoma cells. The adenocarcinoma then pervades all the layers of the uterus and attaches to abdominal organs. The primary tumor may metastasize to the liver, lungs, and brain within a year. These rabbits will present early with hematuria, or frank blood clots in the urine. In later phases, the rabbit will be anorexic, quiet, dull, and may present with mastitis, pale mucous membranes and dyspnea from metastasis. An enlarged, firm uterus can be found on abdominal exam, and the rabbit will likely react from pain during palpation. Radiographs, especially of the chest to look for metastasis, can aid in prognosticating. Complete surgical excision is the preferred treatment, but this may not be an option in the older, unstable rabbit with metastasis. Therapy then becomes focused on palliative pain management and assisted feeding to keep the gastrointestinal tract moving. Oral anti-inflammatories such as liquid meloxicam, and opioids such as tramadol suspension, or buprenorphine are recommended. The rabbit's pellets can be blended with water to create a gruel for hand feeding. Alternatively, Oxbow Animal Health makes a powdered formula (Critical Care®) that most rabbits find palatable. Rabbits with uterine adenocarcinoma often do not want to be picked up, and may avoid their litter box because jumping in and out of the litter box, and the act of urinating, can be painful. Advise rabbit parents to maintain a diligent pain medication schedule and offer petting and attention without picking the rabbit up. A low-sided litter box and frequent bedding changes are helpful to keep the rabbit clean. Humane euthanasia should be performed when the rabbit becomes progressively weaker, dyspneic, or suffers unresponsive gastrointestinal stasis (Quesenberry and Carpenter, 2012).

Renal Failure

Renal failure is a common presentation of the geriatric rabbit, especially chronic renal disease. There are many causes of chronic renal disease described in the literature, with some of the most common being chronic nephritis from damage caused by the parasite *Encephalitozoon cunculi*, lymphosarcoma, calcinosis, nephroliths and fibrosis. These rabbits are often quite thin and lethargic, with a dull poor hair coat. They often present with anorexia, diarrhea or no stool at all, and with seizures or in a comatose or recumbent state. Complete blood count and chemistry values will be consistent with azotemia, as in small animals, with profound hyperphosphatemia (Queseneberry and Carpenter, 2012). If a rabbit in acute crisis with renal failure can be stabilized with diuresis and supportive care, then pet parents can be taught to give regular subcutaneous fluids at home, hand feed, and give erythropoietin injections. These rabbits will also need a low-walled litter box that is easier to get in and out of, as well as and frequent bedding changes. Feeding washed and wet low-calcium containing greens and dandelion greens can help with diuresis. Pain medication, such as tramadol suspension and buprenorphine, are also recommended. These patients will need to be reassessed regularly as their condition can change quickly, and they are labor intensive for pet parents to manage.

Orthopedic Concerns

Osteoarthritis from degenerative joint disease and spondylosis are common musculoskeletal concerns in geriatric rabbits. These rabbits may be no longer getting in the litter box, and not stretching out on their sides. They may also have difficulty grooming, as they may be unable to reach back and groom themselves or reach up with rear legs to clean their ears. Consequently, their fur may become matted, dull, and soiled. They will stop hopping and will often sit hunched in a corner. The degenerative joint changes, bony bridging, and osteophytes on the vertebrae can be seen radiographically (Oglesbee, 2006). These rabbits are treated symptomatically, addressing pain, hygiene, and mobility. Oral meloxicam suspension, together with tramadol or buprenorphine, is widely used. Adequan® injections can also be used for degenerative joint pain. Grooming assistance by shaving the affected areas, regular ear cleanings, initial oral antibiotics and topical medications for the perineal area are needed to restore good hygiene. Over-the-counter moleskin and corn pads can be placed on the bottoms of the feet to provide traction and to protect skin from soiling. Yoga matting in the rabbit's cage or play area may also be used to provide traction. Sherpa wool blankets are good for the rabbit with low mobility to help wick away moisture. These rabbits also need a modified, low-wall litter box and frequent bedding changes. Laser treatments for arthritis pain have grown in popularity and seem to greatly help these rabbits. Laser therapy is non-invasive and often well tolerated (Figure 19.1). Acupuncture is also reported for rabbits with chronic pain, but the author has found few individuals will tolerate this treatment. These rabbits can often be managed with the multimodal therapies described for some time; however, when their mobility significantly declines, or a concurrent geriatric illness develops, then it is time to have the end-of-life discussion.

Vestibular Disease

Many senior rabbits will present with head tilt and symptoms of vestibular disease similar to our aging canine patients. In older rabbits, this is often caused by *E. cuniculi* infection, chronic otitis interna or a brain lesion. In addition to head tilt, these rabbits may have nystagmus and profound rolling. A thorough otoscopic exam and *E. cuniculi* testing are recommended. Treatment aimed at the underlying cause, with antibiotics or anthelmintics, and is described in detail in the literature (Quesenberry and Carpenter, 2012). From a supportive care aspect, these rabbits will need to be confined in a small,

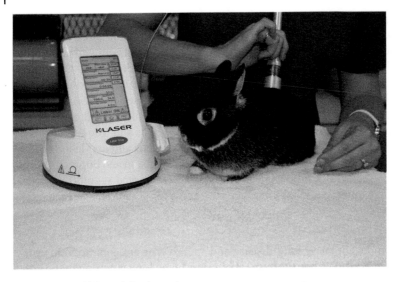

Figure 19.1 Rabbit receiving laser therapy.

well-padded space and monitored for corneal ulcers of the "down eye." Offer fresh, wet, leafy greens or hand feed regularly if needed. Meclizine can be helpful with the rolling and nausea. Anti-inflammatories and opioid pain medication, together with gentle massage of the often-painful neck muscles is warranted. Oral midazolam may be needed if the vestibular signs are severe. If the vestibular signs are mild to moderate, the patient may respond well to treatment. If clinical signs are more severe or if the patient is unresponsive to treatment, then the quality of life will quickly decline and the pet parents should be coached accordingly.

Treatment of any of these common geriatric conditions of rabbits requires maintaining hydration and food intake, as well as gastrointestinal health and movement. Consistent pain support and regular attention to the rabbit's hygiene and mobility are also critical. These cases can be an intensive time and financial investment for pet parents. Therapies can be considered successful if the rabbit's "happiness" can be restored, and if it is able to enjoy petting and interaction once again. Since these can be intense cases, veterinarians will need to work closely with parents of these geriatric rabbits to ensure their quality of life remains optimal in their senior years.

Geriatric Care of the Guinea Pig

Guinea pigs have a reported life expectancy of six to eight years, but are often seen in "geriatric" condition in veterinary practice around three to five years old. They are also a "prey" species, and thus often hide symptoms of illness or pain. This ability to mask early clinical signs means that guinea pigs commonly present in dire condition. Aging guinea pigs may develop osteoarthritis, reproductive tract neoplasia, pneumonia, abscesses, and dental disease. If they can be stabilized, then there are some medical management and supportive care options available for these pets.

Osteoarthritis

Osteoarthritis is caused by degenerative joint disease and/or chronic vitamin C deficiency in the guinea pig. These animals will have swollen, painful joints, and will be reluctant to move. Treatment is symptomatic, with pain management including oral meloxicam and tramadol or buprenorphine (Quesenberry and Carpenter, 2012). These patients should be provided soft, clean bedding to help with pressure sores. The author has also used laser therapy on an arthritic guinea pig and has noticed some pain relief. These patients will need assistance with grooming, as with the arthritic rabbit.

Reproductive Tract Neoplasia

Reproductive tract tumors are common in the unspayed guinea pig. Ovarian cysts can grow so big that the animal will often present with gastrointestinal symptoms. Mammary and uterine tumors are also regularly reported. These patients will have serosanguinous vaginal discharge and swelling and pain of the mammary chain (Quesenberry and Carpenter, 2012). Treatment of choice is ovariohysterectomy, but that is often not an option in the sick, geriatric guinea pig. These patients should be provided consistent pain management with non-steroidal anti-inflammatories and opioids, as recommended in rabbits, and be hand fed with Critical Care or a pellet gruel. Supplemental fluid therapy is also often needed. Guinea pigs with reproductive tract neoplasia can decline quickly, and pet parents should be advised that if quality of life cannot be reached in a reasonable amount of time, then euthanasia, sooner rather than later, is best.

Immunosuppression

Older guinea pigs can become immunosuppressed with age, and thus will be predisposed to pneumonia, abscesses, and dental diseases. One theory is that the immunosuppression stems from chronic vitamin C deficiency, but many other theories are described in the literature. Often, a geriatric guinea pig with pneumonia is in a critical condition. If severely dyspneic on presentation, then the prognosis is grave. If a guinea pig parent is not able to regularly medicate and monitor their pet, then treatment is not advised, and humane euthanasia is best. Dental disease in guinea pigs can also be a significant financial investment and requires a fair amount of nursing care, including regular hand feeding and pain management. Chronic dental disease in guinea pigs often results in permanent bony changes to the jaw, making the condition difficult to manage. The author has found that guinea pigs are often a child's pet or a classroom pet, but medical management must be explained and performed by an adult in order to achieve best compliance. As such, it is also imperative to clearly prognosticate for the adult owner so decisions can be made regarding these difficult to manage geriatric guinea pigs.

Euthanasia of Exotic Pets

When it comes time for humane euthanasia of these exotic pets, the process can be just as peaceful as with dogs and cats, with proper planning. It is highly recommended to give intramuscular sedation to these patients, so that an intravenous catheter can be placed, a pet parent can hold the animal, and aid in smoothness of the entire procedure.

There are a variety of protocols in the literature. Briefly, the author uses butorphanol/ ketamine with rabbits and guinea pigs and tiletamine/butorphanol with ferrets. If an intravenous catheter is not an option, or peripheral venous access is difficult, there are many other suitable options. In an anesthetized rabbit or guinea pig, the intrahepatic injection is recommended. The left liver lobe is bigger than the right, so place the animal in right lateral recumbency for best access. An interrenal injection is also recommended, because the kidneys are often easily palpable, just under the spine, and about grape sized in these small mammals. Intracardiac injections can also be used, as long as the patient is unconscious and anesthetized. The author has used a combination of tiletamine and acepromazine to induce anesthesia via injection for the euthanasia procedure. The intracardiac injection should be made at the point of the elbow on the chest wall. Clay paw prints can be made with these little pets, as for cats and dogs, and provide a cute memento of a beloved pet (Figure 19.2).

Regardless of the exact diagnosis or underlying cause of disease in a geriatric exotic pet, attention to the quality of life, in addition to close communication between veterinarian and pet parent, is critical for proper management. Medical and supportive care interventions are imperative; these patients must have adequate and consistent pain control and nutrition must be assisted if they are unable to eat and drink on their own. Their hygiene needs to be regularly evaluated and maintained. Adaptations should be made in their environment to assist with limited mobility, such as traction surfaces, soft bedding, user-friendly litter boxes, and close availability of fresh, appealing food and water. Lastly, the "happiness" factor for these animals must not be overlooked. Can the patient enjoy petting and interaction with its human and animal family? Can therapeutic intervention bring back some joy and comfort to this pet? Pet parents should be advised that the individual attention and care in the accepting exotic pet has

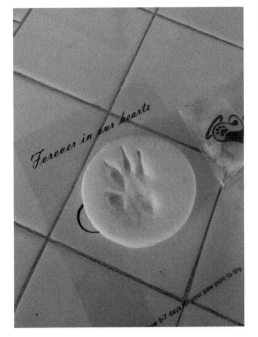

Figure 19.2 Rabbit paw impression and fur clipping.

endless advantages for both animal and person. When the quality of life is declining or no longer present, the veterinarian should be able to move forward and provide a peaceful end-of-life transition for these special pets.

References

Bays, T. B., Lightfoot, T. L., Mayer J. (2006) *Exotic Pet Behavior: Birds, Reptiles and Small Mammals*. Philadelphia, PA: Saunders Elsevier.

Johnson-Delaney, C. (2011) "Geriatrics: What to Do and When to Stop." In C. A. Johnson-Delaney (ed.). *Ferret Medicine and Surgery*, Chapter 27. Boca Raton, FL: CRC Press.

Morrissey, J. K. (2013) "Ferrets." In Carpenter, J. W. (ed.) *Exotic Animal Formulary* (4th ed.), pp. 561–74. St Louis, MO: Elsevier Saunders.

Oglesbee, B. (2006) *The 5-Minute Veterinary Consult Ferret and Rabbit*. Ames, IA: Blackwell.

Quesenberry, K. and Carpenter, J. (2012) *Ferrets, Rabbits and Rodents: Clinical Medicine and Surgery* (3rd ed.). Philadelphia, PA: Elsevier.

Villalobos, A. (2008) "The "HHHHHMM" Quality of Life Scale. Ontario VMA Conference, February 1, 2008. Available at http://pawspice.com/q-of-l-care/new-page.html.

Part III

What Matters Most in the End

"When your friends begin to flatter you on how young you look, it's a sure sign you're getting old."

— Mark Twain

20

Understanding the Behavior of Geriatric Patients to Enhance their Welfare

Carlo Siracusa

The Effect of Aging on the Behavior Body System

The protection of animal welfare and the prevention and relief of animal suffering are core duties of the veterinary profession (American Veterinary Medical Association, 2017). The welfare of an animal is determined by the animal's quality of life, as perceived by the animal itself. Welfare is a function of the degree of adaptation that an animal has to its own environment. Hence, welfare is a changing characteristic of each individual and varies from negative to positive. Positive welfare is characterized by good health and positive emotions. A happy animal is a healthy, fear-, stress-, and pain-free and comfortable animal (Yates and Main, 2008). Strategies for accomplishing these goals with geriatric patients have been discussed in the previous chapters of this book. In this chapter, we focus our attention on the behavior and welfare of geriatric patients, and in particular on their freedom to display normal, species-specific behavioral patterns and adapt to changing living conditions, up to a level that is perceived as positive. The changing equilibrium of an animal adapting to living condition is called "allostasis" (Korte *et al.*, 2007; Ohl and van der Stacy, 2012). Owing to the age-related physical and cognitive limitation of geriatric patients (sensory impairment, pain, cognitive decline, and so on), old dogs and cats are in an allostatic state, often characterized by a narrower regulatory range. They struggle to adapt to changes and challenges of their everyday life, and require a special attention to their needs. Veterinarians should therefore guide and support the caregivers of geriatric pets.

The welfare of household dogs and cats is not always perceived as a concern when compared with the welfare of production animals. We tend to assume that pets live in general a good and comfortable life. However, household pets often experience poor welfare when their caretakers do not have adequate knowledge of their species-typical behavior (Tami and Gallagher, 2009). Moreover, the welfare of geriatric patients can be especially compromised since other welfare-essential freedoms (Yates and Main, 2008) may be difficult to achieve; that is, freedom from discomfort, disease, and pain. Elderly pets experience a loss of brain plasticity and adaptability to environmental changes, which makes it difficult for them to maintain their quality of life. It is therefore pivotal for veterinarians to know about species-typical behavior, body language and communication, social interaction, and space distribution of dogs and cats, and how these are affected by senility. No other professional figure possesses the knowledge necessary to assess, monitor and guarantee the welfare of animals; this is even more true for our geriatric patients suffering pathologies that affect their welfare and that only veterinarians can treat.

It is commonly accepted that the physical health of an individual is determined by the condition of his body systems and organs. However, it is not always so intuitive understanding that also the mental status of an individual is regulated by a body system: the behavior body system. The sensory organs, the central nervous system, and the muscular–skeletal system are involved, among others, in the regulation of animal behavior (Carlson, 2013). Any pathology affecting components of the behavior body system will cause a behavioral change; and behavioral changes are among the most precocious (and often the only) signs of medical pathologies. Geriatric changes that alter, for example, a dog's sight (such as lens sclerosis; Figure 20.1) or joints will cause both physical and behavioral changes. Moreover, improving the welfare of an animal through behavior treatment can ultimately result in improved medical conditions (Landsberg *et al.*, 2013).

When an animal attempts to cope with its environment in presence of a stimulus perceived as a challenge or threat, the stress response is activated to restore the lost equilibrium. This biological response triggers a cascade of hormones, neurotransmitters, and modulators of the immune response (catecholamines, cortisol, cytokines) that will in turn cause behavioral changes. Different dogs and cats respond to the same stressor in many different ways. Some animals are more proactive and "fight", and some are more passive and take "flight"; while others "freeze" or engage in displacement activities ("fidget" response: pacing, self-grooming). Moreover, the same subject may vary its response based on the context (Notari, 2009). Recognizing the behavioral signs of stress is essential to identify a state of poor welfare of canine and feline patients and, therefore,

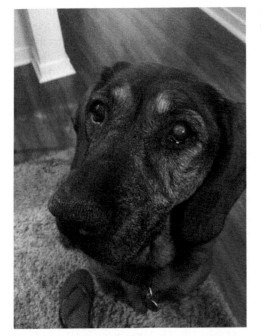

Figure 20.1 Dog with lens sclerosis. Source: Courtesy of Dr. Leontine Benedicenti.

it enables veterinarians to take an appropriate action and improve their quality of life. An overview of stress-related behaviors for dogs and cats is presented in Table 20.1. Many of these behaviors can also be signs of chronic pain, which should be always considered as potential stressor in geriatric patients (Wiese, 2015).

Table 20.1 Stress-related behaviors.

Category	Behaviors	Dog	Cat
Vocalizations	Barking	X	
	Growling	X	X
	Whining	X	
	Yelping	X	
	Hissing		X
	Spitting		X
	Yowl/howl		X
	Purring		X
Facial and oral behaviors	Yawning	X	X
	Lip-licking	X	X
	Self-grooming	X	X
	Panting	X	X
	Biting	X	X
	Licking (another individual)	X	
	Cheek puffing	X	
	Whiskers back		X
	Pupil dilation	X	X
	Teeth chattering	X	
	Showing teeth	X	X
	Grin/smile	X	
Posture	Low posture	X	X
	Reluctance to move or change posture	X	X
	Paw lifting	X	
	Ears back/flattened	X	X
	Piloerection	X	X
Locomotor	Tail chasing	X	
	Circling	X	
	Pacing	X	X
	Digging	X	
	Jumping	X	

(Continued)

Table 20.1 (Continued)

Category	Behaviors	Dog	Cat
	Trembling	X	X
	Escaping	X	X
	Excessive bunting/rubbing		X
	Excessive allogrooming		X
	Self-scratching	X	X
	Mounting	X	
	Swatting/scratching		X
	Restlessness	X	X
	Suckling (on inanimate object or cloth)	X	X
Explorative	Visual scanning	X	X
	Excessive sniffing	X	X
	Staring	X	X

Environmental Enrichment for Geriatric Dogs and Cats

Providing geriatric dogs and cats with an appropriate environment, perceived as safe and comfortable, is an important first step to increase environmental predictability, decrease stress and enhance welfare. Pets of all ages should always have access to safe havens and welfare-enhancing core areas, where all essential resources are available and perceived threats are minimized. For geriatric patients, safe havens and core areas have to be rearranged and the available space redistributed accounting to their needs, in order to guarantee a safe and ready access to low-stress areas. For example, a geriatric cat should be provided with safe havens and hiding spaces that he can easily access without jumping. Environmental enrichment should account for the decreased ability of the geriatric patient to reach for, handle and chew on toys; for the ability to obtain food from food-enhanced toys; and for the accessibility and comfort of resting places and safe spots (Corridane, 2009; Siracusa, 2016a).

Changes in the social dynamic of the household group should be considered in the environmental management of geriatric patients. Old cats and dogs may in fact find it particularly challenging to manage their social interactions, particularly with young and active individuals (Figure 20.2). Affective aggression between household dogs may arise when a young dog is introduced into a household with elderly dogs. Therefore, the possibility to avoid unwanted interactions on a voluntary basis should always be warranted to the geriatric animal. Safe areas to retreat to should be on the same floor level where the animal spends most of his time, and physical obstacles (such as stairs or slippery floors) to their access should be removed (Siracusa, 2016a,b).

Environmental predictability should be maximized for geriatric patients. Old dogs and cats do not easily adapt to environmental changes, even in contexts in which they used to cope well at a younger age. Feeding and walking schedules should be regular and frequent traveling should be avoided. Entrance and exit points should be consistently

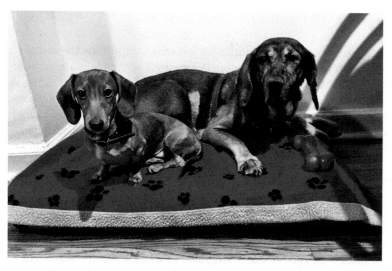

Figure 20.2 Very patient geriatric dog with younger housemate. Source: Courtesy of Dr. Leontine Benedicenti.

Box 20.1 Environmental Enrichment for Geriatric Dogs and Cats

- Predictable schedule:
  - Increase control over environment and reduce stress
  - Consistent feeding schedule
  - Consistent walking schedule for dogs
  - Consistent access to restricted areas of the home environment
  - Consistent use of home access/exit points
  - Consistent access to resting/sleeping areas
  - Regular, consistent and contingent use of basic training
- Safe havens to retreat without disturbances (comfortable room, crate, exercise pen)
  - Multiple spots with different degree of confinement/isolation
  - Increase control over environment and reduce stress
  - Minimize social interaction and conflicts
  - Keep resources safe
  - Readily and easily accessible: remove physical and social barriers (e.g. stairs, other dogs/cats, children)
- Toys and food-enhanced enrichment devices (e.g. KONG, puzzles)
- White noises to muffle threatening noises
- Barriers (e.g. contact paper, curtains, blinds) to obstruct visual threats
- Appeasing and facial pheromones (Adaptil, Feliway)
- Multiple resting spots (beds, blankets, pillows, rubber mats)

---

and predictably used; for example, a dog should be walked outside through the same route, so he does not get disoriented and signal the wrong exit when he needs to go outside for eliminating. Regularly practicing short, reward-based training exercises to help the dog in navigating his environment would enhance predictability and control, while providing mental stimulation (Landsberg *et al.*, 2013). See Box 20.1 for a review of environmental modification strategies for geriatric dogs and cats.

Behavior Management of Geriatric Dogs and Cats

Sensory impairment, chronic pain, and cognitive decline may compromise the ability of a geriatric patient to perform normal behaviors. Nevertheless, an adequate amount of behavioral stimulation should be provided to ensure a good quality of life. Special training protocols should be implemented with the ultimate goal to increase environmental predictability and improve communication. Training exercises should be brief and simple, and should be targeted to the specific skills of the subject. For example, a "sit" cue should be avoided in dogs with chronic pain of the lower back, hips or knees, and a "watch me" cue may be used the get their attention. Conversely, if the vision is impaired a "touch" cue may be preferred to a "watch me" cue to redirect a dog's focus. It is also important to keep in mind that learning skills and memory of a geriatric patient may be impaired, and therefore frequent repetition of the exercise may be beneficial (Landsberg and Araujo, 2005; Landsberg *et al.*, 2013).

The use of verbal cues should be consistently employed to give directions to the dog (such as, "go to your place", "let's go outside"). Regularly practicing short, reward-based training exercises also provides the geriatric patient with mental stimulation. Keep in mind that changes in the behavior body system of an old animal may influence his response to training. For example, a dog that has consistently gotten "off" the bed or couch on cue throughout his life, may refuse to promptly "get off" later in life because of the pain and discomfort this movement may induce in presence of osteoarthritis. In such cases, geriatric patients might also show aggression toward the person giving the cue, if their challenging situation is not understood and adequately treated; providing the animal with a ramp to facilitate the access to favorite resting places may prevent aggressive interactions. Behavioral changes in a geriatric patient should always be considered as potential early signs of non-behavioral pathologies (Landsberg and Araujo, 2005; Landsberg *et al.*, 2013).

Classical and operant conditioning are used for training dogs and cats. These two learning processes need a different level of cognitive engagement. Classical conditioning "spontaneously" happens when two stimuli are repeatedly and consistently presented together, without requiring the animal to do something upon request. Conversely, operant conditioning requires the animal to perform a voluntary behavior (that is, to "operate") and then to associate to the response showing a specific outcome (reward or punishment). This higher level of cognitive engagement required by operant conditioning may make it more difficult for the geriatric patients to respond to trained cues based on operant conditioning; therefore, the use of classical conditioning may be a better choice in this situation. For example, a dog that had reliably responded throughout his life to a "watch me" cue used to get his attention, may be less responsive when older. Hence, when necessary, his attention could be redirected just showing him a positive stimulus (usually food) to give it to him "for free" without expecting an operant behavior (that is, responding to the "watch me" cue; Mills, 2009).

The ability of an animal to remember or reverse a learned association is negatively affected by senility and this is used to measure cognitive decline and improvement; for example, when studying the efficacy of substances in slowing cognitive decline or improving cognitive function (Landsberg *et al.*, 2013, Vite and Head, 2014). Therefore, changes in the response to trained tasks should be monitored for an early detection of sensory or cognitive decline. Clients should be actively questioned about potential changes observed in the behavior and training of their dogs and cats. People may in fact assume that behavioral decline, even severe, is a "normal" and irreversible process of old pets; this lack of action may result in a significant detriment in the welfare of our geriatric patients. If signs of cognitive and/or sensory decline are detected, the behavior management of our patients should be consequently adjusted; if a dog is not responding to a visual stimulus that used to trigger a specific behavior (for example, grabbing the leash to induce the dog to come to the door for a walk outside), then this stimulus should be complemented with a verbal cue (such as "let's go for a walk").

Behavior Problems of Geriatric Dogs and Cats

The behavior of dogs and cats is regulated by a complex and rich body system including the brain, sensory organs, muscles, and bones. Undesirable behaviors of geriatric patients can be abnormal behaviors caused by primary behavior pathologies mainly affecting the brain (for example, disorientation due to cognitive dysfunction) or normal behaviors secondary to medical problems affecting components of the behavior body system (for example, increased aggression secondary to pain or sensory impairment). A separate chapter has been dedicated to cognitive dysfunction (see Chapter 8); here, we focus our attention on primary behavior pathologies other than cognitive dysfunction and behavior problems secondary to medical pathologies of geriatric patients.

Decreased brain plasticity and adaptability can cause the animal to respond with anxiety to environmental changes (such as the birth of a child, or the introduction of a new household dog). Senility can also cause the relapse or exacerbation of previously controlled behavior problems. Anxious and reactive dogs and cats may find it more difficult to manage interactions with distrusted individuals (for example, by quickly retreating to their safe haven), and this may result in increased aggression. Dogs with a history of separation anxiety may experience a relapse of this behavior pathology (Landsberg and Denenberg, 2009).

Changes in behavior are often the first sign of disease, although they often go unnoticed or misinterpreted because of their subtleness or the lack of knowledge about species-typical behavior. The situation may be even more complicated for geriatric patients in which aging processes modify their ability to show normal behavior signs. Unfortunately, behavioral signs of medical conditions and pain are often unspecific and significantly overlap with primary behavioral signs of stress and anxiety (Fatjó and Bowen, 2009). Therefore, collecting a comprehensive and accurate history of the behavioral changes observed will help the veterinarian to understand if they are likely to be caused by a medical pathology, a primary behavior pathology, or both.

Sensory impairment is often the cause of behavioral changes that may be misinterpreted and confused with signs of behavioral pathologies, like cognitive dysfunction. Vision loss and/or decreased amplitude of accommodation may cause increased aggression, fear, changes in social interactions, disorientation, and/or house soiling. Hearing loss may cause increased aggression, decreased attention and responsiveness, increased anxiety and fear, and/or disorientation (Landsberg *et al.*, 2012, 2013). Under the guidance of their veterinarian, owners should modify their way of interacting with their dogs and cats taking in account their sensory capabilities. If a pet has experienced vision loss, using a verbal anticipatory cue before approaching him (such as "it's me!")

may help prevent a startle response and potential consequent aggression. In a similar context, gently tapping with a foot on the floor may help dogs and cats experiencing hearing loss. Interestingly, some behavior problems can improve with aging. Noise fear can improve because of hearing loss, and thunderstorm fear can improve because of hearing and/or vision loss.

Behavioral changes are often the most sensitive sign to detect chronic pain in geriatric patients. Changes can consist of either the presence of a new or exaggerated behavior (for instance, increased aggression towards humans and conspecifics, inappropriate elimination) or the decreased frequency of a typical behavior (for example, decreased level of activity, difficulties in changing posture). Several behavior-based scales and questionnaires to detect pain are available, and a few of them have been scientifically validated. Among the behaviors usually included in these scales, subtle behaviors resulting from altered mobility (for example, reluctance to change body posture, decreased explorative behavior) are useful to detect mild or moderate pain. However, none of them is specific for the detection of pain and can be greatly influenced by the level of stress and anxiety experienced by the animal. This should be appropriately considered when using these tools and, in general, when using behavior as a pain marker; consistently keeping a record of a long-term patient's response to in-hospital stressful contexts (such as confinement in a cage) may help to differentiate stress from pain-related behaviors. When the presence of chronic pain is suspected in an anxious dog or cat, anti-anxiety drugs with a known effect on chronic pain may be used, such as tricyclic antidepressants, clomipramine and gabapentin (Wiese, 2015).

Metabolic diseases are also frequent causes of behavior alterations. Hypertension and hyperthyroidism should be considered in cases of increased vocalization of a geriatric cat (Figure 20.3). Chronic kidney disease and diabetes mellitus are potential causes of inappropriate elimination in a geriatric patient. It is important to keep in mind that old cats have a decreased sensitivity to thirst, so water should be readily available also in

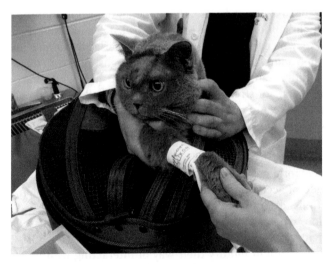

Figure 20.3 Geriatric cat with bilateral retinal detachment and hypertension that was restless and had increased vocalization.

cases of inappropriate elimination. Behavior changes of geriatric patients that do not respond to conventional behavior treatment may also be caused by a neoplasia, which should be therefore listed among their possible differential diagnoses (Little, 2012).

Veterinarians should remember that, owing to low specificity of behavior changes, the association of a certain behavior with a diagnosed medical condition does not prove a causal link between the two elements. Therefore, if the behavior change observed does not respond to the treatment for the diagnosed medical problem other potential medical, behavioral and/or environmental causes should be explored.

References

American Veterinary Medical Association. (2017) "Veterinarian's Oath." Available at https://www.avma.org/KB/Policies/Pages/veterinarians-oath.aspx.

Carlson, V. (2013) *Physiology of Behavior* (11th ed.). Upper Saddle River, NJ: Pearson.

Corridane, C. (2009) "Basic Requirements for Good Behavioural Health and Welfare in Dogs." In D. Horwitz and D. Mills (eds), *BASAVA Manual of Canine and Feline Behavioural Medicine* (2nd ed.), pp. 24–34. Gloucester, UK: BSAVA.

Fatjó, J. and Bowen, J. (2009) "Medical and Metabolic Influences on Behavioural Disorders." In D. Horwitz and D. Mills (eds), *BASAVA Manual of Canine and Feline Behavioural Medicine* (2nd ed.), pp. 1–9. Gloucester, UK: BSAVA.

Korte, S. M., Olivier, B., Koolhaas, J. M. (2007) "A New Animal Welfare Concept Based on Allostasis." *Physiology and Behavior*, 92: 422–8.

Landsberg, G. and Araujo, J. A. (2005) "Behavior Problems in Geriatric Pets." *Veterinary Clinics of North America Small Animal Practice*, 35: 675–98.

Landsberg, G. and Denenberg, S. (2009) "Behaviour Problems in the Senior Pet." In D. Horwitz and D. Mills (eds), *BASAVA Manual of Canine and Feline Behavioural Medicine* (2nd ed.), pp. 127–35. Gloucester, UK: BSAVA.

Landsberg, G., Hunthausen, W., Ackerman, L. (2013) "The Effects of Aging on Behavior in Senior Pets." In Landsberg G, Hunthausen W, Ackerman L (eds), *Behavior Problems of the Dog and Cat* (3rd ed.), pp. 211–35. Philadelphia, PA: Elsevier Saunders.

Landsberg, G. M., Nichol, J., Araujo, J. A. (2012) "Cognitive Dysfunction Syndrome: A Disease of Canine and Feline Brain Aging." *Veterinary Clinics of North America Small Animal Practice*, 42: 749–68.

Little, S. E. (2012) "Managing the Senior Cat." In *The Cat: Clinical Medicine and Management*, pp. 1166–74. St. Louis, MO: Elsevier Saunders.

Mills, D. (2009) "Training and Learning Protocols." In D. Horwitz and D. Mills (eds), *BASAVA Manual of Canine and Feline Behavioural Medicine* (2nd ed.), pp. 49–64. Gloucester, UK: BSAVA.

Notari, L. (2009) "Stress in Veterinary Behavior Medicine." In D. F. Horwitz and S. D. Mills (eds), *BSAVA Manual of Canine and Feline Behavioural Medicine* (2nd ed.), pp. 136–45. Gloucester, UK: BSAVA.

Ohl, F. and van der Staay, F. J. (2012) "Animal Welfare: At the Interface Between Science and Society." *Veterinary Journal*, 192: 13–19.

Siracusa, C. (2016a) "Creating Harmony in Multiple Cat Households." In S. Little (ed.), "*August's Consultation in Feline Internal Medicine*, Vol. 7, pp. 931–40. Philadelphia, PA: Elsevier.

Siracusa, C. (2016b) "Status-Related Aggression, Resource Guarding, and Fear-Related Aggression in Two Female Mixed Breed Dogs." *Journal of Veterinary Behavior*, 12: 85–91.

Tami, G. and Gallagher, A. (2009) "Description of the Behaviour of Domestic Dog (Canis Familiaris) by Experienced and Inexperienced People." *Applied Animal Behaviour Science*, 120: 159–69.

Vite, C. H. and Head, E. (2014) "Aging in the Canine and Feline Brain." *Veterinary Clinics of North America Small Animal Practice*, 44: 1113–29.

Wiese, A. J. (2015) "Assessing Pain: Pain Behaviors." In J. S. Gaynor and W. W. Muir (eds), *Handbook of Veterinary Pain Management* (3rd ed.), pp. 67–97. Philadelphia, PA: Elsevier Saunders.

Yates, J. W. and Main D. C. J. (2008) "Assessment of Positive welfare: A Review." *Veterinary Journal*, 175: 293–300.

21

Environmental Enrichment and Senior Pets: The Next Best Thing to the Fountain of Youth

Steve Dale

Zoos have known about enriching the environments and the lives of captive animals for decades. Many of today's larger zoos even have a full-time employee dedicated to the task of inspiring lives of their residents, ranging from cheetahs, to polar bears to Savannah monitor lizards. A zoo lizard may arguably enjoy an environment that is more enriched than even the most "spoiled" of pets. Spoiling pets is oftentimes a part of the problem. Up to 69% of the feline pet population is now living indoors only (American Pet Products Association, 2016), and because of this, being run over by a car or run down by a coyote is not too likely. However, despite an indoor-only existence, cats are born with a hard-wired prey drive, and they continue to have the need to chase, pounce and kill – even if it is only a mouse toy (Overall, 2013). If we do not properly enrich their environments and satisfy these primal feline needs, we run the risk of bolstering a nation of fat, brain-dead cats.

According to the Association of Pet Obesity Prevention, 58% of cats are overweight or obese (Association of Pet Obesity Prevention, 2015). Many of them only get off the sofa for their meals, which is obviously not healthy. In fact, according to Karen Overall (personal communication), many of these overweight and obese cats are clinically depressed, owing to their inability to be able to pounce, hunt and activate their prey drives. And many of these cats are "senior citizens." Furthermore, in cats, there is a correlation between unenriched environments and interstitial cystitis, often dubbed idiopathic feline lower urinary tract disease (FLUTD) or "Pandora's syndrome" (Westropp and Buffington, 2004; Herron and Buffington, 2010; Buffington *et al.*, 2014). This uncomfortable or painful condition combined with anxiety may prompt them to eliminate outside their litter boxes. Having "accidents" is a significant cause for breaking of the human–animal bond, and ultimately owner relinquishment. In general, it turns out that enriching the environment is an effective treatment for FLUTD, and this appears to be true no matter how old a cat may be (Westropp and Buffington, 2004; Herron and Buffington, 2010; Buffington *et al.*, 2014). Of course, in older cats arthritis, feline cognitive dysfunction syndrome and underlying kidney disease and or/other medical issues may contribute to inappropriate elimination, and require appropriate medical attention.

Treatment and Care of the Geriatric Veterinary Patient, First Edition. Edited by Mary Gardner and Dani McVety.
© 2017 John Wiley & Sons, Inc. Published 2017 by John Wiley & Sons, Inc.
Companion Website: www.wiley.com/go/gardner/geriatric

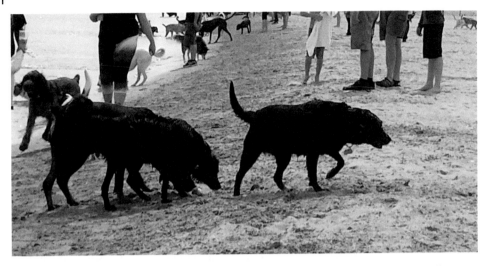

Figure 21.1 Most dogs love going to the dog park, lake or beach – often times it is just to sniff and make friends with other humans but at other times it is to play with others of their own kind.

By any definition, many of today's dogs are "livin' the good life." After all, millennials barely even know what a dog house is, and today, 50% of dogs share our beds (American Pet Products Association, 2016). It seems wonderful – and in many ways it is. However, few dogs were bred to live their lives on beds and do little else. Most dogs were bred for a purpose, from retrieving waterfowl to herding sheep to guarding property. And having a purpose in life seems to be healthful in dogs (Figure 21.1), as it may be in people (Boyle *et al.*, 2012).

We live in a nation filled with unemployed dogs. Often, retrieving dogs do not even get to fetch a tennis ball. With no other outlet to herd, herding dogs may wind up chasing children and are admonished or even relinquished to shelters. Guard dogs are discouraged from doing what may come naturally because that behavior might be inappropriate for high-rise living, as an example. Oftentimes, dog owners do not realize that it is important to support dogs in having a purpose, or have the time to allow natural behavioral outlets. Like cats, too many dogs are overweight or obese, at about 53% (Association of Pet Obesity Prevention, 2015). The American Zoological and Aquariums Association Behavioral Advisory Group has described enrichment:

> Environmental enrichment is a process for improving or enhancing zoo animal environments and care within the context of their inhabitants' behavioral biology and natural history. It is a dynamic process in which changes to structures and husbandry practices are made with the goal of increasing the behavioral choice available to animals and drawing out their species-appropriate behaviors and abilities, thus enhancing their welfare. As the term implies, enrichment typically involves the identification and subsequent addition to the zoo environment of a specific stimulus or characteristic that the occupant(s) needs but which was not previously present.
>
> *(American Zoological and Aquariums Association*
> *Behavioral Advisory Group, 1999)*

A simpler but true enough definition is: "Manipulating the environment to suit animals' (normal) behavior" (Dale and Briere, 1992). These definitions also apply to companion animals as much as they do to captive wild animals at zoos or sanctuaries. Before examining enrichment for pets, it may be helpful to better understand enrichment by offering examples of enrichment at zoos. Zoo enrichment might include PVC piping filled with food, which a giant anteater uses its long sticky tongue to probe for goodies. Cheetahs are inspired to chase and catch a dead chicken pulled across the exhibit on a pulley at a high speed. Talk about your ultimate fish 'n chips, a polar may chip away at a giant ice cube floating in an exhibit with a fish frozen inside it (Steve Ross, personal communication; Shepherdson, 1989, 1998; Schulz, 2004; Baker, n.d; Markowitz, 1982).

Decades ago, primatologist Jane Goodall discovered that chimpanzees use sticks as tools to poke into termite mounds, and then lick the bugs off for a meal. Using this knowledge, zoos often provide an artificial log with holes, and in each is filled a condiment. Chimps can use debris in the exhibit, such as straw, to poke into a hole for the condiment of their choice. One important component of enrichment is to offer individual choice or preference (Dale and Briere, 1992; Steve Ross, personal communication; Shepherdson, 1989, 1998; Baker, n.d; Markowitz, 1982).

Enrichment does not need to be only about food. For example, zoo animals can be offered old rags or burlap sacks infused with different odors. Enriching an environment may also mean offering different textures, and/or varying items to investigate. Orangutans enjoy investigating and methodically taking items apart (Dale and Briere, 1992; Baker, n.d; Markowitz, 1982).

Thus far, studies on enrichment in zoo animals have not specifically focused specifically on benefits to geriatric animals and the role enrichment may play in maintaining physical health and/or brain health. However, anecdotal evidence and studies in people and dogs support that notion. I recall one zookeeper telling me about an older orangutan who was living alone for several months after his "spouse" passed away. Veterinarians said his health was declining, and arthritis was a problem as well. He seemed "depressed." One day, the keeper went to a toy store and purchased several plastic puzzle toys, the kind where plastic circle pieces fit into circle holes, and triangles fit where the triangle holes are. The great ape perked up. The keeper rotated different types of puzzle toys, and encouraged climbing merely by placing the pieces all over the exhibit. I was told, "If I made it too easy to find the puzzle pieces, he (the orangutan) would look at me as if to say, 'really, this is too easy.'" No doubt the non-steroidal anti-inflammatory drug also eased the orangutan's arthritis, but increased activity likely also played a role. Most important, the big guy seemed "like his old self," according to the keeper, who, over time, purchased various toys and continued to rotate them for nearly all the rest of the great ape's life.

A myriad of studies demonstrates that zoo animals benefit physically and mentally from the stimulation provided by an enriched environment (Dale and Briere, 1992; Steve Ross, personal communication; Shepherdson, 1989, 1998; Baker, n.d; Markowitz, 1982). Numerous studies of zoo animals demonstrate that living in unenriched and uninteresting environments is unhealthy, potentially leading to various abnormal behaviors and can play a role in weight gain and general ill health (Dale and Briere, 1992; Steve Ross, personal communication; Shepherdson, 1989, 1998; Baker, n.d; Markowitz, 1982). Also, with less anxiety, there is generally less stress on immune systems, which may contribute to preventing disease onset, who knows – could even slow the aging

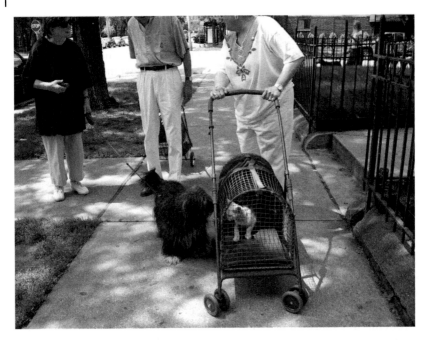

Figure 21.2 Roxy, 13, gets a weekly walk in her special stroller where she enjoys sniffing the air, as well as passers by.

process (Dale and Briere, 1992; Steve Ross, personal communication; Shepherdson, 1989, 1998; Baker, n.d; Markowitz, 1982).

While there is certainly a correlation between zoo animals and companion animals, few clients live with anteaters or cheetahs. More relevant is how enrichment may be used to enhance lifespan and quality of life of our pets, particularly senior pets (Figure 21.2). For dogs and cats of all ages, enrichment may alleviate boredom, and provide "brain exercise". It may be a source of physical activity, and may offer an appropriate outlet for natural behaviors. It may assist in dealing with or even preventing behavior problems, and it is simply fun for the pet – and for pet owners (Seksel, 2006; Virga, 2004; Ohio State University, n.d.).

Offering food or treats from toys and food puzzles is one example of enriching companion animals' lives (Overall, 2013). It turns out that the eagerness to work for food and a preference to problem solve has been studied, although not very much specifically for dogs or cats (Figure 21.3). Studies do indicate that rats, grizzly bears and other animals will choose to work for their meal over a "free meal". This phenomenon, called "contrafreeloading", does contradict the basic tenant that animals are hard-wired to expend the least possible energy for meals to enhance their odds of survival (McGowan *et al.*, 2014; Inglis *et al.*, 1997). While there are no specific data regarding contrafreeloading in dogs and cats, much less in senior pets, it appears to be a very real phenomenon for many individuals.

At the age of 13 or so, our Brittany Spaniel, Chaser, was clearly showing typical aging dog signs, increasingly moving only when she absolutely wanted to. I suspect that arthritis played a role. However, she remained motivated by food, and continued to eat from treat dispensing toys. Was she truly enjoying working for her meals? Of course, it is impossible to say for sure, but on the rare occasions when food was offered from a

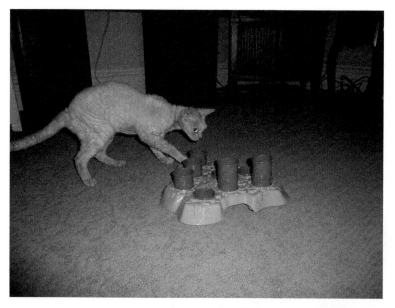

Figure 21.3 Roxy, 13 years old, using the Aikiou food puzzle toy to search for treats.

Figure 21.4 Ethel, 11 years old, with enrichment toys with foods and treats, encouraging her prey drive.

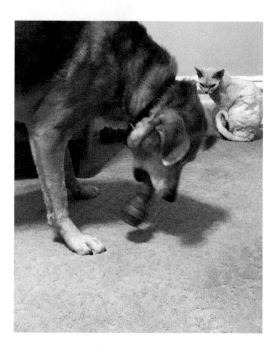

bowl, she seemed less enthusiastic about scarfing it down, compared with "working" for the meal. What's more she was attending a "stretch" free class each time she was fed. She would voluntarily move in ways she otherwise might not, as she moved the food dispensing toys around, especially when they might roll underneath furniture she would reach in to poke them out (Figure 21.4).

Often, I would also hide treats for her. Instantly, a spark returned to her previously "old lady walk," as she sprinted around the house with her little tail wagging seeking whatever we had hidden. Perhaps, a part of this behavior was to "compete" with our other much younger dog. In this case, it was clear that her brain was working, and she was moving, voluntarily, although I concede her actions were enticed by food. Cats are born with a hard-wired prey drive, to seek and kill. Hiding food in various places and at various heights may motivate older cats to climb and also to stretch (Figure 21.5). They also need to think about where those morsels may be hiding. All reasonably healthy cats retain a prey drive and benefit by having an outlet for that drive (Overall, personal communication). Kibble may be hidden in a multitude of treat dispensing toys or food puzzles for dogs and cats, and they are available anywhere pet products are sold (Figure 21.6). Clients can

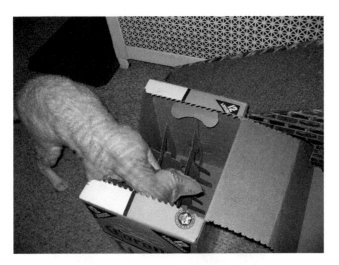

Figure 21.5 Roxy's owners used an empty beer box with different compartments to put treats in.

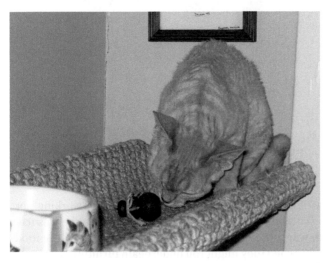

Figure 21.6 Feeding Roxy on top of a cat tree not only encourages her to climb but also putting treats up there a part of her daily 'hunt for treats' game.

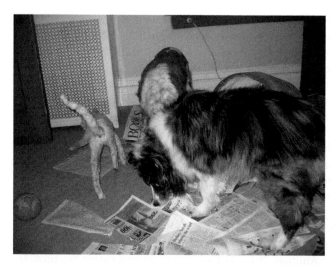

Figure 21.7 Newspaper enrichment – hide treats in layers of newspapers and let the pets hunt.

easily make their own, such as folding both sides of a toilet tube roll and cutting holes in the center for food to tumble out when it is rolled around. Large dogs may prefer an empty plastic milk carton with a couple of holes cut out to allow kibble to fall out. The ideas are only limited by pet owners' creativity.

Hiding "ordinary food," or providing it in toys may not be stimulating enough for geriatric pets with a compromised sense of smell and taste (Dodman and Lidner, 2012). Bringing out the "good stuff" may be necessary to entice, such as using yogurt, tuna or favorite manufactured treats (Figure 21.7). Of course, it is not advisable to force an elderly hungry dog or cat to search for food, or to be fed out of food toys if they're absolutely uninterested, or physically unable. The NoBowl Feeding System™ was developed by Liz Bales, VMD for cats to seek and even pounce on "prey," that look like little mice which kibble is deposited into. When cats maneuver the NoBowls kibble tumbles out. The idea is to teach cats to seek the individual hidden NoBowls. For some elderly cats, this is far too challenging, for others it's a great means to keep cats engaged using their hard-wired skills.

Throughout their lives, many dogs enjoy chewing. However, older dogs may be even more inclined to break teeth and/or items may cause stomach upset. Instead of leaving products like antler ears, hooves, hard bones or even rawhide, there are countless "squishy" treats which require some chewing but are not as likely to break teeth or cause damage to the delicate gums our geriatric pets often have, because of inflammation from dental disease. Other possibilities include apple slices (which can be frozen for a "better chew"), mini-carrot sticks, Virbac® C.E.T.® Oral Hygiene Chews or prescription dental diets, are some examples. Of course, veterinary advice of what applies to individual pets is always suggested.

Cognitive enrichment starting early in life may help to protect against the development of early cognitive decline and dementia in some dogs and in people (and therefore one may assume cats as well; Milgram *et al.*, 2006). Enrichment is important for dogs and cats as puppies and kittens, why would it be any less important as they age? Based on personal observations, many people do seem to take their older pets for granted – although I am not suggesting they are loved any less. Often owners assume, "Well, they're old – let them be," or because they're moving less, truly motivating these older animals may require more effort. Sometimes that motivation happens as a surprise but pet owners may not recognize it. A zookeeper told me how she often would rotate with various animals when she first joined the zoo, filling in wherever she was needed. She maintains that her old little terrier mix was happy to see her return home before she accepted that job, as nearly all dogs are happy to see their people. But once she began at the zoo, the hello consisted of intense and lengthy sniffing, as if to discoverer, "So today you worked in the bird house?" She told me her new job seemed to give a new purpose to her old dog's life.

While this dog seemingly enjoyed the new odors, some animals may not – and likely most cats would not appreciate those new outrageous smells. Come home to your stable, old, cat smelling like a cheetah, and you may be sprayed on by an agitated cat. And while enrichment is about stimulating natural behaviors, and about changing things up – little disturbs cats more than too much change. The secret is finding that right balance.

Since pets live by their noses, and even with failing eyesight their sense of smell remains the primary sense, introducing new scents may be fun, or not. For example, anecdotally some cats enjoy lavender, while others actually appear to be disturbed. It turns out the lavender plants may be dangerous, and so are the oils in the potpourri (American Society for the Prevention of Cruelty to Animals, 2017). For most (not all) cats, catnip can provide a fun release, and valerian root can have calming affects for many cats, although not all cats (Houghton, 1999). Spritzing odors, such as just a little cologne or perfume near a cat or dog bed or along a baseboard, may be "interesting," although at least one study suggests that cats in particular do not much care (Wells and Ellis, 2010). For dogs (not cats), you can create a foreign exchange program, where clients can borrow a friend's soft dog toy. It may be more fun to sniff the toy than it is to play with it. If your pet sleeps away from you, placing a worn t-shirt near the pet may be comforting. If there is some suspected uneasiness, pheromonal products, such as Adaptil or Feliway, may lessen anxiety.

We have all heard stories about how adding a second pet provides a new spark, and older pet begins to play like a young one. Beware, because adding another pet to a household may be an example of far too much change for a geriatric pet to deal with. A seriously ill pet or a pet in declining health is unlikely to benefit from having another member of their same species. In fact, sometimes such a change may cause that pet to go downhill faster. A pet who has no previous experience living with another pet might have done fine if that other pet had been introduced at a younger age, but the timing might not be right. Also, new cats, in particular, must be introduced very gradually into a home with an existing older cat. Having said that, a second pet may be positively enriching.

There is no doubt that stimulation resulting from an enriched environment may delay or even prevent onset on canine or feline cognitive dysfunction syndrome (Overall, 2013; Studzinski et al., 2006). For individually social dogs and for people, there is research that demonstrates that socialization, including exercise-derived from walks, may help to delay or even prevent deleterious cognitive changes (Overall, 2013; Johnson et al., 2011; Studzinski et al., 2006).

Aging dogs have been used as model for older people, and it turns out that there are real and similar benefits for both species. For example, walking turns out to be just as beneficial for older dogs as it is for older people (Overall, 2013; Johnson et al., 2011; Milgram et al., 2006). In fact, a simple walk, especially exploring new neighborhoods, may be the most enriching activity for any dog. Think of all those new and exciting smells (Dodman and Lidner, 2011; Johnson et al., 2011). And social dogs benefit by meeting new people and new dogs. While some older dogs may be too impaired for a walk, the walk does not need to break speed or distance records. Or debilitated dogs may even be pushed in a carrier or wagon (Johnson et al., 2011).

Motor learning (as opposed to mere motor activity) may increase synapse formation in the cerebellar cortex in rats (Milgram *et al.*, 2006). One might assume the same is true for dogs and cats – learning does not need to ever stop. For years, independent living centers for seniors have encouraged adult continued education, such as learning a computer program or how to play chess, as well as encouraging movement through exercise classes. Studies support that these activities are beneficial for both the mental and physical health of residents (Winsted *et al.*, 2013, 2014). In many ways, dog and cat brains operate in a similar way to human brains, and age similarly (Landsberg *et al.*, 2013). New challenges are important. That old axiom from grandpa turns out to be right, when he said, "if you don't use it, you'll lose it." No wonder, so many facilities continue to support funding for these activities because of the results they witness.

There are numerous studies to support the notion that laughter is, as the old expression goes, the best medicine (Mayo Clinic, 2016). If that is the case in people, might the same be true for dogs or cats? Perhaps an antidote to illnesses associated in aging pets is simply to encourage them to have a good time with a tug toy or squeaky mouse.

References

American Society for the Prevention of Cruelty to Animals. (2017) "Toxic and Non-Toxic Plants: Lavender." Available at http://www.aspca.org/pet-care/animal-poison-control/toxic-and-non-toxic-plants/lavender.

American Pet Products Association. (2016) *2015–2016 National Pet Owners Survey.* Greenwich, CT: APPA.

American Zoological and Aquariums Association Behavioral Advisory Group (1999). Workshop at Disney's Animal Kingdom.

Association of Pet Obesity Prevention. (2015) "2015 Obesity Facts and Risks." Available at http://petobesityprevention.org/pet-obesity-fact-risks.

Baker, M. (n.d.) "Manufacture, Selection, and Responses to Habitat Enrichment Items for Captive Nonhuman Primates." Available at http://faculty.ucr.edu/~maryb/enrichment.htm.

Boyle, P., Buchman, A., Wilson, R., Yu, L., Schneider, J., Bennett, D. A. (2012) "Effect of Purpose in Life on the Relation Between Alzheimer Disease Pathologic Changes on Cognitive Function in Advanced Age." *Archives of General Psychiatry*, 69(5): 499–505.

Buffington, T., Westropp, J., Chew. D. J. (2014) "From FUS to Pandora Syndrome: Where are We, How did we get Here, and Where to Now?" *Journal of Feline Medicine and Surgery*, 16: 579–98.

Dale, S. and Briere, A. (1992) *American Zoos.* New York, NY: Mallard Press.

Dodman, N. and Lidner, L., eds. (2012) *Good Old Dog: Expert Advice for Keeping Your Aging Dog Happy, Healthy and Comfortable.* Boston, MA: Mariner Books.

Herron, M. E. and Buffington C. A. T. (2010) "Environmental Enrichment for Indoor Cats". *Compendium of Continuing Education for Practicing Veterinarians*, 32(12): E4. PMCID: PMC3922041.

Houghton, P. J. (1999) "The Scientific Basis for the Reputed Activity of Valerian," *Journal of Pharmacy and Pharmacology*, 51(5): 505–12.

Inglis, I. R., Forkman, B., Lazarus, J. (1997) "Free Food or Earned Food? A Review and Fuzzy Model of Contrafreeloading." *Animal Behavior*, 53: 1171–91.

Johnson R. A., Beck A., McCune, S. (2011) *The Health Benefits of Dog Walking for People and Pets: Evidence and Case Studies.* West Lafayette, IN: Purdue University Press.

Landsberg, G., Hunthausen, W., Ackerman, L. (2013) *Behavior Problems of the Dog and Cat* (3rd ed.). St Louis, MO: Elsevier Saunders.

McGowan, R., Rehn, T., Norling, Y., Keeling, L. "Positive Affects and Learning: Exploring the 'Eureka Effect in Dogs," *Animal Cognition,* 17(3): 577–87.

Markowitz, H. (1982) *Behavioral Enrichment in the Zoo.* New York, NY: Van Nostrand Reinhold.

Mayo Clinic. (2016) "Healthy Lifestyle: Stress Management. Stress Release from Laughter? It's No Joke." Available at http://www.mayoclinic.org/healthy-lifestyle/stress-management/in-depth/stress-relief/art-20044456.

Milgram, N. W., Siwak-Tapp, C. T., Araujo, J., Head, E. (2006) "Neuroprotective Effects of Cognitive Enrichment Aging Research." *Aging Research Reviews,* 5(3): 354–69.

Ohio State University (n.d.) College of Veterinary Medicine. "Indoor Pet Initiative." Available at https://indoorpet.osu.edu.

Overall K. (2013) "Normal Feline Behavior and Ontogeny: Neurological and Social Development, Signaling and Normal Feline Behaviors." In *Manual of Clinical Behavioral Medicine of Dogs and Cats,* pp. 312–59. St Louis, MO: Elsevier Mosby.

Schultz, C. (2004) "Behavior Techniques in Zoo Animals." In Proceedings North American Veterinary Conference Post Graduate Institute, United States Department of Agriculture.

Seksel, K. (2006) "Environment Enrichment in Cats." Proceedings AVMA 2006.

Shepherdson, D. (1998) "Introduction: Tracing the Path of Environmental Enrichment in Zoos" In D. J. Shepherdson, J. D. Mellen, and M. Hutchins (eds). *Second Nature: Environmental Enrichment for Captive Animals,* pp. 1–14, Washington, DC: Smithsonian Institute Press.

Shepherdson, D. (1989) "Stereotypic Behaviour: What is it and How Can it be Eliminated or Prevented? *Ratel,* 16: 100–5.

Studzinski, C. M., Christie, L. A., Araujo, J. A., Burnham, W. M., Head, E., Cottman, C. W., *et al.* (2006) "Visuospatial function in the beagle dog; an early market of cognitive decline in a model of human aging and dementia," *Neurobiology of Aging,* 86(2): 197–204.

Virga, V. (2004) "Environmental and Social Enrichment for Indoor Cats." Proceedings AVMA.

Wells, D. and Ellis, S. (2010) "The Influence of Behavioural Enrichment on Cats Housed in a Rescue Shelter." *Applied Animal Behavior Science,* 123(1–2): 56–62.

Westropp, J. L. and Buffington, T. (2004) "Feline Idiopathic Cystitis: Current Understanding of Pathophysiology And Management." *Veterinary Clinics of North America Small Animal Practice,* 34: 1043–55.

Winsted, V., Anderson W. A., Yost, E., Cotton, S. R., Warr, A., Berkowsky, R. (2013) "You can Teach an Old Dog New Tricks: A Qualitative Analysis of how Residents of Senior Living Communities may use the Web to Overcome Special and Social Barriers." *Journal of Applied Gerontology,* 32: 540–60.

Winsted, V., Yost, E., Cotton S, Berkowsky, R, Anderson, W. (2014) "The Impact of Activity Interventions on the Well-Being of Older Adults in Continuing Care Communities." *Journal of Applied Gerontology,* 33: 888–911.

22

Where Are all the Grey Muzzles?

Marketing and Caring for Geriatric Pets in your Practice
Mary Gardner

Introduction

Many believe that since I perform euthanasia on a daily basis (carrying out an average of 60 euthanasias each month), I would suffer greatly from depression or compassion fatigue. In fact, my feelings are quite the opposite; I experience the utmost fulfillment and satisfaction in the niche I have dedicated my career to. Although I am helping families through that dreaded moment, the receipt of a warm hug, and hearing through tear-streaked cheeks and choked-up voices, the most kind and sincere "thank you," makes it all worth it. Yes, indeed it is sad, and sometimes I cry right alongside the families, knowing first-hand how it feels to experience those final moments of a pet's life. Nonetheless, being able to honor a pet and comfort a family in an unparalleled way is absolutely remarkable. By the end of the day, I am overflowing with compassion because I have delivered peace to a pet, and eventually to the family, by fully empathizing with the struggles of saying goodbye.

Compassion requires the recognition of suffering, the desire to reverse it, and taking appropriate action – regardless of the outcome. With that being said, the one thing that frustrates me is seeing pets that could have benefitted from help, but failed to receive it. Not to blame the family or their primary care veterinarian, it is just an unfortunate state of affairs. Many families simply stop providing formal care to their pets at a certain stage for a variety of reasons. Here are some common explanations as to why:

"My vet just wants me to spend hundreds when the result will be nothing I don't already know – he has arthritis/kidney failure/etc."

"I don't want to go to extreme measures and do more harm than good."

"He is an old dog and I don't want to spend money on him when he is just going to die soon anyway." (Not my favorite but I do hear it.)

"He doesn't seem to be in too much pain."

"There isn't anything that can be done – he is just getting old."

After many years of seeing and hearing these remarks, I became curious, wondering just how many pets could benefit from additional care during their geriatric stage of life.

In December 2015, Lap of Love Veterinary Hospice performed a survey and analysis of our patients. Keep in mind that we only provide veterinary end of life services in the

Treatment and Care of the Geriatric Veterinary Patient, First Edition. Edited by Mary Gardner and Dani McVety.
© 2017 John Wiley & Sons, Inc. Published 2017 by John Wiley & Sons, Inc.
Companion Website: www.wiley.com/go/gardner/geriatric

home and we currently help approximately 3,000 pets per month nationwide. During the period of the study, we saw 3,120 patients spanning the country and covering a wide range of financial and cultural demographics. The pets were classified as either "geriatric" or "not geriatric" based upon their age, weight, size and fragility; 88% (2,746) of the patients seen were categorized as geriatric. The others were either younger pets with an imminent disease, senior pets, or pets that were difficult to categorize. Additionally, as part of the survey, our veterinarians questioned how long it had been since the pet was seen by a veterinarian. Thankfully, 55% of the pets had been to their regular vet within the last six months. Alarmingly, however, 22% had not seen their veterinarian in over a year, with the remaining 23% having seen their vet 7–12 months ago.

Our veterinarians provided their subjective opinion about those geriatric pets that had exceeded six months since their last veterinary appointment (1,208 pets). We asked our vets, "based on the exam findings and symptoms reported, would the pet have benefitted from seeing a veterinarian," and "considering the length of time that the pet was dealing with the symptoms, would therapies such as pain management, anxiety management, or hygiene management have helped?" For purposes of this study, we excluded those needing surgery (that is, limb amputation, tie-back for laryngeal paralysis, and so on) or other extensive treatment, such as radiation or other cancer treatments outside of prednisone.

Almost 45%, or 544 pets, did not receive basic care and treatment for their ailments, yet they could have benefitted from some form of veterinary care. Instead, these pets were left to struggle for many months. To summarize, approximately 17% of the patients we see for euthanasia at Lap of Love are geriatric, have not been to a veterinarian in six months, and could have benefited from care. Being mindful that we are not their primary care provider, just imagine the abundance of patients a general practice has that could benefit from a geriatric wellness exam and treatment.

In 2007, the American Veterinary Medical Association reported that 14% of dogs were over the age of ten years. Based on this statistic, the number of qualifying geriatric pets and potential gross revenue for a single geriatric exam can easily be calculated (see Box 22.1). The amount listed in the example may not appear overly significant, but the benefits to the pet, the family, and even to the staff are priceless; thus, representing an

---

Box 22.1 Example Calculation

• Total number of dogs seen at clinic	7,000
• Percentage of dogs over the age of 10 years	14%
• Total number of dogs over age of 10 years	7,000 x 0.14 = 980
• Percentage of those dogs that have not been to the clinic in 1 year	20%
• Number of dogs over the age of 10 years that have not been to the clinic	980 x 0.20 = 196
• Percentage of clients that came to your clinic after marketing	25%
• Total number of dogs seen that may have otherwise not been seen	196 x 0.25 = 49
• Average client transaction fee for geriatric wellness	$65
• Total possible gross revenue for one visit per year	49 x $65 = $3,185

opportunity for both pets and veterinarians. The trust invested in and garnered from the family will remain with them for years to come; therefore, establishing a long-lasting relationship.

When our veterinarians were asked if they had compassion fatigue from euthanasia, not one of them answered "yes"; however, many reported suffering from compassion fatigue as a result of seeing pets that could have been helped sooner. One way we, as an industry, can help with the emotional state of our team members is to encourage families to have their pets seen regularly and create opportunities for geriatric pets to have better care. The price we pay on our emotional wellbeing is not easily calculated; but, then again, adding services that support the mission of caring for pets will help bring us out of compassion debt.

Developing a Geriatric Service in the Clinic

Most clinics provide services for senior pets. But do you target and have policies in place for the fragile geriatric pets as well? Setting up your clinic to best care for the geriatric patient, educating the staff, creating bundled service offerings and properly marketing, tracking and following up with the families will increase the grey muzzles in your practice.

Education

Educating staff on the process of aging is the first step in developing a geriatric service in the clinic. The staff's complete understanding of the most common symptoms that plague our grey-muzzled patients is key. Moreover, their ability to use this knowledge towards instructing pet owners on tips and tricks for managing their pets identified symptoms is imperative.

Section II of this textbook offered an in depth look at the body systems and the symptoms developed by common ailments with advancing age. Every clinical team member should take the time to learn, at the appropriate level for their position, these changes that occur. Ultimately, the greater the understanding from the clinical team, the better the education extended to the client.

Client education is paramount. Offering literature to a client or referring them to an online source will assist them with the understanding of the disease process and symptom management. Stating to an owner that "old age is not a disease" is contraindicated. Instead, taking the time to listen to the problems the pet and caregiver are facing, then reviewing the causes and providing possible treatment options are essential in helping to manage the aging pet.

Clinic Visits and Environment

Geriatric patients are extremely fragile, many in a chronic state of pain. It is important to realize that a system already in pain, is more sensitive than a naïve one. The same concept remains for anxiety. Simple actions such as gentle holding can greatly reduce physical and emotional stress. Practicing Fear Free techniques (fearfreepets.com), or other methods used for establishing a calm and stress free environment, is encouraged. The Fear Free Initiative aims to "take the 'pet' out of 'petrified'" and get pets back for veterinary visits by promoting considerate approach and gentle control techniques used in calming environments. Use of Fear Free methods and protocols leads to reduction or removal of anxiety triggers, which creates an experience that is rewarding and safer for all involved, including pets, their owners, and veterinary health care teams. The whole veterinary team needs to know the expectations the clinic has for caring for geriatric pets and a well-defined policy should be put in place (see Appendix 22.1). A few additional ideas to provide a wholesome environment for the geriatric pet at your clinic are:

- Provide a dedicated parking spot near the front for the "grey muzzles."
- Lay out yoga mats as a runway for the pet to the exam room.
- Perform tasks and sample collection in the exam room to prevent the pet feeling stressed in the treatment room or being removed from the caregiver's presence.
- Careful handling techniques are essential during any procedure. Pets are fragile and even the slightest awkward movement could leave them sore the next day.
- Fast track those patients out of the clinic! There is no place like home for a geriatric pet. Have them in and out of your clinic as quick as you can. If they must stay for a procedure or boarding, encourage the owners to bring something from home to help with any anxiety.

Additionally, providing in-home evaluations, or asking owners to film videos, are principal methods toward gaining insight to how the pet fares in their home environment and how the owner manages the pet.

Examination and Conversation

When people bring their advanced aged pets to your clinic, it is important to realize that not only are the pets nervous, but the owners are as well. They are worried about the results and prognosis, uneasy about their pets' reactions to the procedure and clinic (feeling scared, pained, anxious, and so on), and most often anxious about being judged, wondering "Did I wait too long to bring my pet in?" You need to earn their trust and have them know that you have their (and the pet's) best interest at hand.

Based on the conversation with the pet owner, veterinarians should garner a list of challenges the family is dealing with and what they are concerned about most. This list can then be prioritized and the most pressing issue addressed first. For example, an owner might know that their pet has horrific teeth, but that may not be the principal problem – instead, the sleepless nights take precedence in the household's perceived quality of life. As a vet, listening to owners with the intention of identifying what is important to them, then tailoring your focus to their needs is key. Once solving the primary issue, the secondary and tertiary can then follow. In reference to the above example, once identifying and correcting the sleepless nights, the teeth can then be addressed. By taking into consideration and tailoring treatment towards the owners' needs, a healthy veterinarian–client–patient relationship is formed, thus resulting in the owner building trust, establishing consistency, and obeying recommendations.

Lap of Love has created a Geriatric Questionnaire that caregivers can fill out before they are seen by the veterinarian. This provides a means of comprehensively reporting problems and symptoms their pet may be experiencing by helping to identify those that

---

Box 22.2 Suggested Retail Products

- Accessories for blind dogs (halosforpaws.com)
- Books on pain, such as *Dr. Petty's Pain Relief for Dogs* by Michael Petty
- Customized wheelchairs, such as Walkin'Wheels™ (walkinwheels.com)
- Harnesses, such as the Help'EmUp™ harness (helpemup.com)
- Mesh beds (handicappedpets.com)
- Ramps for beds, cars and stairs (inthecompanyofdogs.com)
- Rubber-soled booties, such as Ruffwear® (ruffwear.com)
- Self-adhesive traction pads for paws (inthecompanyofdogs.com)
- Toe grips, such as Dr. Buzby's ToeGrips™ (toegrips.com)

---

the owner may not have known to report. One great example is a change in the dog's bark, which is often a precursor to laryngeal paralysis. Although this is extremely important information to a veterinarian, the lay client may not understand the significance, which is where the questionnaire exhibits its relevance (see Appendix 22.2).

Geriatric Wellness Plan

Similar to wellness plans for younger patients, clinics can create geriatric wellness plans to encourage owners to consistently bring their pets in for exams. Bundling services and avoiding services that may not be necessary at this life stage is the foundation. An example of bundling services is offering four visits per year for a discounted rate (for example, if your typical office visit cost is $45, offer four visits for a discounted rate of $135 instead). At the geriatric stage, diseases and symptoms progress fast; thus, warranting the need for multiple visits in a year. Bundled service discounts are a great way to maximize compliance for pets in need by incentivizing for a visit every quarter.

Offering unique services is another component of a geriatric wellness plan. For instance, geriatric pet sitting, monthly "sanitary shaves", Fear-Free nail trims, laser therapy, physical therapy, and geriatric boarding or day care are a few ideas that can be incorporated into the plan.

At this stage in life, many pets will also need specialized accessories or products to help to manage their daily activities. This can be done by offering a retail space within the clinic, or if that is unfeasible, simply by providing information sheets to clients on useful items and where to order them. Box 22.2 offers a sample list of products, and the clinic may also add local companies that carry similar products.

Nursing Care in Hospital

Providing an ambient environment helps to reduce stress for the patient. Selecting a cage or kennel in a particular location can be a challenge – what irritates one pet may bring joy to another. Some pets like peace and quiet, while others like activity.

It is important to learn your patient's preference and provide that level of service. Even though our patients cannot speak, their appreciation will show through their actions and body language. Additionally, allowing pets to have items from home, such as a toy or blanket, with a familiar scent, also aids in providing comfort.

Mobility and weakness are common for the geriatric patient. Creating a slip-free floor, with yoga mats or rubber flooring, allows for a safer and more comfortable environment for the pet. Furthermore, offering low rider stretchers to assist those commuting a farther distance is a prime recommendation in geriatric care. For those suffering from urinary incontinence, a mesh sling bed will help prevent urine scaling and keep the patient dry and clean. Lastly, if a patient must stay overnight, establishing visiting hours for the caregiver offers comfort to both the patient and the owner. If the caregiver is unable to offer this time, sending text messages, with pictures and updates, as displayed in Figure 22.1, is a viable alternative. This line of communication works wonders for reducing anxiety and building a trusting relationship with clients.

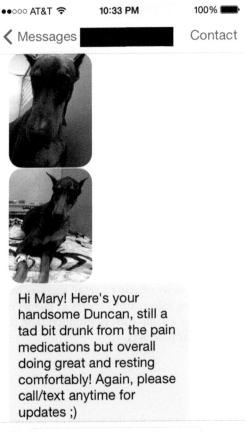

Figure 22.1 The text message that the veterinary specialist sent to me when my Doberman had a laryngeal tie back. I cannot put into words the feeling of relief I felt when I received this message.

Follow-Up and Tracking Advanced Aging Pets

Too often, when pets hit their golden years, families are reluctant to bring them to their veterinarian. It is the clinic's duty to flag those geriatric patients so that they do not slip through the cracks. Create a procedure of running reports every six months to target certain age ranges and ailments, and those "lost clients" then allot the time to follow up with them. Through targeted marketing campaigns, you can easily remind owners of all the benefits offered to their pet by scheduling a visit, while also highlighting the techniques incorporated into your practice to make for a pleasant trip.

In Summary

As a profession, we have been well educated and equipped for marketing and caring for the senior pet. For those fragile, advanced aged geriatric pets there is an opportunity to provide better care as they enter their golden years, and support the families as they struggle alongside their pet. Marketing specifically to this group helps to highlight the symptoms the pet will encounter while also focusing on the challenges the caregiver may face. Overall, this confirms to the caregiver that you empathize with their plight, gains their trust, and encourages them to reach out for assistance with their pet when needed.

Appendix 22.1

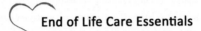

End of Life Care Essentials

The end of life stage is a delicate time for pet parents and involves a myriad of questions, concerns and emotions. Please use this fundamental checklist while creating your clinic's End of Life Care program:

Geriatric Care
Every practice should:
- ❑ Train entire staff on the aging process, including challenges pets may experience
- ❑ Routinely follow up and track advanced aging patients
- ❑ Identify and discuss the owner's feelings and challenges that arise when caring for a geriatric pet
- ❑ Ensure all pets are being treated for pain, anxiety or any other symptom associated with aging

Hospice Care
Every practice should:
- ❑ Educate and train staff on veterinary hospice, including services they can offer their clients
- ❑ Create and deliver a hospice handout package for clients including: disease information, euthanasia information, quality of life assessment tools and local ancillary services
- ❑ Ensure all pets in the hospice program are managed appropriately in a relaxed environment

Assessing Quality of Life
Every practice should:
- ❑ Have dedicated team members thoroughly educated in quality of life discussions
- ❑ Provide Quality of Life scales and guide owners on how best to use them
- ❑ Discuss with owners their concerns and wishes for end of life care

Euthanasia
Every practice should:
- ❑ Provide entire team training on all aspects of the euthanasia appointment
- ❑ Cultivate an environment that recognizes the importance of the euthanasia appointment and embraces ways to make it as peaceful and painless as possible
- ❑ Ensure the staff answering the phones are comfortable and fluent with how to handle the call
- ❑ Clearly communicate with owners about the euthanasia process and what to expect – even before the appointment is made
- ❑ Create a peaceful space for these appointments
- ❑ Use the best medicine possible to ensure a relaxed, pain-free and anxiety-free experience for the pet
- ❑ Treat every pet, even drop offs, with respect and dignity
- ❑ Provide memorial items at the time of appointment
- ❑ Follow up with a phone call to every family the next day

Aftercare
Every practice should:
- ❑ Partner with a reliable and trustworthy crematory
- ❑ Schedule annual visits to the crematory to ensure your highest standards are met
- ❑ Know exactly what happens with each type of cremation option (private, individual or communal)

Pet Loss
Every practice should:
- ❑ Provide information to owners about local pet loss groups or national hotlines
- ❑ Educate staff on how to recognize and handle anticipatory grief and bereavement
- ❑ Encourage staff to speak up if they are experiencing any emotional difficulty with end-of-life care

Lap of Love
VETERINARY HOSPICE
& In-Home Euthanasia

Appendix 22.2

GERIATRIC QUESTIONNAIRE

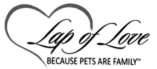

Lap of Love
BECAUSE PETS ARE FAMILY™

The effects of the natural aging process can slowly take a toll on companion animals. It can be difficult to notice these changes unless you look for specific clues. Since you know your pet better than anyone, you may be best to notice the subtle changes in your pet's behavior, habits, and activities. This checklist will provide your veterinarian a roadmap to help diagnose conditions – many of which can be managed, providing a better quality of life for your pet, even in their advanced age.

Pet's Name: _____   Male❑ | Female❑

Dog❑ | Cat❑   Breed: _____   Weight (lbs):_____   Age: _____

SLEEP PATTERNS:

How many hours sleep does your pet average per day? _____

Do they have a peaceful sleep throughout the night? YES ❑ | NO ❑

> *If No:* Do they get up during the night to (mark all those that apply):
> ❑ Urinate | ❑ Defecate | ❑ Drink Water | ❑ Pant | ❑ Pace | ❑ Whine | ❑ Bark | ❑ Other

HOUSE TRAINING: Has there been...?

❑ increase in urination | ❑ urinary accidents | ❑ leaking urine where they lay | ❑ changes of fecal appearance
❑ fecal incontinence | ❑ awareness of fecal incontinence

> *If Any:* Please explain: _____

EARS/EYES/NOSE/THROAT: Have you noticed...

❑ a change in hearing | ❑ change in their bark or meow | ❑ meowing/moaning more | ❑ coughing more
❑ a cough that sounds like throat clearing | ❑ bad breath | ❑ panting more frequently | ❑ vision problems

> *If Vision Problems* (mark all those that apply): ❑ in bright light | ❑ in dim light | ❑ at night | ❑ up close

SKIN: Have you noticed...

❑ nails longer than normal | ❑ itching | ❑ shivering | ❑ masses | ❑ smell bad | ❑ licking or chewing body

For Cats: Does your pet still groom him or herself? ❑ YES | ❑ NO

Is your pet's skin: ❑ flaky | ❑ dry | ❑ oily | ❑ unkempt

Does your pet seek out areas that are: ❑ hot | ❑ cold | ❑ soft | ❑ sunny| ❑ hard

MENTATION: Does your pet do any of the following?

❑ pace during the day | ❑ stare off into space | ❑ show increased aggression | ❑ experience any seizures
❑ exhibit less interaction with family | ❑ act disoriented or distant during the day | ❑ show agitation certain times of the day | ❑ find themselves stuck in odd locations

How long is your pet left by him or herself during the day? _____

Does your pet have a favorite game? ❑ YES | ❑ NO

> *If Yes:* Please explain: _____

---

1 | *Content developed and prepared by Lap of Love for clinic use

EATING/DRINKING: Has there been...?

❑ increase in thirst | ❑ weight loss | ❑ weight gain

What is the diet your pet is currently on, including treats? _____

MOBILITY: Check all of the following that pertains to your pet?

❑ needs assistance to get up | ❑ dragging feet/toes | ❑ change in gait/walk | ❑ has difficulty jumping

❑ must navigate up/down stairs in or outside the home | ❑ need assistance climbing stairs

What floor type do you have at home: ❑ tile | ❑ wood floor ❑ laminate | ❑ rug | ❑ other

What is your pet's exercise schedule? _____

Has this changed in the past year? YES ❑ | NO ❑

MISCELLANEOUS QUESTIONS: *Please discuss the following items in detail with your veterinarian*

Are there other pets in the home – if so – what kind/how old? _____

Are there any major concerns you have? _____

Describe what a good day is like for your pet? _____

List your pet's top 5 favorite things: _____

List 3 things your pet hates: _____

What quality of life do you think your pet has right now (1-10 with 10 being the greatest)? _____

HOW OLD IS YOUR PET IN PEOPLE YEARS?

Years	1	2	3	4	5	6	7	8	9	10	11	12	13	14	15	16	17	18	19	20
Small Breed / Cats (1-20 lb)	7	13	20	26	33	40	44	48	52	56	60	64	68	72	76	80	84	88	92	96
Medium Breed (20-50 lb)	7	14	21	27	34	42	47	51	56	60	68	69	74	78	83	87	92	96	101	105
Large Breed (50-90 lb)	8	16	24	31	38	45	50	55	61	66	72	77	82	88	93	99	104	109	115	120
X Large Breed (>90 lb)	9	18	26	34	41	49	56	64	71	78	86	93	101	108	115	123	131	139		

■ Adult ■ Senior ■ Geriatric

Chart courtesy of Fred L. Metzger, DVM, DABVP.
The above ages are intended as general guidelines only.

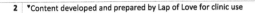

23

Veterinary Hospice in Your Practice
Mary Gardner and Dani McVety

As veterinary medicine continues to grow and new treatment options are discovered, pets are living longer and are able to live quite comfortably, even with some life-limiting diseases. But there comes a time when our treatment options either run out or they are not keeping the symptoms at a level that can be tolerated by the pet or family. As with human hospice, there is a growing demand for veterinary hospice care, both within our practice and in general practitioners' offices. However, veterinary hospice is still misunderstood, even within our profession. We are often asked, "What is veterinary hospice? Isn't that prolonging the inevitable (or suffering)?" Because of this misunderstanding, hospice is still underused in our profession.

What Hospice is NOT

I believe it is necessary to first understand what hospice is NOT: It is not prolonging suffering, nor is it euthanasia or natural dying.

Hospice Definition

Hospice is a medically supervised service dedicated to providing comfort and quality of life for the pet (and support for the owners) until euthanasia is elected or natural death occurs.

I find it interesting that still so many in our profession (as well as the general public) view veterinary hospice as something negative, going too far, or prolonging the inevitable. Yet, we widely recognize the wonderful service hospice provides for humans. Why the double standard? Is it because we have the option of euthanasia? I suggest that veterinary hospice patients may not be in a hospice program as long as a human hospice patient probably because we do have the treatment option of euthanasia – but hospice is still a service that has a place in veterinary medicine, albeit slightly different.

Treatment and Care of the Geriatric Veterinary Patient, First Edition. Edited by Mary Gardner and Dani McVety.
© 2017 John Wiley & Sons, Inc. Published 2017 by John Wiley & Sons, Inc.
Companion Website: www.wiley.com/go/gardner/geriatric

A few years ago I ran into an old vet school professor and Chief of Surgery at the University of Florida, Dr. Gary Ellison. He hugged me and said, "Mary – I'm so proud of you! I love what you're doing for pets and families. You see – last year my father battled with pancreatic cancer and when in the hospital, they took blood every three hours for sugar levels (as he was diabetic). Then when he became worse and we knew his time was limited, they moved him to hospice. On the first day, the nurse came into his room. With a sour look on his face, he held out his arm and said 'You're here for blood?' She smiled broadly and said 'NO Mr. Ellison! I'm here to find out what your favorite flavor of ice cream is!'" Dr. Ellison told me that his father's face lit up! He was thrilled to not worry so heavily on numbers but just enjoy what is important in the end. Dr. Ellison said to me, "That is what veterinary hospice is about." Coming from a surgeon, I was impressed and humbled at the same time. He got it. Now, I am not saying to give your next terminally ill patients ice cream … but maybe on the last day!

This chapter gives a high-level overview of bringing hospice into your clinic. There are wonderful veterinary hospice books available, as well as an organization dedicated to veterinary hospice (IAAHPC.org) where you can get a more granular look into the world of hospice.

How to Start Adding Hospice to Your Practice

Hospice is not just for the old. It is for any pet that is facing end of life, regardless of life stage. It is needed for the puppy with parvovirus, a six-year-old dog with unmanageable diabetes or the sixteen-year-old cat with cognition issues that meows all night and is in a constant state of confusion.

When you have a client that is facing the end of their pet's life, you should be willing to discuss and offer hospice services within your clinic. Using the word "hospice" to describe this care will help families to realize that their pets are at the end of their lives and that curative options are no longer being pursued. Many times, just the use of this word is a relief to pet owners, and in other times they start to think about humane euthanasia.

If an owner choses to not do diagnostics or if they want to cease treatment or decide against it, avoid making pet owners feel guilty and instead support them in this difficult decision. For example, if an owner decides against having his or her pet's blood work checked every six months (to evaluate long-term non-steroidal anti-inflammatory drug administration), do not threaten to cease medical treatment. Instead, take measures to ensure the family feels supported, comforted, prepared, and not financially burdened.

- Educate the owner on potential adverse effects, highlighting the importance of presenting the pet for treatment if any adverse effects are noted.
- Have the owner sign a liability waiver refusing blood work, to protect you and your practice.
- Help the owner to plan a compassionate approach to end-of-life care for his or her pet.

As soon as a pet enters your hospice program or is deemed hospice worthy, mark their chart "hospice". Within your clinic, agree between doctors and support team that if a case is marked as "hospice", the family can elect euthanasia at any time without the need to go through the entire history with the attending doctor. They should feel supported by the entire team without the requirement to defend the choice to say goodbye.

Education and Consultation

Often, when owners are considering euthanasia but not ready to commit to the decision – I know that the pet is not well (so much so euthanasia is looming) and could probably benefit from some sort of service. Or the owner could benefit from a conversation about the disease the pet has and how best to manage the symptoms as they progress over time. This is when I suggest a "consultation" first. It is a softer approach to lead them into the hospice mindset and is more often accepted by the clients. You may be surprised at how appreciative the client is for 30 minutes with a veterinarian discussing what to expect and how to manage their pet's disease and progression. Communication, preparation, and more communication is the hallmark of a successful hospice case.

A great deal of families, as would I for my own pet, wish to keep their pet alive for as long as possible, while also maintaining a good quality of life but simply do not know how, they feel helpless. They may not have the tools, time or support to handle their aging or terminally ill pet. When dealing with a hospice patient and their family, we must have a mutual understanding that we are willing to help extend life as long as pain and anxiety are controlled, but this is always preceded by a lengthy discussion on the progression of the disease process and a clear "stop point" which we agree is the ending of a good quality of life. The most important thing that clients need to know is what they risk if they wait too long, which is why education about their pet's disease progression is crucial. I often tell owners that "It will always seem to early – until it is too late". Below are some actual examples of stop-points we have used with families. They can be used as individual points or combination of one or more:

- When he cannot stand up for more than 30 minutes straight.
- When his resting respiratory rate is more than 60 breaths per minute three times during the day.
- When he does not sleep more than three hours in a row.
- When she refuses her favorite treat.
- When he does not try to attack the mailman and has refused French fries in the same day.

Hospice Handouts

A detailed end-of-life information package should also be available for the hospice family, in the same manner that veterinary clinics provide pet owners with a puppy/kitten package. Some things to include are:

1) Daily diaries that describe appetite, thirst, urination, defecation, mobility, and clinical signs of disease, which are important things to monitor while a pet is in hospice care as they help to determine overall quality of life.
2) Disease sheets with detailed information about the illness affecting the pet, including end-stage clinical signs.

3) Quality-of-life scales help to give a measurable value to owners; the pet can be evaluated daily or weekly, and ideally by more than one person in the family, which provides a more accurate evaluation of the pet. Make sure to teach the owner(s) how to accurately use the scale.

4) Adjunctive services that you support and trust (preferably mobile) in the area, such as acupuncture, massage, mobile grooming, in-home pet sitting (great opportunity for technicians).

5) Local pet loss groups or grief counselors (your local human hospice is a wonderful referral source).

6) Emergency clinics in the local area, if your clinic does not offer 24-hour emergency care.

7) Information on what natural death may look like.

8) Specific euthanasia information, including:
   - when and how to schedule euthanasia at your clinic, and if your clinic offers euthanasia in the home;
   - how to handle an emergency situation, such as nights or weekends, when a veterinarian may not be available. for example, "rescue" pain medication to get the pet through the night if emergency is care is not available or possible;
   - aftercare information (owners need to plan ahead), including services your clinic provides and prices;
   - local pet crematories or cemeteries, services that will pick up the pet at the home after it has passed, and so on.

Palliative Care

Palliative care for the hospice client is a key component to providing this type of service. The five most common areas of care are:

- pain management
- anxiety control
- nutritional support
- nausea control
- hygiene maintenance
- infection control.

Pain Management

Providing adequate pain medication is vital, and evaluating its effectiveness is just as important. We also equip the owner with "emergency intervention" or a "comfort kit" they can do themselves. For example, the client with a dog with osteosarcoma or severe degenerative joint disease should leave your clinic with a dose of injectable pain medication and the knowledge of how to administer it in case of a pathologic fracture. That way, the pet can have some relief while the next steps are organized. Teaching owners to recognize pain can be challenging; Colorado State University provides pain scales to help in assessing both acute and chronic pain (Hellyer, 2006a,b).

Anxiety Control

Many dogs are up all night, panting and pacing, with many owners awake as well. Providing medication that helps them to sleep through the night helps the anxiety level and is appreciated by everyone in the house. In addition, anxiety and distress change pain perception and pain threshold, which can exacerbate the pet's level of pain and then managing it is even more difficult.

Nutritional Support

Some diseases will lead to a decrease in appetite. While appetite stimulants are useful at times, often their effectiveness decreases quickly. Many owners are willing to cook for their pets so providing nutritious recipes with alternating protein sources can be helpful (Figure 23.1).

Nausea Control

Often, pets dealing with certain illnesses or on some medications will become nauseous. It is best to control nausea proactively so that the pet does not go off their food and cause even more issues.

Hygiene Maintenance and Infection Control

Urinary and fecal incontinence is usually an ailment that geriatric pets succumb to. Although incontinence may not affect quality of life too drastically, some pets do become anxious when they have accidents in the house, the human–animal bond is tested, and infection or urine scaling can occur. It is important to keep the pet clean with sanitary grooming/shaving, baby-wipes, diapers, waterproof bedding, low litter boxes and frequent walks.

Figure 23.1 Hospice patient Andy enjoys his meals when they are mixed with baby food.

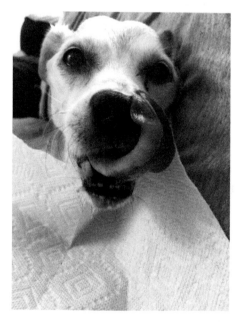

Follow-Up

Do not let these patients slip through the cracks! They need to have a plan for follow-up. Based on the pet's ailment and current quality of life, you can give a good estimate of length of time in hospice. If we have a patient in the early stages of hospice, we request monthly updates via email or phone. However, if the pet is advanced, weekly, even daily updates are needed. This allows consistent monitoring of the effectiveness of treatment, the progression of the disease, overall quality of life, and the owners wishes. Some owners reach out via emails with updates, videos or pictures while others may want the veterinarian to reassess every few weeks.

The American Veterinary Medical Association's policy on hospice care states:

> Veterinarians or veterinary hospitals that are unable to offer hospice care should be prepared to refer clients to another veterinarian who can offer these services.
>
> *(American Veterinary Medical Association, 2017)*

Conclusion

While offering veterinary hospice may not provide the largest avenue of revenue, the long-term benefits are immeasurable. The satisfaction your clients will have with the full circle of veterinary care at your clinic will be priceless. This will lead to positive word of mouth, referrals, and repeat business with other pets from that client when necessary and most importantly, it is what is best for the pet.

When families have a better end of life experience with their pets, they heal more quickly from the debilitating emotional loss. They are better able to cope with their decisions, feel confident in their ability to care for their pets, and more quickly open their homes and hearts to pet ownership again.

References

American Veterinary Medical Association. (2017) "Guidelines for Veterinary Hospice Care." approved by the Executive Board 04/2001; reaffirmed 04/2007; revised 04/2011. Available at https://www.avma.org/KB/Policies/Pages/Guidelines-for-Veterinary-Hospice-Care.aspx.

Hellyer, W., Uhrig, S. R., Robinson, N.G. (2006a) "Canine Acute Pain Scale." Colorado State University Veterinary Medical Center. Available at https://www.biomedcentral.com/content/supplementary/s12917-015-0338-4-s2.pdf.

Hellyer, W., Uhrig, S. R., Robinson, N.G. (2006b) "Feline Acute Pain Scale." Colorado State University Veterinary Medical Center. Available at https://www.csuanimalcancercenter.org/assets/files/csu_acute_pain_scale_feline.pdf.

Further Reading

Shanan, A., Pierce, J., Shearer, T. (eds.) (2017) *Hospice and Palliative Care for Companion Animals: Principles and Practice.* Hoboken, NJ: John Wiley & Sons, Inc.

Shearer, T. S. (ed.) (2011) "Palliative Medicine and Hospice Care." *Veterinary Clinics of North America Small Animal Practice*, 41(3): 477–702.

Resources

International Association for Animal Hospice and Palliative Care: iaahpc.org
Emerging group for all members of a pet hospice team.

Lap of Love Veterinary Hospice: www.LapofLove.com/Education/Common-Diseases
End-of-life information on common diseases seen in hospice practice.

24

Quality of Life Assessment and End of Life Decisions
Mary Gardner

Bogey

The early December phone call from Sharon started off as most of our calls do, with lots of heartfelt tears and a pause in the initial sentence to help swallow that knot in the throat. It was clear that Sharon and the entire family were struggling and desperately needed support and additional education through this tough time. Bogey, their 13-year-old male Golden Retriever was diagnosed with lymphoma a month prior. Bogey had been to the best oncologist in Southern California but his disease was aggressive and they did not have much time. He was on prednisone, pain management, and gastro protectants. But the family was in the great abyss of uncertainty and needed help.

I rang the door bell and could hear a loud but croaky bark followed by the sound of Bogey's nails on the tile floor that could be heard through the front door. As the door opened, I was greeted by a big jolly mass of beautiful light golden hair, soulful eyes and a smile that lit up the room. I exchanged some kisses, he sniffed my bag and then he turned and guided me to the living room where everyone was waiting. He was a big boy – definitely a healthy eater! It was easy to see his mobility issues and increased panting (my medical mind started to go through the list – "could be from the pred, pain, anxiety, possible lar par or enlarged lymph nodes...").

The family went over Bogey's life history (Figure 24.1), shared some stories and then began to talk about the last few months and his cancer diagnosis. His mobility was definitely an issue and he struggled to get on his favorite couch, but he was also having a difficult time sleeping through the night and was keeping the whole house up with the constant panting and pacing. They loved Bogey immensely and did not want to prolong his life just for them, but they did think he still had some time (and I agreed). They also hoped he would be able to make it to Christmas. Bogey was a huge part of the family tradition and had graced the Christmas card for the last 13 years. "Doc – how long do you think we have? This may sound silly but we don't know if we should put him on the Christmas card as we don't want to upset anyone if he passes before. We just want him to be happy and as pain free as possible."

Before I got to the medicine and assessing quality of life, I addressed one of their concerns, one which many in veterinary medicine may shrug off as insignificant.

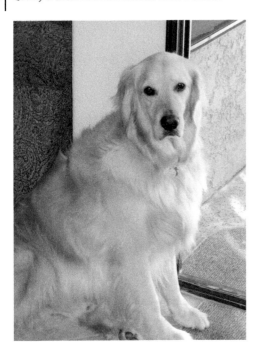

Figure 24.1 Bogey at four years old.

"Bogey SHOULD be on the Christmas card – regardless of what may happen, he will be your Christmas angel whether it is here on earth or watching from above – Bogey has to light up people's faces this year." They all smiled, nodded in agreement and we then started to discuss quality of life.

The Million Dollar Question: When will I know It's "Time?"

One of the most common questions care givers will ask their veterinarian is, "How will I know when it's time?". This question comes with a heavy heart and is not one that can be quickly answered or given a stock answer such as "You will know," or "When they stop eating" – often the answer can be more convoluted than that. Although, at times, those stock answers can be good indications of it being time, often they are not. The 13-year-old Labrador with osteoarthritis may still be eating and looking excited when his owner comes home, yet he can barely get up, falls down the stairs and is sitting in his own feces half the day. People will tell care givers, "You will know – they will give you a look." And I agree – sometimes they will give a pathetic look but if you think carefully, they are giving you a look because they are suffering – and isn't that what we want to avoid? Therefore, waiting for a look – may be waiting for suffering.

Assessing quality of life is an important part of helping families navigate the end of life stage. And this discussion is not something to avoid or belittle – it requires no less skill than performing surgery but requires more delicacy than you will ever realize you need.

The Three Core Components to Evaluating Quality of Life

Figure 24.2 illustrates the three core components to evaluating quality of life, and shows how they are interlinked.

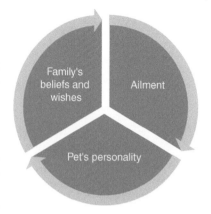

The Pet's Disease or Ailments

Each disease or ailment a pet faces will carry a different set of struggles, pain, anxiety, or even suffering. A thorough discussion of the symptoms the pet is currently facing, what they will face in the short term, and maybe what they will face during the dying process, is needed. The quality of life for the German Shepherd with hip

Figure 24.2 The three components of quality of life.

dysplasia may be within an acceptable level if they are still maintaining nutrition, hydration, pain control, and interaction with family. However, the cat in heart failure that struggles with respiratory distress everyday may have an unacceptable quality of life and intervention may be needed sooner than later.

When discussing the pet's disease, one must cover what the disease process means in terms of how it feels to the pet and how it progresses over time. Often owners with cats in kidney failure are told it is not painful; however, dehydration, toxin buildup, ulcers, nausea are not without discomfort. Outlining the most common future problems, time frame and expectations can help a family navigate through the assessment process and also create a "stop point" for when they should consider intervention.

The Pet's Personality

One must consider how the pet deals with different situations such as pain, anxiety, medications, tools, and just like humans, every pet will handle things a little different. So much so that where one pet may easily tolerate a harness, the next pet will do everything in its power to get out of it. Giving medications to some pets can be very difficult whether it be orally, sublingually or subcutaneously. It may be easy for the veterinary team to administer, but to the family it can be a struggle, which can cause a pet to grow weary of their family consequently straining and compromising the human–animal bond.

What the pet enjoys in life is also important. If a dog enjoys laying around being a couch potato (Figure 24.3), then a disease that limits mobility may not be as quality crushing as a herding dog whose "job" in life is to herd the flock or family. The very quality that we love in pets – individuality – can be a limiting factor when trying to manage a chronic disease.

Owner's Abilities, Beliefs and Wishes

The ability and desire to care for an aging or terminally ill pet can impact the quality of life for the pet as well as the owner. Some owners may seek treatment until all options have been exhausted, while others will opt for a more simple approach to keep them as

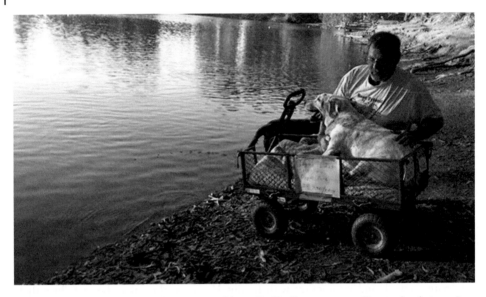

Figure 24.3 Hospice patient Yogi in a cart used for walks. Yogi's owner was willing to do whatever it took to allow Yogi to enjoy his final days.

comfortable for as long as possible, without going to the medical 'extremes'. Since pets are unfortunately seen as property and there is not an unlimited supply of funds, we cannot force a caregiver to partake in medical treatment for the pet. We can step in as the pet's advocate but in chronic cases, that would typically mean euthanasia or forcing treatment. The quality of life of a pet can be altered by the family's ability to care for the pet, their beliefs of what is right and what they wish for the pet near the end. What one person considers good "quality" can differ from the others.

We Can All Agree on One Thing

Most people will agree on one thing – that they do not want their pet to suffer, but suffering can still be subjective. This is where assessing quality of life quantitatively can help. But what do you measure? The most commonly used objective measurements for quality of life by veterinarians are mobility, appetite, pain, and proper voiding. I certainly do not disagree with any of these but the presence of quality of life based on these items should not be answered with a "yes or no," but rather "if or then".

Quality of Life Assessment Tools

There are many tools available that can assist owners and the veterinary team with evaluating quality of life; some are very simple and others are complex. Selecting the right tool for the family will enable them to monitor the quality progression. There is no perfect tool for all situations, pets and families but finding a tool that covers the most significant concerns is best. This chapter describes some of the commonly used tools.

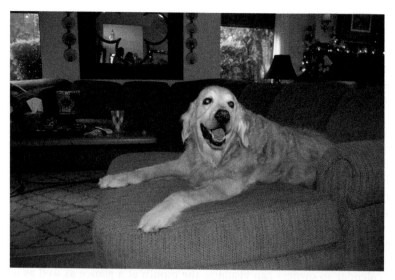

Figure 24.4 Bogey on his favorite couch. It was important to the family that Bogey was still able to get on his couch – even with assistance. And they wanted this final moments to be on the couch.

Basic Quality of Life Assessment Tools

Rule of Five

A common suggestion that veterinary team or friends of the family will tell an owner is to pick the pet's five most favorite things to do. When the pet no longer does three or more of those, then it is time to consider intervention. This may be eating, going for walks, interacting with family, toys, or other things (Figure 24.4). The one drawback to this is that the pet may actually still be doing those five favorite things, yet their quality of life is clearly not well. For example, cognition issues: While a pet is "alert" they may act, eat, play normally – but when they are in a cognitively impaired state, they are pacing uncontrollably or staring frozen into space until they become physically exhausted. I have witnessed pets that are in a "trance"-like state for up to18 hours a day and the rest of the time they are eating, playing or sleeping comfortably.

If this method of evaluation is used, I also suggest including something a pet does *not* like. If they have passion for hating something and they lose that passion – they may not be well. For example, if the dog hates the doorbell and eventually does not have enough energy to make the smallest bark when it is rung, then the quality of life may be poor.

Good Days or Bad

Ensuring that the good days outweigh the bad may seem like a logical way to evaluate quality however most people do not actually record the number of good days. A suggestion I make with all my clients who want to use this method of evaluation is to simply use a calendar to mark and track the bad days. Actually seeing the bad days accumulate helps owners to visualize the severity of the situation. It also prevents them from inadvertently forgetting how bad previous days or weeks were when the cherished "good" day comes around. Lap of Love has developed a calendar for owners to use (http://lapoflove.com/Pet_QoL_Calendar.pdf).

Pennies in a Jar

Another uncomplicated way to track quality of life is to get two jars – one labeled "good day" and the other "bad day". Have the owner put a penny in the appropriate day jar based on the pet's behavior, habits, daily functions, and so on. After a few weeks, you can see if the pet is having more bad days than good and can signal an appropriate time to recommend euthanasia.

Grey Muzzle Application (iPhones and Android)

Developed by Lap of Love, Grey Muzzle is the first electronic application to journal a pet's days on an iPhone/iPad and Android devices (Figure 24.5). A pet owner simply downloads the Grey Muzzle application from the app store and creates their pet's profile. Then every day they mark whether the pet had a good day, bad day, or neutral day. This way they can keep track of those bad days.

Owners should mentally prepare for when the pet has more bad days than good, and speak to their veterinarian about intervention. Or they may decide as a family that if the pet has 30% bad days (for example), that it is appropriate to say goodbye. The Grey Muzzle app has a calendar so owners can visualize the month at a glance as well as a summary page to see a pie chart of the pet's progress.

Advanced Quality of Life Assessment Tools

HHHHHMM Scale

Developed by Dr Alice Villalobos, the HHHHHMM Scale was one of the first tools that veterinarians could instruct a client to use to evaluate clinical signs with a more objective lens. This scale takes into consideration hurt, hunger, hydration, hygiene, happiness, mobility, and more good days than bad. Owners score those symptoms with a 1–10 (1 being worst and 10 being best) and add the values up to create a grand total. If the pet is above or below a certain mark, then they may be in an acceptable state or

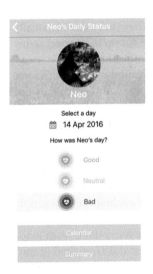 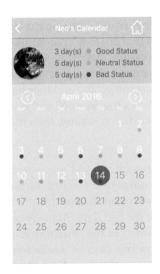 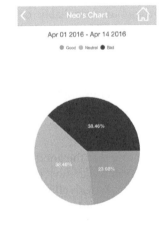

Figure 24.5 Grey Muzzle App screens.

in need of intervention. It can be downloaded by following this link: http://pawspice. com/clients/17611/documents/QualityofLifeScale.pdf.

Lap of Love Quality of Life Scale and Daily Diary

This scale's concept is similar to the HHHHHMM scale in terms of scoring and meeting an acceptable threshold but has six criteria (mobility, nutrition, hydration, interaction/ attitude, elimination, and favorite things). It also has space dedicated to daily notes so that the owners can jot down any significant changes in their pet that day. It is available at lapoflove.com/Pet_Quality_of_Life_Scale.pdf.

Lap of Love Pet's Quality of Life and Family Concerns

This scale is a tool that also asks questions for the family, to make sure their needs are addressed (Box 24.1).

Interactive Quality of Life Assessments

Pet Hospice Journal

The Pet Hospice Journal is a free online quality of life scale. It is the first interactive assessment tool developed by Lap of Love. The biggest concern with most quality of life scales is that they do not take into consideration the disease the pet has and what symptoms they will experience with that particular disease. The dog with arthritis may score a "0" for mobility but their eating gets a "3", as does doing their favorite things. This will falsely elevate the quality of life score. The Pet Hospice Journal was developed so that a caregiver could create a profile for their pet and based on the disease they selected, the criteria for assessment would change as well as the "weight" each answer earned. This tool is free for vets and pet owners and can be found at pethospicejournal.com.

Suggestions When Using Any Quality of Life Scale

1) Complete the scale at different times of the day, note circadian fluctuations in wellbeing. (We find most pets tend to do worse at night and better during the day.)
2) Request multiple members of the family complete the scale; compare observations.
3) Take periodic photos of the pet to help remember their physical appearance.
4) Keep detailed notes.
5) Create a stop point for when intervention will be sought.
6) Do not get frustrated – this is not an easy time and there is no black-and-white answer.
7) Pick the tool that best fits the pet's ailment and family's personality. Not everyone is willing to do the interactive tool, yet some people want more than a jar of pennies.

Other Questions to Explore

Conversations with owners are vital to help them uncover their own thoughts, feelings, and boundaries for their pet surrounding end of life decisions. I use the following questions to help me gauge the family's time, emotional, physical and (when appropriate, financial) budgets:

1) Have you ever been through the loss of a pet before? If so, what was your experience (good or bad, and why)? Side bar: "Have you ever been through this before?" is usually the first thing I ask. I find that families experiencing quality of life evaluation

---

Box 24.1 Pet's Quality of Life

Score each subsection on a scale of 0–2:
0 = agree with statement (describes my pet)
1 = some changes seen
2 = disagree with statement (does not describe my pet)

1) Social Functions
   a. Desire to be with the family has not changed.
   b. Interacts normally with family or other pets (i.e., no increased aggression or other changes).
2) Natural Functions
   a. Appetite has stayed the same.
   b. Drinking has stayed the same.
   c. Normal urination habits.
   d. Normal bowel movement habits.
   e. Ability to ambulate (walk around) has stayed the same.
3) Mental Health
   a. Enjoys normal play activities.
   b. Still dislikes the same things. (i.e., still hates the mailman = 0, or doesn't bark at the mailman anymore = 2)
   c. No outward signs of stress or anxiety.
   d. Does not seem confused or apathetic.
   e. Nighttime activity is normal, no changes seen.
4) Physical Health
   a. No changes in breathing or panting patterns.
   b. No outward signs of pain (see Resources below).
   c. No pacing around the house.
   d. My pet's overall condition has not changed recently.

Results:
0–8 = Quality of life is most likely adequate. No medical intervention required yet, but guidance from your veterinarian may help you identify signs to look for in the future.
9–16 = Quality of life is questionable and medical intervention is suggested. Your pet would certainly benefit from veterinary oversight and guidance to evaluate the disease process he/she is experiencing.
17–36 = Quality of life is a definite concern. Changes will likely become more progressive and more severe in the near future. Veterinary guidance will help you better understand the end stages of your pet's disease process in order to make a more informed decision of whether to continue hospice care or elect peaceful euthanasia.

Family's Concerns
Score each section on a scale of 0–2:
0 = I am not concerned at this time.
1 = There is some concern.
2 = I am concerned about this.

Box 24.1 (Continued)

I am concerned about the following things:

1) Pet suffering.
2) Desire to perform nursing care for your pet.
3) Ability to perform nursing care for your pet.
4) Pet dying alone.
5) Not knowing the right time to euthanize.
6) Coping with loss.
7) Concern for other household animals.
8) Concern for other members of the family (i.e., children).

Results:

0–4 = Your concerns are minimal at this time. You have either accepted the inevitable loss of your pet and understand what lies ahead, or have not yet given it much thought. If you have not considered these things, now is the time to begin evaluating your own concerns and limitations.

5–9 = Your concerns are mounting. Begin your search for information by educating yourself on your pet's condition; it's the best way to ensure you are prepared for the emotional changes ahead.

10–16 = Although you may not place much value on your own quality of life, your concerns about the changes in your pet are valid. Now is the time to prepare yourself and to build a support system around you. Veterinary guidance will help you prepare for the medical changes in your pet while counselors and other health professionals can begin helping you with anticipatory grief.

---

for the first time generally need more hand-holding and more direct language about the process ahead. They tend to wait for that handwritten letter from their pet saying "I'm ready now, Mom." This is not just my observation, it is what I hear from these pet owners time and again after the loss of their pet; "I can't believe I waited that long."

2) What do you hope the life expectancy of your pet will be? What do you think it will be?
3) What is the ideal situation you wish for your pet's end of life experience (at home, pass away in her sleep, and so on)?
4) Do you hold any stress or anxiety about any of these issues? (This section is meant to help in identifying the main concerns the family has):
   - pet suffering
   - desire to perform nursing care for pet
   - ability to perform nursing care for pet
   - pet dying alone
   - not knowing the right time to euthanize
   - coping with loss
   - concern for other household animals
   - concern for other members of the family (children).

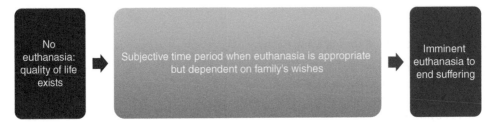

Figure 24.6 Three categories for quality of life and intervention.

Ideally, every family's budgets and boundaries align with the disease process at hand. The family that places greatest weight on both the happiness of the pet in addition to avoiding an emergency situation at all costs needs to understand the significant risk they run by waiting too long with imminent conditions. Each disease process has it's own set of clinical signs that should be weighted most heavily.

If the pet is declining in health and there are no additional diagnostics or treatments, the family is either willing or able to explore, then quality of life is either an imminent concern or will be at some point soon. If the family's emotional, time, physical, or financial budgets are being drained, there is a subjective time period during which euthanasia is an appropriate decision to make. This period could be hours, days, weeks, or even months. Before this specific period, I will refuse to euthanize, since there is clearly a good quality of life. After this period, however, I will insist on euthanizing due to suffering of the pet. During this larger subjective time however, it is truly dependent on the family to make whatever decision is best for them under the guidance of a supportive medical team (Figure 24.6). Some owners need time to come to terms with the decline of their pet while others want to prevent any unnecessary suffering at all. Everyone is different. After all, owners know their pet's personality better than anyone, even the vet!

Pain and Anxiety

Pain in animals is another important topic that all pet owners should be well versed in. It is the main topic I discuss during my in-home hospice consultations. I, and many other professionals, believe that carnivorous animals, such as cats and dogs, do not "hide" their pain, rather, pain simply does not bother them in the same way it bothers humans. Animals do not have an emotional attachment to their pain like we do. Humans react to the diagnosis of cancer much differently than Fluffy does! Fluffy does not know she has a terminal illness, so it bothers us more than it bothers her. This is vastly different than prey animals like rabbits or guinea pigs, who must hide their pain to prevent carnivorous attacks. If you are interested in learning more about pain and suffering in pets, grab Temple Grandin's (2005) book *Animals in Translation* and read chapter 5.

When discussing the decision to euthanize, we should be just as concerned about anxiety in our pet as we are about pain. Personally, I feel that anxiety is worse than pain in animals. Think about the last time your dog went to the vet. How was his behavior? Was he nervous in the exam room? Did he give you that look that said "this is terrible!"? Now think back to when he last hurt himself. Perhaps scraping his paw or straining a muscle after running too hard. My dog rarely looks as distraught when she's in pain as she does when she is anxious. It is the same for animals that are dying. End-stage arthritis patients begin panting, pacing, whining, and crying, especially at night time. Owing to hormonal fluctuations and other factors, symptoms can usually appear worse at night. The body is telling the carnivorous dog that he is no longer at the top of the food chain; he has been demoted and if he lies down, he will become someone else's dinner. Anti-anxiety medications can sometimes work for a time but for pets that are at this stage, the end is certainly near.

"Pets do not fear or anticipate death – but they do fear and anticipate pain."
(Robin Downing, DVM during a presentation
at a veterinary conference)

Suffering

Pain is an obvious condition owners and veterinarians want to avoid for the patient. Suffering however is also talked about but not completely easy to define. As with pain – no one wants their pet to suffer. I tell owners that suffering, for me, is when I can't think or do anything but concentrate on the physical or emotional discomfort I am in. I cannot be my true self nor can I achieve happiness. I feel that some diseases bring a level of malaise that leads to suffering and can be worse for a pet when compared with a painful condition (like arthritis).

Waiting Too Long

An interesting trend that I did not expect when starting my hospice practice is that the more times families experience the loss of a pet, the sooner they make the decision to euthanize. Owners experiencing the decline or terminal illness of a pet for the first time will generally wait until the very end to make that difficult decision. They are fearful of doing it too soon and giving up without a good fight. Afterwards, however, most of these owners regret waiting too long. They reflect back on the past days, weeks, or months, and feel guilty for putting their pet through those numerous trips to the vet or uncomfortable medical procedures that did not improve their pet's quality of life. The next time they witness the decline of a pet, they are much more likely to make the decision at the beginning of the decline instead of the end.

What About a Natural Death?

Yes, there are those pets that peacefully fall asleep and pass naturally on their own, but just as in humans, this is rare. Many owners fear their pet "passing alone" while others do not. Occasionally I am asked to help families through the natural dying process with their pet. For different reasons, these families are against euthanasia. I explain everything I possibly can, from how a natural death may look, how long it may take, what their pet may experience, and so on. Inevitably, almost all of these families regret doing this.

Most of them comment afterwards "I wish I would not have done that, I wish she didn't have to suffer." A natural death can be difficult to watch, especially for non-medically oriented people. Most people can watch a human family member in pain much more easily than they can their pet. To an extent, we can talk other humans through physical pain or discomfort. Humans can perceive an ending to their pain (via medication or even death) but there is little emotional comfort we can offer a pet that is suffering, they simply cannot perceive an ending to that pain. Families take this guilt difficultly and I do my very best to not only readily suggest euthanasia when appropriate, but prepare families for a "worst-case" scenario should they chose to wait.

Weigh Your Options Carefully

If the most important thing to the family is waiting until the last possible minute to say goodbye to their pet, they will most likely be facing an emergency, stress-filled, sufferable condition for the pet. It may not be peaceful and they may regret waiting too long. If a peaceful, calm, loving, family-oriented, in-home end of life experience is what they wish for their pet, then the decision will have to be made a little sooner than desired. Making that decision should not be about ceasing any suffering that has already occurred, but about preventing suffering from occurring in the first place. Above all, our pets do not deserve to hurt.

I have heard from countless pet owners that the death of their pet was worse than the death of their own parents. This might sound blasphemous to some, but to others it is the cold truth. Making the decision to euthanize a pet can feel gut-wrenching, murderous, and immoral. Yes, those are strong words, but that is what our pet families experience. They feel they are letting their pet down or that they are the cause of their friend's death. They forget that euthanasia is a gift, something that, when used appropriately and timely, prevents further physical suffering for the pet and emotional suffering of the family. Making the actual decision is the hardest part of the experience and I am asked on a daily basis.

Using any method to help evaluate quality of life of the pet in conjunction with the family's quality of life has helped many owners feel empowered over their decisions – whether to continue with treatment/care or euthanize their pets. How I wish the answer to the question of "When is it time?" was simple and clear cut. I believe that it is our duty to assist owners with end of life decisions and to help end and prevent suffering of animals. There are many ways to help families explore quality of life questions but the one way that is an injustice to our profession is if you simply say, "Call me when it's time". Owners need more than this and animals deserve more.

Bogey Continued

After a lengthy conversation with the family, and evaluation of Bogey's condition, we decided to start Bogey in our Hospice Program, provide palliative care and assess his quality of life on a daily basis. For Bogey's family, it was best to place large sticky piece of paper on the wall in the kitchen (Figure 24.7). That way everyone in the family could write notes about how Bogey was doing, how he ate, if he had a good night's sleep, etc.

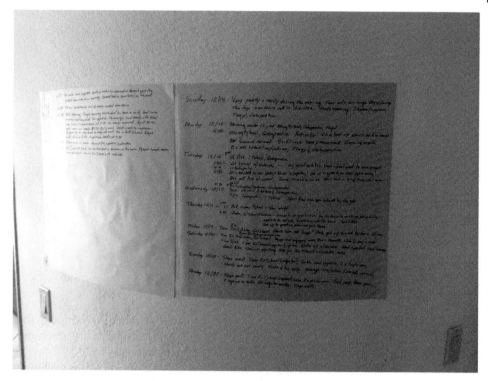

Figure 24.7 Bogey's quality of life scale on the wall.

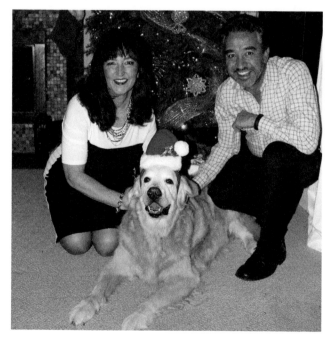

Figure 24.8 Bogey gracing the 2014 Christmas card.

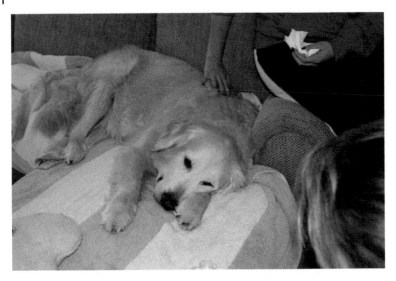

Figure 24.9 Bogey's passing on his favorite couch.

Bogey did really well for a few weeks. He started to sleep better, and even through the night. He was enjoying time with the family, playing with toys, getting on his couch and maintained his appetite. And he even made it to Christmas (Figure 24.8).

A week later, on New Year's Eve, Bogey's family decided it was time. He was declining but still having good days. They wanted him to go on a good day. So, with all of those who loved him close by, Bogey passed peacefully on his beloved couch (Figure 24.9).

References

Grandin, T. and Johnson, C. (2005) Animals in Translation. New York, NY: Scribner.

Villalobos, A. (2011) "The "HHHHHMM" Quality of Life Scale. Pawspice. Available at http://pawspice.com/clients/17611/documents/QualityofLifeScale.pdf.

25

Anticipatory Grief and Preparation for Pet Loss
Shea Cox

Anticipatory Grief

Anticipatory grief refers to the process whereby survivors rehearse the bereaved role and initiate working through the emotional changes associated with a death. Hospice and palliative care situations allow for families to be forewarned about an impending death, permitting their preparation for the impending loss. Anticipatory grief has many of the same symptoms as the grief experienced after a death, and includes all of the thinking, feeling, cultural, and social reactions felt by the individual. It is generally thought that anticipatory grief mitigates the intensity of the grief reaction following the actual death, leaving the survivor less vulnerable to maladaptive reactions. However, the evidence on the adaptive value of being forewarned that a death will occur is inconsistent (Siegel and Weinstein, 1983). Some investigations have shown that bereaved people who have had an opportunity for anticipatory grief adjust better to their loss, while other research has not demonstrated any benefit (Parkes and Weiss, 1983).

Preparing Families for Loss

When preparing families for an impending loss, it can be helpful to involve all family members in end of life discussions, whenever possible. Involving all caregivers in communications allows for a better assessment of the family's overall understanding, as well as helping to determine what a family's specific needs may be. Additionally, when everyone is involved in conversation, it can lessen the potential for misunderstandings or disagreements with regards to the decisions of care offered at end of life, preventing unnecessary guilt, anger or prolonged grief. It is important to educate family members that anticipatory grief is different for everyone, and each family member may experience or cope in different ways.

Encourage caregiver self-care. The stress associated with anticipatory grieving affects all aspects of a person's being, including one's mental, physical, emotional and spiritual states. In a short period of time, a person can use up the majority of their energy

Treatment and Care of the Geriatric Veterinary Patient, First Edition. Edited by Mary Gardner and Dani McVety.
© 2017 John Wiley & Sons, Inc. Published 2017 by John Wiley & Sons, Inc.
Companion Website: www.wiley.com/go/gardner/geriatric

resources, becoming overwhelmed and exhausted from the stress of grief. It is important to give families "permission" to practice their own self-care, in addition to the care they are providing for their dying pet, to help sustain them on their grief journey.

Provide information. The more information that an individual is provided with, the more they can prepare themselves for what is to come; knowledge of what to expect at a pet's end of life can lessen fears by taking away elements of the unknown. Therefore, all aspects relating to an impending death should be discussed, including what to anticipate as disease progresses, what options are available to manage disease, discussion of what makes for a good quality of life for that particular pet, the euthanasia process and what to anticipate during the dying process, options for ceremony or memorial services, aftercare considerations and common aspects of grief experienced.

Offer the opportunity to honor and spend time with the deceased pet afterwards, if wished for. All family members should be offered the opportunity to partake in ceremony or memorial services, as well as be allowed to spend as much time as needed with their deceased pet's body (Figure 25.1). This not only allows the opportunity to appropriately mourn, but affords the individual the emotional freedom to say goodbye in a way that is needed, allowing one to fully accept the finality of death.

Emphasize that grief is normal and provide a safe environment for the expression of grief. A common question asked by people is, "How can the death of my pet hurt as much as that of a family member?" Individuals may feel that they cannot, or should not, grieve the same over the loss of a pet as that of a person, which may inhibit them from fully and appropriately grieving the loss of their pet when it dies. Having discussions about the "normalcy" of the intense grief that can be felt with the loss of a pet can be helpful in validating feelings of impending loss and the grief that may be experienced during this time.

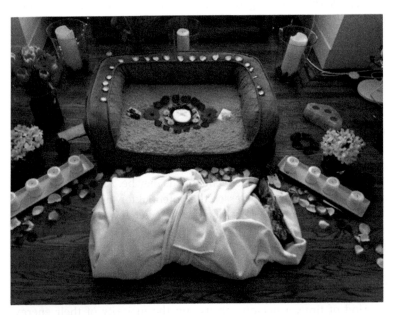

Figure 25.1 All family members should be offered the opportunity to partake in ceremony or memorial services.

Offer bereavement support and counseling resources proactively. Individuals can benefit from services that can provide additional sensitive listening, reassurance and help with managing all the changes posed by bereavement. There are an increasing number of resources available to help people through their grief process, including when they are anticipating the loss of their pet. Local, national, and online support service information should be provided proactively in every end of life situation. Such resources enable individuals to safely test out their feelings, questions, and thoughts when facing the impending loss of a pet.

What if Families are Reluctant to Discuss Grief?

Individuals may resist engaging in end of life discussions, and one prevalent reason includes implementing denial as a coping mechanism. If a family member is reluctant to talk about death and dying, exploring the reasons behind that reluctance may allow the health care provider to discover a way to approach the topic that feels more comfortable, and can be an indirect way to obtain additional information about their preferences in a manner that is more emotionally safe to that individual.

Special Considerations: Children and Grief

Well-meaning adults often wish to protect children from painful events, but doing so can often leave children feeling excluded from events that are important to them. Children begin to develop an understanding of aspects of death and bereavement as early as two or three years. By the age of five, over half of children have full understanding, and virtually all children will by the age of eight (Figure 25.2). How early a

Figure 25.2 By the age of eight, children have full understanding of aspects of death and bereavement.

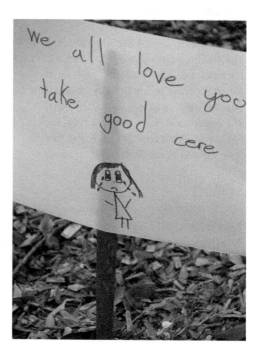

child develops such understanding depends primarily on whether adults have given truthful and sensitive explanations during previous experiences pertaining to loss (Sheldon, 1998).

It is helpful to discuss with parents what experiences their children may have previously had surrounding death, as well as what they have already been told and what they currently understand about the situation. When a death is about to occur, it is important to encourage children to ask questions regarding the death, and to continue to do so after the death has occurred.

Parents are the best people to talk to their children, but they may need support and advice from professionals to help them to do so. Parents may also be preoccupied with the practical challenges of caring for their pet that is dying, or overwhelmed with their own grief. In these situations, it may be useful to involve family, friends or teachers. Adolescents struggling to develop their individuality and independence may find members of their peer group to be helpful, particularly if they know someone who has also experienced bereavement (Relf, 2006).

During the grieving process, it can be helpful for children to create memory boxes to store treasured photos and keepsakes, to read storybooks (see Box 25.1), or to use the workbooks on death and bereavement that are now available.

Box 25.1 Pet Loss Book Resources

Child

Cat Heaven; Dog Heaven, Cynthia Rylant
For Every Dog an Angel; For Every Cat an Angel, Christine Davis
I'll Always Love You, Hans Wilhelm
The Kids Book About Pet Loss: Grieving and Healing After Loosing Your Pet, Vicky Taylor
When a Pet Dies, Fred Rogers
When Your Pet Dies: A Healing Handbook for Kids, Victoria Ryan
The Williams Family and Andy Cat: When the Loss of a Pet Really, Really Hurts, Jennifer Foreman de Grassi Williams
When You Have to Say Goodbye: Loving and Letting Go of Your Pet, Monica Mansfield
Saying Goodbye to Lulu, Corinne Demas
The Tenth Good Thing About Barney, Judith Viorst
I Miss You: A First Look at Death, Pat Thomas
Where the Red Fern Grows, Wilson Rawls

Adult

How to ROAR: Pet Loss Grief Recovery, Robin Jean Brown
Parting Words/Parting Ways: Saying Good-Bye to Your Pet, Laura Ritter Carlson
Paw Prints in the Stars: A Farewell and Journal for a Beloved Pet, Warren Hanson
Goodbye, Friend: Healing Wisdom for Anyone Who Has Ever Lost a Pet, Gary Kowalski
When Your Pet Dies: A Guide to Mourning, Remembering and Healing, Alan D. Wolfelt
Saying Goodbye to Your Angel Animals: Finding Comfort after Losing Your Pet, Allen and Linda Anderson

---

(Continued)

Box 25.1 (Continued)

For Adults Helping Children

When Children Grieve: For Adults to Help Children Deal with Death, Divorce, Pet Loss, Moving and Other Losses, John W. James and Russell Friedman
Pet Loss: Thoughtful Guide for Adults and Children, Herbert A. Nieburg
The Grieving Child: A Parent's Guide, Helen Fitzgerald
Children and Pet Loss: A Guide for Helping, Marty Tousley
Remembering Candy: Helping Your Child Cope With the Loss of Their Own Pet, Amanda van der Gulik
When a Family Pet Dies: A Guide to Dealing with Children's Loss, Joann Tuzeo-Jarolmen

---

Conclusion

Families with a pet facing a terminal illness usually begin the grieving process prior to the actual death. Anticipatory grief is sometimes helpful and may result in fewer grief complications later. It is important to understand that each person will experience anticipatory grief in his or her own unique way, and that it is a process that can help individuals prepare for emotional and physical closure, as well as a way to prepare for change.

References

Parkes, C. M. and Weiss, R. S. (1983) *Recovery From Bereavement*. New York: Basic Books.
Relf, M. (2006) "Bereavement." In Fallon, M. and Hanks, G. (eds.), *ABC of Palliative Care* (2nd ed.), pp. 74–7.
Sheldon F. (1998) "ABC of Palliative Care. Bereavement." *BMJ*, 316: 457. doi: https://doi.org/10.1136/bmj.316.7129.456.
Siegel, K. and Weinstein, L. (1983) "Anticipatory Grief Reconsidered." *Journal of Psychosocial Oncology*, 1(2): 61–73.

26

The Look

Faith Banks

[*Editor's note*: This chapter was written by a friend, colleague, and fellow hospice veterinarian from Toronto, Canada. Dr. Banks is also a contributing author in this book but most importantly a pet mom that has gone through the struggles of dealing with an aging pet, deciding when it is time and evaluating quality of life for her dog Smudge.]

I often get "The Look" when friends and family come over to our house. They look at Smudge struggle to rise from her relaxed recumbency, watch her walk straight legged as she makes her way to the door, then wag her tail when they give her a pat hello. "Awwwww, poor thing," is often the next thing that squeaks out of their mouth.

Poor Smudge. The thing is, I don't look at her that way. Does she look like the robust, beautiful Berner she did when she was seven years old? Heck, no! (Figure 26.1). Smudge has basically doubled the average life expectancy of a Bernese Mountain Dog, and lost the equivalent of a medium-sized dog in weight and muscle mass. Sarcopenia, the dreaded common side effect of growing old. Old dogs are not pretty. They are lumpy, skinny and sometimes stiff. They often have accidents in the house. They are not steady on their feet and they can seem spacey due to some degree of doggy dementia. Our almost-14-year-old Smudge has all of the above.

Is it time to say good bye? Give her the blue juice and free her of her mostly broken body? I don't think so. Am I wearing denial goggles? I hope not.

When clients are stuck in this same grey zone of not wanting to say goodbye too early and not waiting until it becomes too late, we discuss and fill out a quality of life scale. Although it does not sit exactly right that I am discussing the life of a much loved pet and reducing that life into a number in each category from 0 (very low) to 5 (normal), it does seem to be a very helpful exercise for pet parents. It helps to put things in perspective.

Smudge's appetite…5, breathing difficulties…5, gives love/takes love…5, accidents in the house…2, mobility…2–3, and the list goes on. I often find owners can get through this questionnaire with dry eyes until I ask them, "Do you think your dog is happy?" Tears begin to flow. They reminisce about chasing balls in the park, swimming

Treatment and Care of the Geriatric Veterinary Patient, First Edition. Edited by Mary Gardner and Dani McVety.
© 2017 John Wiley & Sons, Inc. Published 2017 by John Wiley & Sons, Inc.
Companion Website: www.wiley.com/go/gardner/geriatric

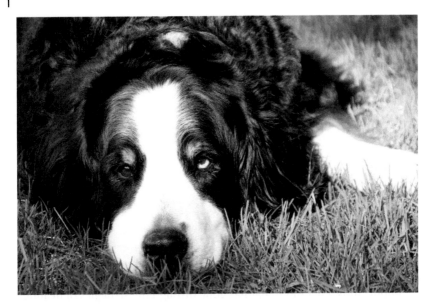

Figure 26.1 Smudge as a healthy senior Bernese Mountain Dog.

off the boat in the summer time, frolicking in the snow (Figure 26.2a), or rolling over for belly rubs. When your dog stops doing their favorite things, it can be a clue that they are not happy and no longer have joy in their life. Smudge typically scores between a 70–75%. Still quite good, but this high score does not come easily. She is on six different medications to treat her pain, hypothyroidism and cognitive dysfunction. I massage her every night, she has had several chiropractic sessions and she just had her first session of acupuncture. She has a special harness for times when she needs extra support. She needs help getting up the two steps from our back deck into our house. Our entire main floor is covered in a crisscross runway of yoga mats for her so she does not splay out on her back legs, and her food and water bowls are now elevated to prevent her neck from stretching down too far to the ground. Did I mention she has fecal incontinence? After a lifetime of no messes in the house, Smudge cannot control her bowel movements. Waking up to an aromatic fragrance is now the norm in our house.

In 2001, early on in our marriage, I surprised my husband with a big furball that came to be known as Smudge (Figure 26.1). When we looked at her nose, it looked like someone took their thumb and smeared the blackness, as if it was smudged. We always knew a dog was going to be our first (fur) baby, and she would help prepare us for the commitment we would eventually make in having our own children. Smudge proved to be a gentle giant with the patience of a saint in her role as playmate for our kids and all other children. She has continued to be an integral part of our family.

She has had a wonderful life. Being loved and loving us in return (Figure 26.2). She deserves a beautiful death. And when we determine it is time for her to leave her failing body, she will leave this world, in her home, surrounded by her family as we shower her with kisses and words of love. If this happens to fall on a warm day, my nine-year-old son has decided we should bring snow from the local hockey arena for her to lie on. One of her favorite things (Figure 26.2b). She will feel no stress or anxiety in her final moments, as

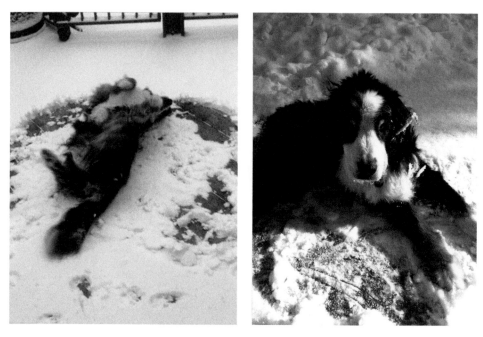

Figure 26.2 Smudge, 14 years old, moments before she was euthanized in the snow, at her home by, her mom, Dr. Faith Banks.

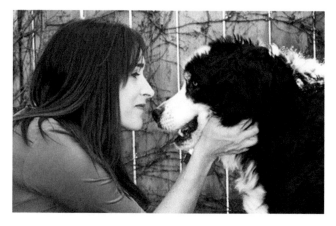

Figure 26.3 Dr. Faith Banks and Smudge.

euthanasia, by my hand, ensures she will pass peacefully and painlessly. That is what she deserves as she heads for the snow covered Swiss mountains in the sky. So the next time you see Smudge, instead of saying "poor Smudge," perhaps give her a pat and say "Lucky Smudge" (Figure 26.3)

27

Convenience and Aggressive Pet Euthanasia
Dani McVety

Introduction

When it comes to euthanasia requests that we consider to be border-line ethical, we have a very important decision to make as veterinarians. We must decide what is best for the pet (our patient), for the client (our customer), and of course, ourselves. We must decide what supports the interest of each party involved, something that is difficult, if not impossible, to do. What follows is an outline of how to handle these difficult cases, together with rules and definitions to help identify, categorize, process, and eventually make a decision based on the "best" outcome for all.

The most common reason that a veterinary professional will use the label "convenience euthanasia" revolve around two words: adoptable and treatable. These are completely subjective words, however. What is adoptable to one person, is not to another. A condition that is treatable to someone with unlimited finances is not treatable to someone on a tight budget. Removing judgment and assumptions like this will set you up to more openly listen to a client, their "budget" (which is different for everyone), and the best outcome possible.

Once judgments and assumptions have been suspended, we need to ask the right questions. Instead of deciding whether or not you are comfortable euthanizing that pet, the question should be "what are the alternatives for this pet." By requesting euthanasia in the first place, the family is communicating to you that the human animal bond is broken. We can either help to change the situation for them (remove the pet from their care via adoption or euthanasia), or do nothing by sending them home because "I just can't do it." And in my opinion, doing nothing is professional suicide; you have now ruined any rapport you had with that family, a small loss that does not create societal trust and respect for our profession. Helping a family, in whatever way, is far preferable than sending them home with a broken human–animal bond. Remember, medicine is not our product in the veterinary world, the human–animal bond is. Without that bond, they are not coming into our clinics. When euthanasia is requested, the family is telling us that there is something wrong with that bond, and they care enough to tell you about it instead of letting the dog or cat go on the side of the road.

So what should be done in these extreme cases of uncomfortable euthanasia requests? Allow me to push the boundaries a bit; in my opinion, we must take responsibility for the pet in some way. As a housecall hospice veterinarian, if I am at a home of a pet that I do not feel comfortable euthanizing, and with an owner that simply cannot go on, the pet will come home with me. Yes, it is happened. And have I euthanized animals that I may not have euthanized if they were mine? Absolutely. Have I euthanized animals that other veterinarians have refused to euthanize? Absolutely. Have I euthanized animals whose owners were completely at a lost, unable to go on for many reasons, and with tears in everyone's eyes (including mine), we knew it was a difficult but good decision? Absolutely. And when those families hug me, knowing that I did not judge them for that tough choice we made together, that I did not force an altruistic or idealistic view on them, and that I partnered with them in opting for the best alternative option for their pet, a new level of respect is earned.

Euthanasia Definitions

Convenience Euthanasia

"Convenience euthanasia" is a very subjective term. We use this phrase when euthanasia is requested for a pet that would otherwise be deemed adoptable under most circumstances and the family is unwilling to explore these options. For example, "My pet doesn't match the decor in my home any more" (yes, I have heard this). Personally, I do not offer convenience euthanasia in my practice, we offer support and resources to rehome these pets (see Box 27.1).

Non-Medical Euthanasia

Non-medical euthanasia is a term I use when describing a request that is not related to the medical stability of the pet. This is a broad term, which includes behavior issues (such as aggression or improper elimination in the home), in addition to emotional

---

Box 27.1 Non-Medical and Convenience Euthanasia Rules to Live By

- Do not euthanize a pet that you do not feel comfortable euthanizing. Period. (But say "No" carefully, keeping these other rules in mind.)
- Always help the family to explore alternative options, and think about how those options will effect the family and the pet down the road. Remember that a shelter is the deadliest place for a pet to be. Write them down, discuss them, think about what effect those alternatives have on OTHER animals in society.
- If you are comfortable euthanizing, even if you do not completely agree, you must help the family understand that although this is difficult for you (and them), you care greatly for them, their pet, and that this is the best decision that can be made given the circumstances. You do not want them to feel judged, which could lead to a lifetime of guilt.
- Do not get involved in cases if you do not plan to help; you will do more harm to our profession by judging and berating clients that if you simply hand them a number to a different veterinarian (preferable), or at least the local shelter or rescue organization.

or lifestyle changes of the family that precludes the pet from experiencing a quality of life (see Box 27.1).

Non-Imminent Medical Euthanasia

Non-imminent medical euthanasia is a term that describes situations like the 12-year-old cat. These conditions may be manageable or even curable under the right circumstances, but for whatever reason, those circumstances do not exist. This includes the parvo puppy that may survive with intensive care, the five-year-old intact female with a pyometra, or the young cat with a broken leg. Without the right resources and conditions (which may be too expensive), this pet would potentially suffer greatly. Rarely will I turn down this type of euthanasia request.

Medical Euthanasia

Medical euthanasia describes most of the euthanasias that occur in our clinics; a choice that is made when the quality of life of the pet is deemed unsustainable by both the family and the veterinarian.

Euthanizing Aggressive Pets

We have all heard the story from a friend about being bitten by a dog, whether as a child or adult. Many times this person has not bonded with an animal since. At best, they are indifferent to these four-legged creatures that we share the earth with, and at worst they cringe when a dog walks into the room. This is the effect undesirable that canine behavior can have on our society; this is what can happen when we see the warning signs and fail to intervene. I address some important concerns here, and I would like you to keep one thing in mind – this is not about how to prevent your dog from biting you or anyone else, there are plenty of resources about that, it is about what to do when you are at the end of the rope. It is written from my personal experience as a mother, my professional experience as a veterinarian, and as an animal lover.

Over the years, I have euthanized hundreds of dogs and cats for a multitude of behavioral issues that made their life with their families unsustainable, and the vast majority of them were young, physically healthy dogs (and cats, even birds) that could have lived years longer had it not been for some very specific issues. These families either tried behavior modifications unsuccessfully, attempted to find a safer home for the dog, and/or spent years adjusting their personal lives around the special needs of their pet (usually at the complaint of other family members). I had one client that spent over $30,000 trying to get his cat to stop urinating outside the litter box, and another that spent over $10,000 on special training for his short tempered Doberman that worked for a while, but two years later cornered his pregnant wife and four-year-old girl in the kitchen with teeth bared. These are extreme examples, but the interesting thing I found in these cases is that the families have a very unique attitude towards the euthanasia; they are exhausted and they feel intense guilt. They are so tired of worrying, mending their schedule around the dog's needs, not having friends over, not going on walks, and so on. They are emotionally defeated and they know that this pet is their responsibility, they do not want to pawn him off on someone else, who many not be aware of his particular needs, and the guilt consumes them. That's when they call me, and I always wish they would have called me sooner.

Being on this side of the syringe and administering life-ending medication forces me to be fully aware of the choices I make, why I make them, the consequences of not making them, and the ramifications for not only the families I help, but for society in general. My emotional path has been soul-searching, to say the least. As a mother, there is nothing you will not do for your kids, including ensuring their emotional and physical safety every day, we all know that. And as a veterinarian, it is also my duty to ensure the safety and well being of the animals I have pledged to protect. Part of their "wellbeing" is the human–animal bond, which is forever broken when the pet is a threat to the family in any capacity.

I have known many dogs in situations like this. I had one, and I euthanized her myself when the threat to my children and their perception of animals was at stake. Not all dogs that have spent her entire life with one family are better in a shelter or being adopted by someone else, sometimes they are worse off. It's equivalent to taking a 50-year-old autistic person and putting them in another country; new environment, new bed, new language, new expectations, new culture – everything. And in my opinion, that is usually not the best thing to do. They are nervous, scared, unsure, and that is when behavior issues like aggression become even worse. I was not willing to do that. And I know that saying goodbye to my little girl in a calm way was absolutely the best, not only for her, but for my family.

The biggest battle these families face is not with their pet, however, it is with themselves. I have helped thousands of families through my practice, but the ones that come to me due to aggression have the hardest time getting through the guilt of euthanasia. They wonder what else they could have done, why their dog has this problem, did they give up too soon, and so on. One woman told me "I have been grieving his loss since he first growled at me five years ago." She knew she would eventually have to make this tough decision, and after years of not having friends or family over, it was a tragic bite to her mother during a car trip to the veterinarian's office that was the final straw. Just as she said, she felt guilty long before she contacted me, and long before her precious boy was put to rest. That's not a way to live, and in my opinion, not what her dog would have wanted for her either, to live in constant stress.

Although it is not what any of us want to do, including the veterinarian, it is sometimes the best choice we have. What happens if we do not? A child gets bit and is physically or mentally scared for life (or worse), an unfriendly stranger is bit and files a complaint that puts your dog in mandatory isolation, you adopt the dog out and because there may not be a strong bond with the new owner, he beats the dog when his child is bitten, or they take him to a shelter in a few weeks because the behavior is unacceptable. Do see where I'm going with this? These are just immediate consequences. The more long-standing consequences include the child that, 20 years ago, was bitten and has now missed out on the intense love of the human–animal bond. This person could have adopted many, many dogs in her lifetime, but she is scared of them instead. The long-term ramifications of our decisions, or lack thereof, are numerous. When I think about what is best for that pet, taking into account the greater needs of mankind, our children, and the thousands of other healthy young dogs out there that are euthanized everyday because they do not have homes, I know that providing a kind and loving euthanasia of an irrevocably aggressive pet is best, much better than euthanasia in a shelter. That is how I handle my own emotions in this tough conversation, by having a "knowingness" within my self that I am doing the kindest thing. More importantly, I hope that my "knowingness" helps the families I work with through their own emotions and, perhaps, helps them open their heart and homes to another dog at some point – because those are the families that any dog (or cat) would be lucky to have.

Below is an email from me to a family after I euthanized their aggressive dog. Pay close attention to the family's response below. (Names have been changed.)

Dear Randy and Anita,

I'd like share my thoughts and feelings, both professional and personal, about the difficult decision we made for Tita. I imagine right about now you need to hear that it was the right thing... it was, 100%. Being on this side of the syringe forces me to be fully aware of the choices I make, why I make them, the consequences of not making them, and the ramifications for not only the families I help, but for society in general. I have euthanized hundreds of dogs and cats for behavioral issues that made their life with their families unsustainable ... and the vast majority of them were just like Tita.

As a mother, there is nothing you won't do for your kids, including ensuring their emotional and physical safety every day, we all know that. And as a veterinarian, it's also my duty to ensure the safety and well being of the animals I've pledged to protect. Part of their "well being" is the human animal bond, which is forever broken when the pet is a threat to the family in any capacity. A 13 year old dog that has spent her life with one family is not better in a shelter or being adopted by someone else, they are worse-off. It's equivalent to taking a 50 year old autistic person and putting them in another country; new environment, new bed, new language, new expectations, new culture... everything. And in my opinion, that's not the right thing to do. They are nervous, scared, unsure, and that's when behavior issues like aggression become worse. I'm not willing to do that, I know that saying goodbye in a calm way is absolutely the best, not only for the pet, but for the family too.

I hope you all feel in your heart that although difficult and intensely challenging the choice was, that it was the best one. I would not have administered that medication if I didn't have that "knowingness" within myself. More importantly, I hope that my "knowingness" helps you work through your own emotions and, perhaps, reduces any negative feels you might have. The one other piece of advice I will give you is to not talk to others about it. Too many people out there feel they know what's "right" for you and your family (and Tita was, and always will be, your family), but they don't, only you do. So find comfort in each other, call me if you need additional support, and know that I would have done the exact same thing in your situation... and I would have done it weeks ago.

Warmly,
Dr. Dani

Hi Dr. Dani,

Thank you so much for taking the time to write and check in on us. I really appreciate it. Yes, it was a very difficult decision but I am so thankful it was handled is such a peaceful and dignified way. As I am sure you gathered from your few minutes with Tita, she was a very special, outgoing and fun-loving dog. Up until about a year ago, when people met her, they were shocked to hear how old she was! She had been with me as my rock and companion through so many tough times – as well as been a huge cheerleader for me on all of the wonderful days!

I know it was the right decision, and I believe in my heart that she was suffering in some way – either mentally, physically, emotionally or all three perhaps. Tita hadn't been herself for years and I kept chalking it up to moving across town/ weather/whatever excuse I had that day because I didn't want to face the fact that she was creeping closer to the end. I truly believe that her wild behavior these past few weeks were a sign that she was ready, that there were worse things to come. She and I "got" each other and I think she was trying to tell me something in her own way.

I can't begin to tell you how settling it was for me to know that someone like you was with her and took care of her for the last few moments of her life. Barrie has spoken so highly of you and I was so grateful that you went above and beyond to handle the situation in the way that was most comforting for me.

Thank you again for your kind words. We are healing and I have come to terms with the decision. I hope to meet you in the future under different circumstances and give you a proper thank you and a hug for all of your help.

Best,
Anita

28

Letting Go – Handling Euthanasia in Your Practice
Mary Gardner and Dani McVety

The Most Difficult Appointment

We are not taught to be good at carrying out death. No one taught us how to walk into an examination room for a euthanasia appointment, what to say to a crying teenager, or whether to hug the elderly man who just lost the pet that was the last link to his late wife. We never receive direct guidance about proper verbal and nonverbal techniques that make this "most difficult appointment" just a bit easier on everyone, including the veterinary professional. From numerous discussions with new graduates, we have found that about 75% of veterinarians graduate without ever administering a life-ending medication. Therefore, it is no wonder that conference lectures about this topic are packed and why our hospice practice has more requests for externs than we can handle. As the only medical profession licensed to euthanize, veterinarians have an incredible privilege and responsibility to handle this procedure properly.

> If there is one thing to think about when approaching the euthanasia appointment, it is, "What would I do for my own pet?" That is the minimum standard of care you should give your patients and their caregivers.

Three most important things to do to improve the euthanasia appointment:

1) Love on the pet.
2) Acknowledge the decision to euthanize by telling the family that, "We are doing the best thing for him."
3) Physically touch the owner. This conveys more empathy than words ever will.

The entire euthanasia process can be broken down into the following five stages:

1) setting up the euthanasia appointment
2) during the appointment
3) memorial items
4) body care
5) following up: ensuring the client's return.

Treatment and Care of the Geriatric Veterinary Patient, First Edition. Edited by Mary Gardner and Dani McVety.
© 2017 John Wiley & Sons, Inc. Published 2017 by John Wiley & Sons, Inc.
Companion Website: www.wiley.com/go/gardner/geriatric

Stage 1: Setting up the Euthanasia Appointment

Be the First to Say the "E" Word

Clients hate to be the first ones to bring up euthanasia. They think you will judge them for not caring about their pets, or that you will be angry at them for giving up too early. So you need to be the first to say it. And even if they are upset about the suggestion, at 2 a.m., when clients are stressed because a geriatric dog has been pacing all night or an elderly cat has peed outside the litter box for the third time that day, they will know that you have given them permission to think about the next step.

Making the Appointment

Many clients feel they are making an appointment that will kill their best friends; there-fore, how your support team handles this scheduling with the client is crucial. The receptionist should have nothing else on his or her mind other than assisting the client: the client should not be put on hold, and the receptionist should not be checking out another client at the same time. If at all possible, background noise should be kept to a minimum. Most important, empathy must be conveyed. Instruct your team to say, "I'm so sorry you're facing this." Support staff should not be scared to show some emotion – clients want to know they care. When scheduling the appointment, support staff should retrieve as much information from the client as possible. This is generally the time when clients are most capable of making difficult decisions – emotions will only get more painful from this point on.

Gathering Information

1) The support team should ask the name of the pet and use it often. Here are some suggestions for how to phrase this important conversation, in this order:

   "I'm so sorry you're facing this, I know it's tough."
   "Tell me what's going on with Max."

2) For this delicate conversation, use open-ended questions, because it invites the own-ers to share information, with no judgment being passed on the pet's condition. It is best to get this information upfront and to record the client's responses. Then, when the veterinarian walks into the appointment to euthanize the pet, he or she has an understanding of the family's interpretation of their pet's condition (because their perception is their reality).

   "How soon would you like to bring Max in?"

3) Get specifics. "As soon as possible" can mean anything from hours to days.

   "Do you know what you would like to do with Max afterwards?"

Notice that the word "body" is avoided. To the family, it's not Max's body, it's still Max.

4) Next you should describe aftercare.

> "There are three options for what to do with Max afterwards: a private crema-
> tion, in which he will be cremated alone and the ashes returned back to you; a
> communal cremation, in which he will be cremated with other pets and their
> cremains scattered at a butterfly garden [know what your crematory does with
> communal cremains]; and lastly, you are welcome to bury him at home. This is a
> very personal decision, and there is no right answer, only what is right for you.
> If it helps with your decision, the private cremation charge is $200 and the
> communal cremation is $50."

5) If a family asks if it's legal to bury at home, we say (see below).

> "I buried my little one in my back yard. You can check your county ordinances
> and do what you feel is best for you."
> "Just so you know, the total charge for the appointment, including cremation,
> is $250. It may be easier for you to write a check out now, so you don't have to
> worry about it when you get here."

Pricing the euthanasia appointment should be carefully considered and not itemized.
Remember, this is a practice building appointment, not a profitable one. For the support
team, collecting payment is one of the most difficult parts of the euthanasia appointment; set everyone up for success by giving the owners the total in advance and gently
preparing them for payment.

A Word on Home Burial and Other Body Care Options

Pets are property. You cannot demand that a pet's body stay at your clinic. Horses and
other livestock are euthanized with barbiturates and buried all the time, and humans
are buried with mounds of chemicals in their bodies every day. It is the clients' choice
to bury, cremate, or otherwise honor their pets in whatever way they see fit and at their
own risk.

Pre-Euthanasia Practice Building Suggestions

- If the pet is still eating, suggest that the owners bring in a favorite treat or something
  special like ice cream or chocolate (or provide this in the examination room). Owners
  are happy to see their pets enjoying something good when they are saying goodbye.
- If there is a calm housemate, invite the owners to bring this pet along. Many dogs and
  cats have some level of grief when they lose a friend, so allowing them to be present
  or minimally sniff the deceased pet after euthanasia may provide closure. This also
  provides company for the caregiver.
- Invite owners to bring a toy or other keepsake to go with their pet for cremation.
- Ask what kind of car the owners will be driving and direct them to park in the desig-
  nated "Love Spot" for geriatric patients near the front of your clinic. If the dog is large
  and you know the family is burying him at home, offer to perform the euthanasia in
  the car (Figure 28.1).

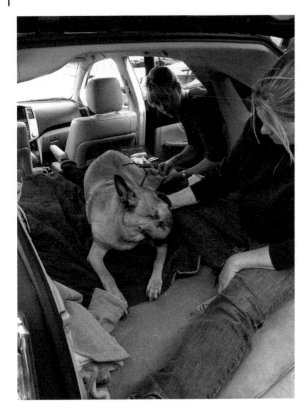

Figure 28.1 This dog loved being in his car and the owner asked if the euthanasia could be done there. There is no reason why this cannot be done. For those large dogs that cannot move, nothing is worse than having an owner struggle to get them into the clinic.

- Do not give the owners too many options. Offer the best from the start. For example:
  - Owners should not decide if their pets should be sedated (we are the ones to make medical decisions, not them, and sedation should always be provided).
  - Have one nice urn chosen for all private cremations and included in your price (your crematorium may have a standard urn option). Only give the owners the option to choose something else if they ask.
  - The most outrageous trend we have heard is that some clinics charge more if the owners want to be present. We understand the thought pattern behind this—the need to provide an indwelling catheter and more room time with the family—but imagine what this looks like to the owner, who thinks, "What are you doing to my pet if I'm not present?" If the owners don't want to be there, they will tell you, so assume they will be.

Stage 2: During the Appointment

The Arrival

When the time for the appointment comes have the paperwork ready, dated, and in the room. Make sure that the room itself is set up properly, and there is someone prepared to assist the client. Have the support team meet the family at their car and help them into the clinic, shuttling them to the room immediately. Paperwork is best completed at this time.

The Room

Whether the room is a separate comfort room or a regular examination room, make it as warm and comfortable as possible (it should not be the cold, sterile environment that owners dread). Here are some tips:

- Put a large fluffy bath rug (with a rubber sole) on the ground or on the table. Soft, pretty blankets and towels specific for euthanasia should be used to wrap the pet in.
- Provide soft background noise, perhaps a water feature, or soft music without words.
- Have a basket ready with items such as tissues, water bottles (dehydration is a common side effect of crying), a small mirror (woman like to check their makeup after they have cried), a small cloth bag for the pet's collar to go in, a container to place a hair clippings in, and material to make a paw print.
- Dim the lights, if you can. If not, have a lamp in the room and turn off the fluorescent lights.

Support Team Presence

The veterinarian should go into the room and preferably not leave again until the pet has passed (unless the owner requests time alone). Go in with the sedation and euthanasia already in syringes in your pocket or give them to your technician. Speak to the client and make a visual assessment of the pet. Do not pass judgement or appear to be uncomfortable with the decision unless you are certain you will not euthanize. Discomfort from you or your support team could leave a family with guilt for years. If you are comfortable with the euthanasia, verbally reassure the owner that "we" are making the best decision.

Explaining the Process

When explaining the euthanasia process, give the owner peace of mind. Explain that euthanasia means "good death" and that the medication is an overdose of anesthesia, in which the pet goes to sleep and does not wake back up. Do not describe every horror that can occur in the dying process. We recommend only saying, "The two things I will prepare you for are that her eyes won't close all the way and her bladder may relax. If anything else happens, I'll explain it at that time."

Giving Them Space

Offer owners some time alone with their pet. If they want time alone, hand them the "ringer" portion of a wireless doorbell. Have the bell portion in the treatment room or give it to the technician assigned to the case. That way, the owners do not have to leave the pet to find someone when they are ready. The human–animal bond should never be broken (Figure 28.2).

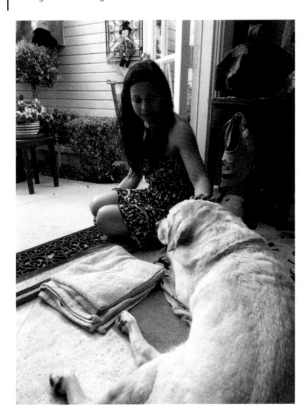

Figure 28.2 Every moment of the euthanasia appointment should take into account the bond between the owner and the pet.

The Procedure

Sedation

Intramuscular or subcutaneous sedation is crucial for the client's experience, and we are always discouraged to learn how many veterinarians do not sedate pets before euthanasia or provide only intravenous sedation (in which their pet rapidly goes from consciousness to unconsciousness, appearing dead). Having five minutes for the pet to slowly relax gives owners time to watch their pet get comfortable.

Euthanasia

When it comes time for the final medication, let the owner know you are proceeding. They should be told that their pet will pass in 30–60 seconds. Whether you use an indwelling catheter, butterfly catheter, or straight needle, do your best to stay out of the way of the owner. Let them hold their pet and instruct them to "keep talking to her; she can hear you." Giving the owners something to do keeps their focus off you and this surreal moment for them.

Alternative Routes for Administration

Common peripheral veins may not be immediately accessible. The medial accessory branch of the down leg on a laterally recumbent pet (good blood pressure), sublingual vein, ear vein, and even tail veins have been used by the author. Cutaneous vessels supplying tumors are also appropriate when visible and perfused. Above all, remain calm and confident in your technical ability. Alternative routes are always available.

The AVMA euthanasia guidelines (American Veterinary Medical Association, 2013) allow for other routes of pentobarbital administration (with unconscious sedation only):

- Intracardiac – if necessary, gently place your hand over the thoracic cavity and say "I'm going to give this in a central vein that will bring it directly where it needs to be." Shield the needle and syringe from the family with your other hand. Aim more cranial and ventral than you think and leave room in the syringe for air and/or blood; 1 ml/10 lb is recommended (Cooney *et al.*, 2012).
- Intrarenal – this is a standard protocol for cats by many in-home euthanasia veterinarians. Say "I'm going to give the second injection through the abdominal cavity into a large vessel, it generally takes anywhere from a few seconds to a couple minutes." Eighty percent will pass before you have finished giving the full injection. Give 3 ml/10 lb in the cortex, even in the smallest of kidneys (Cooney *et al.*, 2012).
- Intrahepatic – if needed, this is a good alternative to the intraperitoneal route, as it causes death in two to five minutes. Explain "I'm going to give the injection near a highly perfused organ, he's going to pass away in just a few minutes." Use 2 ml/10 lb and aim cranially just under the xyphoid process (Cooney *et al.*, 2012).
- Intraperitoneal (pre-sedation not required at this time) – there is some evidence that abdominal irritation from barbiturate injection, but the intraperitoneal route is still a good alternative, especially for fractious cats; 3 ml/10 lb is recommended (Cooney *et al.*, 2012).

After Administration

After administration, listen to the patient's heart and remain silent unless the owner speaks. This is an important moment and must be honored. The statement we like to use when confirming death is, "She has her wings." Stay present in the room for a few minutes as you gather the syringe and supplies. Watch for agonal breath(s), twitching, or any other movements, which generally happen within one to five minutes postmortem. Since we do not recommend warning about all these side effects before administration of medications, this is the time to explain them if/when they occur (see Box 28.1 for phrases to use if this happens).

Box 28.1 Euthanasia Practice Building Suggestions

- Walk in with a gentle smile. Be genuinely happy to see the family and be there with them for this important moment. Greet the pet with a positive statement like "Hi, handsome!" People have been telling this client for a long time how awful their pet looks, so it's a nice change for them to hear someone acknowledge the same beauty in the pet that the owner sees.
- Prime clients for a positive experience. Instead of saying "It doesn't hurt," or "He won't be in pain," both of which use negative words, give the client positive words like "This is a very peaceful process," and "He will be feeling much better than he's felt in a while."

(Continued)

Box 28.1 (Continued)

- You can always change your mind if you're not comfortable euthanizing a pet, but it is hard to make up for guilt the owner may feel. Be aware of the owner's body language when offering alternatives to euthanasia, and only do so if you are certain you will refuse to euthanize and/or if the client specifically asks for these alternatives.
- An alternative for handling paperwork is to have the client sign the consent form after the euthanasia process is explained.
- The last 15–30 minutes the owner has while his or her pet is still alive are precious. You would never want your pet taken from your arms at this moment, so consider not removing them from the room for intravenous catheter placement. Clients appreciate being involved in each part of the process, as well as not being left alone.
- Knowing when to respect silence and let the owners be in the moment is a very important part of the experience for them. As Ghandi once said, "Speak only if it improves upon the silence."
- Hug the owners afterward. If you are not a hugger, a gentle touch on the hand or shoulder will convey more empathy than words ever will.
- Here are some useful phrases for the most common postmortem adverse effects:
  - agonal breath: "This is just a spasm of the diaphragm, like a hiccup; it's uncommon but normal."
  - twitching: "Death is a phase, not a moment, and this is normal as different areas of the body shut down."
  - stretching: "This happens frequently when pets pass on their own; this tells me Max was very close to the natural dying process."

Stage 3: Memorial Items

The paw print is the most traditional and cherished memorial item – sometimes even more than cremains (Figure 28.3). With air dry clay like Crayola® Model Magic®, this is inexpensive and takes very little time. Many clinics make the paw print after the clients leave, but you are missing a huge opportunity to make the owners feel a little bit of joy by giving them one to take home (at no charge). Here's how we suggest providing the paw print.

- As soon as the owners hear their pet has passed, grief washes over them and they typically begin to cry. Give them a few minutes as you quietly prepare to make the paw impression.
- When it is appropriate, let them know that you will be making a paw print for them to keep. As you delicately push each phalange into the clay, the clients focus on the creation in front of them.
- Carefully hand them their new treasure and tell them how to store it.

Post-Euthanasia Practice Building Suggestions

Many owners will want their pet's collar and leash. Have a lovely bag that they can place these in so that they do not have to walk through the clinic with the leash in hand.

Figure 28.3 Veterinarians can help to provide owners with cherished memorials for their beloved pets.

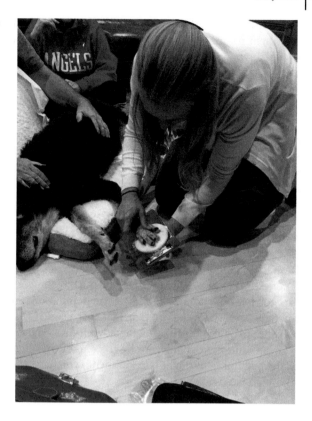

Some owners appreciate a locket of fur. We provide special containers for the clippings that are available at any craft store. The veterinarian preparing these memorial items has a return on the time investment that is priceless. Encourage all the veterinarians in your clinic to provide these few tokens of respect.

How the support team handles the body is a reflection of the respect for the life around us. Everyone should handle the body as if it were his or her own pet. Many veterinary distributors carry colored body bags that steer away from the "trash bag" appearance of black body bags. This is another way to help the veterinary healthcare team feel more respectful of the body and, therefore, more respectful of euthanasia in general.

A call the next day from the veterinarian is a way to exceed clients' expectations. Do not shy away from euthanasia follow-up. This one display of empathy can impact the client enough that he or she never considers using a different veterinary clinic. Ask the family to send a photo and/or memorial for a "Rainbow Bridge" wall in your office. This is a wonderful way to honor the pets you treat and help maintain your bond with the family.

Stage 4: Body Care

If owners need time alone after the euthanasia, allow them that time and hand them the wireless doorbell again. This way, a technician can come back into the room as they leave. Once the owners have left, the team can handle the body. If it is a large pet, always treat the pet respectfully and cover it with a nice blanket. Discreetly carry the pet to the treatment room. No other client should be privy to what is going on and by no means should anyone see a pet in a plastic body bag.

Stage 5: Following-Up and Ensuring the Client's Return

Sympathy cards are a given, and handwritten messages are worth the time. Every support team member who knew the pet and family should have an opportunity to write in the card, not just the veterinarian. Owners like to see that their pets were loved by the veterinary team.

In Summary

If we had to emphasize one thing that improves your end of life care for pets and their families, it is the provision of the best from the get-go. Provide the kind of care that exceeds the expectations of 95% of the population. For example, almost everyone loves the paw print. Yes, one or two may not want it, but that is okay. Provide what you consider to be top notch, and adjust your procedures only if the clients ask. The euthanasia appointment should not be the end of the client relationship, but instead should be the beginning of the next relationship you have with them. And remember, if it were your own pet, what would you want?

A Word on Compassion Fatigue

The veterinary industry is the perfect environment for compassion fatigue, but euthanasia does not need to be a contributing source. Talk to your team about the triggers in the euthanasia appointment that cause them stress or compassion fatigue, because it is different for everyone. See if you can figure ways to avoid those triggers. For example:

- If it is difficult for the receptionist to quote prices for cremation, then do not have him or her do it.
- If the team does not like the way in which the crematory handles the bodies, speak to the owner of the crematory.
- If a veterinarian has a hard time euthanizing the "drop offs," then have a couple of technicians serve as "family" for the pet, and even perform the euthanasia in the comfort room, with the same love, care, and dignity as if the owner were there.

References

American Veterinary Medical Association. (2013) AVMA Guidelines for the Euthanasia of Animals: 2013 Edition. Schaumberg, IL: AVMA.

Cooney, K. A., Chappell, J. R., Callan, R. J., Connally B. A. (2012). Veterinary Euthanasia Techniques: A Practical Guide. Ames, IA: Wiley-Blackwell.

29

The Final Chapter

Mary Gardner

When a family takes in a pet, the last thing they want to think about is when they have to say goodbye. But as the pet ages and shows signs of fragility, it will creep into their minds. Sadness, anxiety and fear will enter as well. Our obligation as their pet's veterinarian is to provide the best care for the pet under the circumstances as well as provide the family the support they need as they navigate through that time. Once we embrace this concept and provide the education and support needed, we are able to provide the level of service and care the pet deserves. And hopefully, over time, the hearts of the family will heal enough to care for another pet and come back to you – since no one else can care for their pets from birth to earth better. The end of life experience for the family can actually be a good one if we hone our communication and medical skills and really listen to the caregivers.

Peak–End Rule

People will evaluate experiences in two ways – the moment they are in it and afterwards. Those two views can be polar opposites. In his book *Thinking, Fast and Slow*, the Nobel Prize winning researcher Daniel Kahneman (2011) explains a phenomenon that occurs, which was proven by an experiment that he and physician Donald Redelmeier performed. They studied 287 patients who were undergoing kidney stone and colonoscopy procedures while they were awake (the procedures lasted anywhere from four minutes to in excess of one hour). They measured their experience of suffering moment by moment, by requesting the patients to rate their pain (via an electronic device) every 60 seconds. A scale of 1–10 was used where a score of 1 would be 'no pain' and a score of 10 would be 'intolerable'.

What they found is that patients reported periods of low to moderate pain, emphasized with periods of significant pain. From the results, most would assume the following: (1) the final results would represent the sum of the moments experienced; (2) having a greater average level of pain is worse than having a lower average level; (3) having a longer duration of pain is worse than having a shorter duration. Surprisingly, this was not the case. The duration of pain was largely ignored. Instead, the results were best

Treatment and Care of the Geriatric Veterinary Patient, First Edition. Edited by Mary Gardner and Dani McVety.
© 2017 John Wiley & Sons, Inc. Published 2017 by John Wiley & Sons, Inc.
Companion Website: www.wiley.com/go/gardner/geriatric

predicted by what Kahneman termed the "Peak–End rule": an average of the pain experienced at just two moments – the single worst moment of the procedure and the very end, meaning that the pain (or lack of pain) at the end was remembered just as much as the moment of maximum pain (Redelmeier and Kahneman, 1996).

Dr Atul Gawande, a human surgeon and best-selling author references the Peak–End rule in his book about human geriatrics and hospice, *Being Mortal*.

> People seemed to have two different selves – an experiencing self who endures every moment equally and a remembering self who gives almost all the weight of judgement afterward to two single points in time, the worst moment and the last one. The remembering self seems to stick to the Peak-End rule even when the ending is an anomaly. Just a few minutes without pain at the end of their medical procedure dramatically reduced patients' overall pain ratings even after they'd experienced more than half an hour of high level of pain. "That wasn't so bad," they'd reported afterward. A bad ending skewed the pain scores upward just as dramatically.
>
> (Gawande, 2014)

What Families Experience

If we think about the end of life experience for the entire family, we can all empathize what they are going through. From the moment they hear about the terminal diagnosis or the first sign of advanced aging, they start to suffer emotionally. How we handle the situation can greatly determine their perceived experience – and make it "not so bad".

If you think about the geriatric life stage on a macroscopic level, this is the "end". What we do to make it better – providing education, pain relief, anxiety relief, environmental changes to improve quality of life and all the other suggestions offered in this book – can change the perceived experience for that family to a more positive one. Looking deeper into the end of life, particularly euthanasia, if we can make the end less painful for the pet and the family they will remember a better experience. And microscopically, looking at the very end, what do most families want to see for their pet? A moment of freedom from pain and anxiety for their pet at the VERY end – and that is what pre-euthanasia sedation provides. To have the family witness their beloved pet experiencing comfort at the end is absolutely vital to ensuring a positive experience.

Endings Matter

We do not view our lives or our pets' lives as an average of all its moments. Life is meaningful because of the stories and the significant moments (good and bad). Our pets are a part of our stories. They are present for many of our significant moments. The geriatric life phase may possess a massive amount of obstacles and ultimately an emotional painful goodbye, but helping families through that time can be the most rewarding part of your career and mean so much to the pets and their families. Although our pets are a part of our stories (an important chapter), their own lives are a story. And in stories, endings matter most. So make the most out of the end and make it good.

Making it GOOD for Serissa

In the summer of 2014, Serissa was now a geriatric pet. But her love for me never aged. Besides having diabetes for seven years, bad hips and cataracts, she was now getting skinnier, her hair was thinning, her bark was weak, and she did not have the sparkle she used to have. Turns out she also had Cushing's. Unfortunately Cushing's and diabetes do not play well together. It became a balancing act to keep her eating, her sugar level stable and her quality of life good.

Late September, I knew her time was soon coming to the end, and that I would have to give heaven back the angel that was simply on loan to me. I made a promise to Serissa that I would not let her suffer, and I wanted her last day to be a good day; one where she was smiling, happy, eating, and enjoying the love from her family. I would not let her die alone, and I certainly would not let her die from anyone's hands but my own. Many ask, "How could you euthanize your own dog?" Veterinarians euthanize hundreds of pets in their careers but have a hard time euthanizing their own pets. We know the process is peaceful and that it can be a kind act. But to take the life of our own pet – most cannot do it.

Since I euthanize many pets in my current career, people assume that I am immune to the idea of death. It is actually quite the opposite. Because of my focus on end of life care, I have become more comfortable in the medicine and the dying process allowing me to be more involved in the family and the colorful stories of their beloved pet. I believe euthanize embodies compassion and thus I see it differently than most.

Serissa was going to die one day – and I was going to make it good. The day was planned – Wednesday October 1st at 4 p.m. I was returning from a trip the week before, so that gave me some time with her when I came back. I picked 4 p.m., as that gave me the day with her. The whole process would take less than an hour. Then I would cry the whole evening and fall asleep in my grief. That was the plan.

Well, my anxiety was full blown the Wednesday before "the day". It was too hard to focus, with "the day" a constant in my head and heart. Every day, I thought, this is my last Thursday, my last weekend … my last Tuesday. When it was Tuesday at 4 p.m., all I could think of is, "this time tomorrow". The anxiety of the upcoming event was numbing and I knew saying goodbye to my girl was going to rip my heart out. But, I rested on the knowledge that it was the best thing for her.

Wednesday morning came and as promised – we made it a great day! She ate whatever she wanted. We walked, laughed, played, and took a million precious pictures and videos. I fought back the tears poorly. Boy, was I going to miss my girl (Figure 29.1).

The veterinarian in me knew exactly what I was going to do. I do this every day. I was going to give her the first medication which is a lovely cocktail of pain relief and mild sedation – to make her feel awesome. The second medication is simply an overdose of anesthesia. This medication first puts the pet into a nice deep sleep. Then, their respiratory and cardiac function slows down and stops – and they die in their sleep. And that is what I wanted for Serissa. To feel really good before she passed in her sleep. And with euthanasia – that is what I can guarantee for her.

The second medication is typically given into a vein, although alternate routes can be used. For Serissa, I gave this step a lot of thought. You see, I wanted to be hugging my girl as she left this world. I wanted to be whispering to her how much she was adored and how much I will miss her. But I could not be in two places at one time.

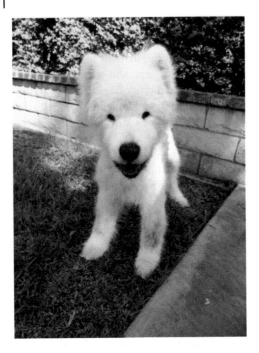

Figure 29.1 Serissa, October 1st 2014 at 3 p.m. – having fun!

I could not be injecting the medication into her leg vein and be spooning her at the same time. So I decided to go with an alternate route and inject the second medication into her abdominal cavity. The only difference with this route, is that it would take longer – about 30–45 minutes. But I thought, "Death doesn't have to be instant. Death is a phase anyway, so she will sleep like a princess and slowly drift off."

Four o'clock came around too quickly! As planned, I gave Serissa the first medication and in about five minutes she started to get sleepy and her perfect chocolate brown eyes got drowsy. She quietly lay down and began to peacefully snore. How I would miss that snore! She laid there in absolute perfection while I simply loved on her. Then I gave her the second medication. Oddly, the act of pushing the plunger was not hard as I thought it would be since I knew I was helping her. I knew that no one else needed to do it but me. I knew she was no longer in pain. I knew she knew I loved her. I knew she loved me unconditionally. So it was an honor for me to help her earn her angel wings that day.

I put my syringe away and I laid down behind her. I snuggled her for one last time. I just closed my eyes and felt her breathing ... and then it began to slow down. Thirty minutes after giving her the final medication, she stopped breathing. Her death could not have been more peaceful and beautiful. She had a good life and I was able to give her a good death (Figure 29.2).

I made a paw impression and clipped some fur. I made a little casket for her, wrapped her in a pretty blanket and surrounded her with flowers. I also put some pasta in there for her – because boy, did she love pasta! Looking down at her, I realized that I was no longer crying. I was actually smiling. I knew she was no longer suffering – she was OK now. The anxiety I was carrying around was instantly lifted. All I could do was smile and be thankful for such an amazing co-pilot in life.

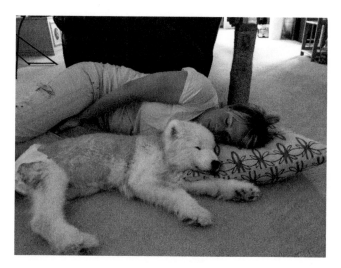

Figure 29.2 October 1st 2014, our last snuggle.

I know she is watching over me from above and when I see my shadow, I think of her. On October 1st 2014, heaven became much brighter with my angel up there. October 1st was a good day.

References

Gawande, A. (2014) *Being Mortal: Aging, Illness, Medicine and What Matters in the End.* New York, NY: Metropolitan Books, Henry Holt.

Kahneman, D. (2011) *Thinking, Fast and Slow.* New York, NY: Allen Lane.

Redelmeier, D. A. and Kahneman, D. (1996) "Patients' Memories of Painful Treatments: Real-Time and Retrospective Evaluations of Two Minimally Invasive Procedures," *Pain,* 66: 3–8.

Index

Note: Page number followed by '*f*' denotes Figure and '*t*' denotes Table

Treatment and Care of the Geriatric Veterinary Patient, First Edition. Edited by Mary Gardner and Dani McVety.
© 2017 John Wiley & Sons, Inc. Published 2017 by John Wiley & Sons, Inc.
Companion Website: www.wiley.com/go/gardner/geriatric

Printed and bound by CPI Group (UK) Ltd, Croydon, CR0 4YY

27/10/2024

14580246-0001